Monoclonal Antibodies

METHODS IN HEMATOLOGY

Volume 13

Monoclonal Antibodies

EDITED BY

Peter C. L. Beverley MB, BS, BSc

Senior Scientist, ICRF Human Tumour Immunology Group,
School of Medicine, University College London, London, UK

CHURCHILL LIVINGSTONE
EDINBURGH LONDON MELBOURNE AND NEW YORK 1986

CHURCHILL LIVINGSTONE
Medical Division of Longman Group Limited

Distributed in the United States of America by
Churchill Livingstone Inc., 1560 Broadway, New York,
N.Y. 10036, and by associated companies, branches and
representatives throughout the world.

First published 1986

ISBN 0 443 02990 3

British Library Cataloguing in Publication Data
Monoclonal antibodies.—(Methods in hematology,
ISSN 0264–4711; v10)
  1. Antibodies, Monoclonal
  I. Beverley, Peter C. L.   II. Series
  612′.118223   QR186.85

Library of Congress Cataloging in Publication Data
  (Methods in hematology, ISSN 0264–4711; v. 14)
  Includes index.
  1.   Antibodies,   Monoclonal.   2.   Hematology—
Technique.
I. Beverley, Peter C. L.   II. Series. [DNLM:
1. Antibodies, Monoclonal.   2. Immunologic Technics.
W1 ME9615L v.14/QW 575 M7469]
QR186.85.M6564   1986   616.07′93   85–19512

Printed in Great Britain
at the University Printing House, Oxford

Preface

The publication of this volume in the *Methods in Hematology* series is an acknowledgement of the important role which monoclonal antibodies have come to play in haematology since the description of the hybridoma methodology by Kohler and Milstein, only ten years ago. Immunologists and haematologists recognised early on that reagents which could accurately identify individual molecules present on or in a cell, would be invaluable tools for studying normal haemopoiesis and immune function, as well as for identifying, classifying and understanding leukaemia. This has proved to be the case and much of this volume deals with methods for analysis of haematological samples as cell suspensions, smears or sections.

Although monoclonal antibodies are already finding a place in routine laboratories their greatest impact, in the long term, may be in elucidating the function of cells and molecules. A part of this volume is therefore devoted, not to current methodology, but to reviews of several aspects of the use of monoclonal antibodies in the analysis of cellular and molecular function. In the future these investigations may provide new therapeutic strategies which will improve on those currently in use, including monoclonal based methods reviewed here.

I should like to acknowledge the excellence and patience of the contributors to this volume, who have combined scientific rigour and clarity of presentation in their contributions. I am grateful also to the staff of Churchill Livingstone for their help. The printing of the colour illustrations was made possible by a donation from Dako.

London, 1986   P.C.L.B.

Contributors

Peter C. L. Beverley MB, BS, BSc
Senior Scientist, ICRF Human Tumour Immunology Group, School of Medicine, University College London, London, UK

Fred J. Bollum PhD
Professor of Biochemistry, Department of Biochemistry, Uniformed Services, University of Health Sciences, Bethesda, Maryland, USA

Dario Campana
The Royal Free Hospital, London, UK

Michael Ronald Clark BSc, PhD
Postdoctoral Research Scientist, University of Cambridge, Cambridge, UK

Rosemarie Dalchau
Blond McIndoe Centre, Queen Victoria Hospital, Sussex, UK

Paul A. W. Edwards MA, PhD
Research Scientist, Ludwig Institute for Cancer Research, London Branch, Surrey, UK

W. N. Erber
John Radcliffe Hospital, Oxford, UK

John W. Fabre MB, BS, BMedSc, PhD
Director, Blond McIndoe Centre, Queen Victoria Hospital, Sussex; Honorary Research Professor, Royal College of Surgeons of England, UK

B. Falini
John Radcliffe Hospital, Oxford, UK

K. C. Gatter BM, BCh
John Radcliffe Hospital, Oxford, UK

James D. Griffin MD
Assistant Professor of Medicine, Harvard Medical School, Boston, Massachusetts, USA

George Janossy MD, PhD
Professor of Immunology, The Royal Free Hospital, London, UK

Lewis L. Lanier
Becton Dickinson Monoclonal Centre, Mountain View, California, USA

David Linch
Department of Paediatric Oncology, Sidney Faber Cancer Institute, Charles A
Dana Cancer Centre, Boston, Massachusetts, USA

Michael J. Loken PhD
Senior Scientist, Becton Dickinson Monoclonal Centre, Mountain View,
California, USA

Andrew J. McMichael PhD, MB, BChir, MRCP
Department of Surgery, John Radcliffe Hospital, Oxford, UK

David Y. Mason DM, MRCPath
Lecturer in Haematology, University of Oxford, Oxford, UK

H. S. Micklem
Immunobiology Unit, Department of Zoology, University of Edinburgh,
Edinburgh, UK

Michael J. O'Hare MA, PhD
Research Scientist, Ludwig Institute for Cancer Research, London Branch,
Surrey, UK

John H. Phillips
Becton Dickinson Monoclonal Centre, Mountain View, California, USA

H. Stein
John Radcliffe Hospital, Oxford, UK

Herman Waldmann MB, BChir, PhD, MRCPath
Lecturer, University of Cambridge, Department of Pathology, Addenbrooke's
Hospital, Cambridge, UK

Noel L. Warner
Becton Dickinson Monoclonal Centre, Mountain View, California, USA

Contents

1
Production of murine monoclonal antibodies

Mike Clark Herman Waldmann

HISTORICAL BACKGROUND

The hybrid myeloma technique developed as a spin off from research into the structure and synthesis of immunoglobulins and on the mechanism for generation of antibody diversity. The clonal selection hypothesis[1] and the subsequent observation that each B-cell or plasma cell is committed to the production of antibodies with a single specificity[2], suggested that a single clone of cells would secrete antibodies of a monoclonal nature. However this property could not be exploited in vitro for the simple reason that B-cells and plasma cells could not be maintained for long periods in tissue culture.

Tumours of immunoglobulin secreting cells arising spontaneously or induced in certain strains of mice[3,4] were a source of monoclonal immunoglobulins but in general these are of undefined specificity. The adaptation of some of these tumours to in vitro culture[5] prompted studies using cloned cell lines of the role of somatic mutation in the generation of antibody diversity[6,7,8]. Such studies of myeloma cell lines in vitro led to the observation that cell fusion between two immunoglobulin producing cell lines results in the co-dominant expression of the immunoglobulin chains[9,10]. Following this observation Kohler & Milstein[11] fused myeloma cells with lymphocytes from a mouse immunized with sheep red blood cells, and obtained hybrid cell clones, some of which secreted antibody specific for the immunizing antigen. Thus by cell fusion continuous cultures of cell hybrids can be derived secreting antibodies of predetermined specificity. The technique has now been adopted so widely that it seems justifiable to say that it is possible to raise monoclonal antibodies against any antigen for which an antibody response can be generated in mice and rats.

METHODOLOGY

In this chapter we will provide detailed accounts of the methodology involved in the production of mouse and rat monoclonal antibodies (the derivation of human monoclonal antibodies being the subject of a separate chapter) drawing chiefly upon our own experience but also making comparisons with alternative techniques used by other workers.

The performance of cell fusion to produce monoclonal antibodies against a given antigen involves a complex series of manipulations. The many variables of the system, for example batch variation in media, sera and reagents, are difficult to

1

control, even within a single laboratory and for this reason it is often difficult to make judgements about the merits of alternative protocols reported from other laboratories. We therefore strongly recommend that laboratories attempting to produce hybrid myelomas for the first time follow a well established protocol, and only once the basic techniques are working routinely within the laboratory should alternative procedures be experimented with.

The detailed methods we will provide here are on the whole taken from our own laboratory 'cook books' and can therefore be regarded as tried and tested techniques. The methods will be provided within a general discussion of the strategies involved in production of monoclonal antibodies. By breaking the whole technique down into a number of different steps, each involving various simple choices, we hope to simplify the overall complexity of the technology.

CULTURE FACILITIES

Production of monoclonal antibodies against a given antigen is likely to involve a considerable amount of commitment in time and in cost. Practical knowledge and experience of basic tissue culture techniques are essential as is access to suitable tissue culture facilities. The following is a list of equipment required in the tissue culture facility:

Incubators ($37°C$) with and without controlled atmospheres of humidity and CO_2 (to maintain the pH of medium in open containers at pH 7.2). Sterile work cabinets or work stations, supplies of autoclaved or disposable sterile pipettes, culture flasks and culture plates, an inverted microscope, refrigerated centrifuge, liquid nitrogen cooled storage vessels and $-70°C$ freezer space. The production of media from powder requires a source of high quality, deionized, double glass distilled water. As mouth pipetting is to be avoided we would recommend the use of a pipette aid (e.g. Bellco Glass Inc., Cat. No. 1225-80122). Sterile universals (Sterilin, Teddington, England, Cat. No. 128A) are convenient and cheap as centrifuge tubes for handling up to 25 ml volumes of cultures.

MEDIA AND ADDITIVES

The most commonly used media for hybrid myeloma production is Dulbecco's modified Eagle's medium (DMEM) supplemented with Fetal Calf Serum (FCS). We have also used Iscoves Modified Dulbecco's Medium (IMDM) for our routine maintenance and cloning of hybrid myeloma cultures but recommend caution in its use in the early culture period following cell fusion as problems can sometimes be encountered with over growth of the hybrid cells by primary cultures derived from the spleen. For all of the methods that follow we will describe the use of DMEM, however if IMDM is used as an alternative media it is usually possible to halve the quantity of FCS used as a supplement.

Media can either be purchased as complete media 1 × DMEM (Flow Laboratories, Irvine, Scotland, Cat. No. 12-332-54; Gibco Europe, Glasgow, Scotland, Cat. No. 041-1965) or 10 × DMEM concentrate (Flow Laboratories, Cat. No. 14.330-49; Gibco Europe, Cat. No. 042 2501) to be diluted with tissue culture grade water.

Certain additives such as sodium pyruvate and L-glutamine may need to be added as indicated by the manufacturers instructions.

If facilities are available we recommend that media be prepared from powder (Flow Laboratories, Cat. No. 10-331; Gibco Europe, Cat. No. 074-2100) following the manufacturer's instructions. Prepare both 1 × media for general culture and a supply of 2 × media for semisolid agar cloning.

HAT selective media can either be purchased in complete form (Gibco Europe, Cat. No. 041-1530; Flow Laboratories, Cat. No. 16-436-54) or alternatively concentrates can be bought (50 × HAT Flow Laboratories, Cat. No. 16-808-49) or prepared as follows:

Methods

Stock 100 × HT. Hypoxanthine (Sigma, Poole, England, Cat. No. H9377) 136.1 mg and thymidine (Sigma, Cat. No. T9250) 38.75 mg are dissolved in 100 ml of tissue culture grade water. It may be necessary to keep the mixture in a waterbath at 70°C for 10 to 20 minutes and/or add a small amount of 0.1 M NaOH to dissolve. Store at –20°C. On thawing warm to 70°C for a few minutes until redissolved.

Stock 1000 × Aminopterin. Aminopterin (Sigma, Cat. No. A2255) 17.6 mg dissolved in 100 ml of water with warming, store in the dark at –20°C and thaw at 70°C for a few minutes.

Stock 50 × HT. Prepared by diluting 100 × HT with an equal volume of DMEM. Filter sterilize and store in aliquots at 4°C.

Stock 50 × HAT. 50 ml of 100 × HT plus 5 ml of 1000 × Aminopterin, are added to 45 ml of DMEM. Filter sterilize and store in aliquots at 4°C.

To prepare 1 × HAT or 1 × HT medium dilute the 50 × stock solutions 1 in 50 into media supplemented with FCS.

Stock 100 × 8-Azaguanine. This additive which can be added to 1 × media for the selection of HGPRT deficient lines is prepared by dissolving 8-Azaguanine (Sigma, Cat. No. A1007) 300 mg in 100 ml of tissue culture grade water with warming. Filter sterilize and store in aliquots at –20°C. Thaw by warming to 37°C until redissolved.

Fetal calf serum (FCS). It is important for success in the production of hybrid myelomas that the medium is supplemented with a suitable batch of serum. Although horse serum was used for the original hybrid myeloma work horse serum antibodies generally contribute a high background in many screening procedures. At present the most reliable serum source is FCS. Batches of FCS should be selected for their ability to support hybrid growth at limiting dilution conditions in DMEM with 20% FCS. To do this dispense cells, ideally a newly established hybrid cell line but alternatively any hybrid cell line or the parental myeloma, in logarithmic phase into the wells of flat bottomed 96 well microtitre plates (Sterilin, Cat. No. M29 ARTL) at cell concentrations giving on average 20, 10, 5 and 1 cell per well. Incubate at 37°C in a humid CO_2 incubator for 7 days and then score for cell growth. In some circumstances it may be useful to culture the hybrid myeloma cells in a completely defined media without added serum,[12,13] however for most current applications of the hybrid myeloma technique the addition of FCS causes no complications and is cheaper and more convenient.

IMMUNIZATION

The first consideration for hybrid myeloma production is the immunization of a suitable animal. At present the only suitable laboratory animals for hybrid myeloma production are rats and mice. The important criteria are that the animals should make a good immune response to the particular antigen and that the final boosting injection guarantees localisation of antigen specific B-cells to the spleen. In rats this necessitates the intravenous route while in mice both intravenous or intraperitoneal injections are suitable. In general spleens are suitable for fusion 3–4 days after the last booster injection. A number of strategies have been used to improve immunization ranging from adoptive transfer of primed spleen cells to irradiated recipients, the injection of small amounts of antigen directly into the spleen[14] or in vitro boosting prior to fusion[15]. In practice one has to modify the immunization protocol to suit the antigen in question. Some laboratories monitor spleen cell sizes to identify the presence of B-cell blasts as a predictor of fusion efficiency[16].

Another factor influencing the choice of animal to be immunized is a consideration of the useful biological properties of the antibodies. For example in deriving rat monoclonal antibodies for therapeutic use in humans we have observed that many rat antibodies are very efficient at lysing human cells using human complement[17,18] and that rat IgG 2b subclass antibodies are effective in antibody dependent cell mediated cytotoxicity using human effector cells[19].

MYELOMA CELL LINE

The choice of myeloma line is partly dependent upon the species immunized. Both mouse[11,20,21,22,23] and rat[24,25,26] myeloma cell lines are now available (for list see Table 1.1) and whilst it is possible to make interspecific hybrid myelomas between rat and mouse cells it is usually more convenient to have hybrids which can easily be passaged in vivo for production of large amounts of antibody as serum or ascites. Our personal recommendations are, if the immunized animal is to be a rat the rat myeloma line Y3/Ag1.2.3 should be used and if the immunized animal is to be a mouse one of the mouse lines derived from X63Ag8 should be used e.g. NS1/1Ag4.1, NS0/u or X63Ag8.653.

The next difference between the myeloma cell lines is in their own intrinsic immunoglobulin production. As mentioned above the fusion of two immunoglobulin producing cells results in the codominant expression of the immunoglobulin chains from each parental cell. Thus if the parental myeloma cell is producing an immunoglobulin heavy and light chain a complex mixture of chains is found in the hybrid cells. Within such cells the heavy and light chains can assemble to give mixed immunoglobulin molecules not found in either parental cell. The chains do not associate totally at random and in general it seems that the light chains may associate with any heavy chain class or subclass but that heavy chains only combine with other heavy chains of the same class (e.g. $\mu + \mu$ or $\gamma 1 + \gamma 2$ but not $\gamma + \mu$). In certain combinations a deviation from an expected random distribution of mixed molecules between heavy and light chains may be observed[27] and it seems likely that this is because of differences in the association between chains with different sequences and structures (e.g. isotype and variable region associated differences).

Table 1.1 Some cell lines suitable for hybrid myeloma production

Species	Cell line	Compatible strain	Immunoglobulin expression	Reference
Mouse				
	P3-X63/AG8	BALB/c	MOPC21 IgG$_1$	11
	NSI/1Ag4.1	BALB/c	kappa chain	20
	X63/AG8.653	BALB/c	none	21
	NSO/u	BALB/c	none	22
	Sp2/OAG14	BALB/c	none	23
Rat				
	Y3-AG1.2.3	LOU	kappa chain	24
	YB2/3.OAG20	(LOU × AO)F1	none	25
	IR983F	LOU	none	26

The presence of such mixed molecular species in any hybrid myeloma product means that specific antibody represents only a proportion of the total immunoglobulin. In addition to this quantitative variation in the proportion of specific antibody there are also variations in the valency of some of the antibody molecules. There are two ways to avoid the problem of mixed molecules. It is possible to use a parental myeloma line that does not express any immunoglobulin chains of its own, the resulting hybrids can therefore only express the spleen cell derived immunoglobulin chains. Alternatively if a myeloma has been used which expressed immunoglobulin chains the number of combinations can be reduced by selecting for chain loss variants of the original hybrid. These variants usually arise spontaneously during continuous culture of the cell lines and are then isolated from the original culture by single cell cloning. The order of loss of chains is not totally random and the expression of an immunoglobulin heavy chain is usually lost before the expression of an immunoglobulin light chain[28]. It is thought that the reason for this is because excess heavy chain production is toxic to the cell.

It may be that for some applications of monoclonal antibodies there is an advantage in using myeloma cell lines which produce their own immunoglobulin light chain. Recent work has shown that the mixed molecules containing the antigen specific immunoglobulin light and heavy chains and a myeloma light chain can be purified from the culture supernatant and are functionally monovalent[29]. These monovalent antibodies fail to modulate cell surface antigens (a desirable property in serotherapy) and seem to be more efficient in promoting complement mediated cell lysis. The therapeutic value of such reagents underlines the value of such light chain secreting myeloma variants.

The different myeloma lines also differ in their efficiencies for rescue of the spleen cell derived immunoglobulin phenotype. In a study using a number of rat and mouse myeloma cell lines fused with either rat or mouse spleen cells it was found that the proportion of hybrid cells expressing spleen cell derived immunoglobulin was dependent upon the particular combination of myeloma and spleen cells[22] (see data summarized in Table 1.2). The proportion of immunoglobulin secreting hybrids in these fusions is considerably higher than the proportion of immunoglobulin secreting spleen cells and this suggests that the use of a myeloma line results in the selective survival of hybrids with cells of the B-cell lineage. The most extreme example is in the case of the rat myeloma line Y3/Ag1.2.3 fused with rat spleen cells where more than

Table 1.2 Immunoglobulin secreting phenotype in mouse and rat hybrid myelomas[22]

Myeloma	Spleen cells	Percentage of hybrids secreting spleen cell derived immunoglobulin
mouse	mouse	40–80
mouse	rat	15–40
rat	rat	>90
rat	mouse	50–90

90% of the resulting hybrid cells secrete a spleen cell derived immunoglobulin. This higher proportion of immunoglobulin expressing hybrids when using the rat myeloma line Y3/Ag1.2.3 compared with the mouse myeloma lines seems to be as a result of the greater stability of the resulting hybrids for immunoglobulin expression. This stability can be usefully exploited in the production of rat × rat hybrids[17] as described later.

CELL FUSION

The act of fusing the cells is perhaps the simplest part of the procedure but also gives rise to the most difficulties.

Basically the process involves mixing the two cell types and then treating the cells with an agent that promotes membrane fusion and the formation of heterokaryons. The first successful fusion to produce hybrid myelomas used sendai virus as a fusing agent[11], however this has in most circumstances been superceded by use of polyethylene glycol (PEG) because of ease of handling and storage. However protocols differ in the exact details of the use of PEG. Different laboratories vary in the use of PEG of different average molecular weight, concentration of solution and length of time of treatment[30]. Certain batches of PEG seem to be more toxic to cells than others even to the extent that some batches are reported to be toxic only in the presence of calcium ions in the solution[31]. It has also been reported that addition of DMSO to the solution allows the PEG concentration to be reduced, thus lowering the toxicity but maintaining the same fusion efficiency[32]. In our laboratory we use PEG 1500 (BDH Chemicals Ltd, Poole, England, Cat. No. 29575; BDH Chemicals Ltd, MERK, Cat. No. 807469) made up in either culture medium (DMEM or IMDM) or PBS (including phenol red as an indicator) by adding 1 g of PEG to each 1 ml of Medium. The pH of the PEG solution has also been shown to influence cell fusion[33] and we usually adjust our PEG solution to a pH between 6.8–7.0 as judged by the phenol red indicator. The length of time the cells are treated with PEG is also a critical factor, too short a time and few hybrids result, too long and the toxic effect of the PEG becomes too great. We treat the cells for a period of between 1.5 to 2 minutes before diluting out the PEG by addition of medium.

The other aspect of the cell fusion is in the preparation of the cells. The spleen cells are prepared as a single cell suspension by disrupting the spleen in medium, some protocols then go to the trouble of removing the red cells. We regard this extra step in preparing the spleen cells as an unnecessary manipulation which may increase the risks of cell damage and losses or of contamination.

Preparation of spleen cells

Materials
Handling medium (DMEM + 2%FCS), 250 ml of 70% ethanol, centrifuge tubes (e.g. disposable universal), a 90 mm Petri dish, a tissue culture washed autoclaved plunger from a disposable 10 ml plastic syringe, an autoclaved stainless steel tea strainer and sterile dissection instruments.

Procedure
All at room temperature.
1. Kill the rat or mouse (e.g. by using CO_2, breaking neck or terminally anaesthetizing with ether).
2. Dip the animal in the 70% alcohol. Place on dissection board and then using sterile instruments and aseptic techniques dissect out the spleen and transfer it intact to the petri dish containing 10 ml of handling medium.
3. Transfer the spleen into the stainless steel strainer over the petri dish and make several cuts using a sterile pair of scissors. Then using the plunger from a disposable syringe gently break the spleen up releasing a single cell suspension.
4. Transfer the cell suspension to a universal and allow large clumps to settle out for 1–2 minutes. Transfer the remaining cell suspension to a second tube and spin the cells down for 10 minutes at $400 \times g$. (At this point it is best to start preparing the myeloma cells as below).
5. Resuspend the spleen cell pellet in 20 ml of fresh handling medium and centrifuge again.
6. Resuspend the cell pellet in 10 ml of handling medium and count the viable nucleated cells. Mouse spleens give approximately 10^8 cells (enough for one fusion) and rat spleens give approximately 2×10^8 (enough for two fusions).

Myeloma cell preparation
1. From a culture of myeloma cells in logarithmic growth pellet at $400 \times g$ for 10 minutes enough cells for the fusion (see numbers as below).
2. Resuspend the cell pellet in 10 ml of handling medium and count viable cells.

Cell fusion

Materials
1. Sterile pipettes 1, 10, 25 ml capacity, a 250 ml beaker for use as a waterbath in the sterile cabinet, centrifuge tubes (e.g. universals), medium without added protein, i.e. no FCS (otherwise the protein will be precipitated by the PEG).
2. 50% PEG: Polyethylene glycol (10 g) MW 1500 (BDH Chemicals Ltd, Poole, Dorset, England, Cat. No. 29575) is autoclaved and then allowed to cool slightly, whilst it is still liquid 10 ml of sterile medium (containing no FCS) is added and the solution is thoroughly mixed. Using the phenol red as a guide adjust the pH to approximately pH 7 (this can usually be achieved either by gassing with CO_2 to lower the pH or by leaving the container open to the atmosphere in a sterile hood to raise the pH).

3. A 37°C water bath. The PEG solution should be equilibrated at this temperature prior to the fusion.

Procedure

All at room temperature except for the PEG treatment.

1. The parental cells prepared as described above should be mixed together, 10^8 spleen cells to 10^7 mouse or 6×10^7 rat myeloma cells and resuspended to 25 ml with medium without added protein in a plastic universal and are then spun down for 10 minutes at $400 \times g$. Resuspend the cells in serumless medium and pellet again at $400 \times g$ for 10 minutes.

2. Remove all the supernatant to avoid dilution of PEG and then disrupt the cell pellet by gentle tapping and transfer the tube to the beaker containing water at 37°C (this is used as a convenient water bath in the sterile cabinet).

3. Carefully over a period of 30 seconds add 0.8–1.0 ml of 50% PEG and continue stirring the cell suspension with the pipette until 60 seconds have elapsed.

4. During the next 30 seconds take up a 25 ml pipette full of medium and then dilute the cell suspension to 25 ml. Spin down the cells at $400 \times g$ for 10 minutes.

CULTURE AND SELECTION FOR HYBRID GROWTH

Selection

Following fusion the cells are plated out and additives are used in the medium to select against the parental cells. Nearly all the myeloma cell lines used for hybrid myeloma production have been selected so that they are unable to grow in medium supplemented with hypoxanthine, aminopterin and thymidine, called HAT medium[34,35]. The cells have been selected for a mutation in the enzyme hypoxanthine-guanine phosphoribosyltransferase (HGPRT) enabling them to survive in the presence of the toxic guanine analogues 8-azaguanine or 6-thioguanine. The enzyme HGPRT is part of a salvage pathway for the production of precursors of nucleic acids, a pathway which is not essential provided de novo synthesis of nucleotides is possible. However aminopterin is an inhibitor of certain steps in the de novo synthesis of nucleotides such that only cells making use of the salvage pathways for synthesis from the precursors hypoxanthine and thymidine will survive. In order for hybrids to survive in HAT medium the enzyme HGPRT has to be present and can only be provided by the spleen cell partner.

Culture

An important consideration following cell fusion is the number of individual culture wells into which the cells should be seeded. This decision may be a crucial factor in determining success or failure in obtaining the required monoclonal antibody producing hybrid myelomas. Depending upon the efficiency of fusion up to about 1000 individual hybrids may be generated from 10^8 spleen cells. Clearly if the fused cells were distributed into very few culture wells (e.g. 50) then multiple hybrids would grow up in each well. This would inevitably result in the loss of some hybrids because of overgrowth by faster growing hybrid clones (termed 'clonal competition').

The alternative is to distribute the cells so that only one or less hybrid clones per well are achieved (e.g. by distributing the 1000 clones into twenty 96 well plates). However the seeding efficiencies may not necessarily be linear with dilution and it is often found when the cells are plated at low concentration that 'feeder layers' or 'conditioned media' are required.

Various other considerations influence the seeding out of the fusion products. If cells are distributed into a large number of cultures then this increases the effort in maintenance and assay of cultures. However because under these conditions the hybrids are in general growing as single colonies per well, once a positive well is scored the positive clone is more easily isolated. The most widely adopted approach follows this policy of plating the cells into a large number of cultures, assaying the supernatants as soon as the hybrid cultures grow up, and then selecting just a few of the culture wells of interest whilst the other cultures are discarded. This approach requires that the assays are simple and that the results can be obtained fairly quickly, otherwise it is possible that desirable positive wells will be lost during prolonged culture prior to freezing and cloning.

The main experience of our laboratory has been in the production of monoclonal antibodies to human and mouse cell surface antigens[18,36,37]. This work has often involved the use of assays such as fluorescence activated cell sorting followed by in vitro culture of haemopoietic colony forming cells for the identification of the subpopulations of cells recognized. Such biological assays are often lengthy and difficult to scale up precluding analysis of many individual supernatants simultaneously. For this reason we tend to distribute cells from fusions into a relatively smaller number of culture wells (e.g. four 24 well plates). Using the rat myeloma line Y3/Ag1.2.3 and immunized rat spleen cells we have found that the resulting cultures containing several hybrid clones can be grown up and the cells frozen in liquid nitrogen. Sufficient supernatant can then be collected to perform numerous assays at leisure. We then adopt assay systems which on average detect only one hybrid in each culture well. For example with use of subclass specific reagents or by screening for particular biological functions such as complement mediated cell lysis or antibody dependent cell mediated cytotoxicity, it is possible to distinguish the many individual reactivities within a given well[17,19,38]. Once all the results are collated it is possible to select culture wells containing hybrids of interest and to take these cultures up from storage and then separate out the individual hybrids by cloning. We have with this approach been able to use quite lengthy and complex assays to identify wells containing clones of interest and have been able to isolate such clones some 3 years following the original fusion. We have had less success in adopting this approach with mouse myeloma × mouse spleen cell fusions and it seems that the difference may be attributable to the greater stability for immunoglobulin expression in Y3/Ag1.2.3 × rat spleen cell hybrids as mentioned above. It seems that when the uncloned rat hybrids are thawed from liquid nitrogen storage they still all continue to secrete antibody. In contrast many non-secreting mouse hybrids arise probably by clonal instability and by clonal competition during the freezing and thawing of uncloned cultures.

The other advantage gained by freezing down all of the cultures from a successful fusion is that the supernatants represent a monoclonal antibody bank derived from the immunization. This bank can then be screened at later dates when new assays are available and may save considerable time and effort by avoiding the need to immunize a new animal to obtain a new specificity which may have been overlooked in the screening of an earlier fusion.

Our recommendations are then, to use seeding at limiting dilutions in circumstances where a simple straightforward assay exists or when making mouse hybrids to simplify the isolation of positive cultures. In situations where assays are lengthy and complex it may be better to use the rat myeloma Y3/Ag1.2.3 and to make rat spleen cell hybrids. It is then possible to seed the hybrids into a limited number of cultures which can be frozen, allowing the assays to be performed on the supernatants at a more leisurely pace.

Methods

The number and type of culture well into which the cell fusion products are to be distributed depend on the considerations mentioned above. If limiting dilution is to be achieved it will be necessary to plate the cells out into a large number of culture wells. Although 96 well culture plates holding approximately 0.2 ml/well are favoured by many workers our personal preferences are for the use of 24 well (Nunc. Cat. No. 1-43982) or 48 well (Costar. Cat. No. 3548) culture dishes. These offer the advantage of providing larger volumes of supernatants for assay and in addition because of the better separation between culture wells there is less risk of cell cross contamination or the spread of infection and feeding is also easier.

The cells are initially plated out overnight in medium (DMEM) supplemented with 20% FCS. The following day the plates should be observed under the microscope, many live cells should remain. Remove half the volume of medium from each culture well and replace with DMEM + 20% FCS supplemented with HAT. Repeat this procedure for 2 more days and during this time the myeloma cells should be observed to die. Thereafter observe the culture wells under a microscope and change half the volume of media in each well at least once every 3 to 5 days (this is because components of the media like glutamine break down during prolonged periods at 37°C).

The time before hybrid growth is observed can be between one week and one month after the fusion and varies from fusion to fusion. Once a hybrid colony approaches confluence in a well and the medium has turned slightly acid as judged by the colour of the medium, it is possible to collect the supernatant for assay following which a decision must be made about the future of the hybrid cells. To minimize the chances of loss of any culture well it is worthwhile to split each culture into a second duplicate plate or expand the cultures into a larger culture well or a culture flask. Alternatively the present culture may be maintained by removing about $\frac{1}{2}$ to $\frac{3}{4}$ of the cells by vacuum suction and feeding with fresh media. It is recommended for less experienced laboratories that a duplicate culture of each growing well be prepared and that the two cultures are fed with different bottles of media reducing the risks of loss of cultures due to contamination. At the stage of splitting it is possible to replace the HAT in the medium by HT for about 3 or 4 feeds (for a period of at least one week) thus diluting out the aminopterin, subsequent culture can then be continued in ordinary medium plus FCS without any HAT or HT.

Based on the assay results, selected cultures can be expanded into small culture flasks, cells frozen, and larger volumes of supernatants collected. At the same time cloning of positive cultures should prevent loss of the antibody through clonal competition or clonal instability.

Once the hybrid cultures are growing well and particularly after cloning when they are well stabilized the percentage of FCS in the media can be reduced. We find DMEM or IMDM supplemented with 2.5% FCS adequate for long term maintenance of cell lines.

Feeder layers and conditioned media

During the early stages of a cell fusion when the cultures are being selected in HAT medium, or when cloning hybrid myeloma cultures at low cell densities it is often found that seeding efficiencies of the cells are non-linear. This implies that the cells growing at higher cell densities are possibly benefiting from a conditioning of the culture medium. Hybrid myeloma cells seeded at low densities will often grow better if feeder layers of other cells are used or if the culture medium is supplemented with supernatant conditioned by another cell line. If feeder layers are to be used it is essential that they are themselves unable to outgrow the hybrid myeloma cells. This can either be achieved by using normal rat or mouse spleen cells, peritoneal macrophages or thymocytes, which have a finite life time in culture, or alternatively by using fibroblast cell lines which have been inhibited from cell division with irradiation or mitomycin C treatment.

Conditioned media

Perhaps the easiest way of improving cell cloning efficiencies is to supplement the growth medium with a suitable source of conditioned medium. This is prepared by collecting the supernatant from a culture in exponential growth phase (suitable cultures being for example a fibroblast cell line such as 3T3 or a non-producing myeloma cell line such as NSO/u). Any cells and debris are removed by centrifugation at $400 \times g$ for 15 minutes and the supernatant should then be filter sterilized through a 0.22 micron filter and stored sterile at $-20°C$. This 'conditioned' medium can then be used to supplement the growth medium for cell fusion or for single cell cloning by adding it at 10 to 20% (v/v).

Mitomycin C treated fibroblasts

3T3 fibroblast cells in log phase in 75 cm^2 culture bottles are treated with mitomycin C (Sigma, Cat. No. M 0503) at 0.04 mg/ml in DMEM for 45 minutes at 37°C. The cells are then removed from the surface of the bottle by removing all the medium followed by addition of 4 ml of Trypsin/EDTA solution (Gibco Europe, Cat. No. 043-5400) for 20 minutes at 37°C. Wash the cells out with 20 ml DMEM 5% FCS and spin down the cells for 10 minutes at $400 \times g$. The cells can be stored frozen in liquid nitrogen or used immediately by distributing $1-3 \times 10^3$ cells into about four 24 culture well plates. It is worth checking each batch of treated cells prepared for lack of growth in case the conditions of treatment were inadequate.

CLONING AND FREEZING OF CULTURES

Having identified the cultures of interest it is necessary to isolate the hybrid cell clones from those culture wells (which are potentially mixtures of multiple hybrid cell clones) by single cell cloning. There are three main ways of cloning hybrid myeloma cultures. The method we routinely adopt is to make dilutions of the cells and then to mix them with a liquid agar or agarose. The agar is then allowed to set as a thin semi-solid layer above a much thicker nutrient agar layer. Colonies grow up over a period of about 1 week and these can either be assayed for their antibody secretion in situ where appropriate or more commonly they can be transferred to liquid culture by picking individual colonies into each well of a multi well culture dish.

The second method of cell cloning routinely used is to plate the cells out into many culture wells at a suitable dilution such that on average there is less than one cell per culture well. In practice it is found that many hybrid cell lines do not clone linearly with dilution suggesting that single cells may not survive to give colonies. The cloning efficiencies can be improved by using feeder layers or conditioned medium. It is here that semi solid agar cloning has an advantage because the colonies are growing physically isolated from each other but are able to help each other grow because of the diffusion of factors and media components.

The third method of cloning used for hybrid myeloma cells is single cell manipulation. Single cells are placed in culture wells either by manual manipulation of cells using micropipettes by observation under a microscope or alternatively it is possible to adapt cell sorting machines such as fluorescence activated cell sorters to place single cells with chosen properties into individual culture wells of a multi-well dish.

Some workers have adopted the policy of cloning the fusion products immediately in semi-solid media containing HAT to select for hybrid cell growth[33,39]. This approach is very useful when the assay can be adapted to detect the positive clones in situ, for example some of the first monoclonal antibodies isolated were assayed in agar monolayers for antibody dependent lysis of sheep red blood cells[11]. A later development involves overlaying the clones with filters coated with antigen or antiglobulin, the filters can then be developed with a labelled second antiserum or antigen[40].

Protocol for semi-solid agar cloning

Materials
Difco Bacto Agar, tissue culture grade water, double strength medium (2 × DMEM), FCS, tissue culture grade petri dishes (e.g. Falcon 35 mm × 10 mm Cat. No. 3001) and a sterile pyrex flask. A waterbath pre-equilibrated at 45°C. Sterile pipettes, 25 ml, 10 ml and 1 ml volumes.

Procedure
1. Prepare 1.1% mass/vol. agar in tissue culture grade water by boiling in the sterile flask over a bunsen burner (avoid boiling for too long to prevent increasing the ionic strength through evaporation of water or scorching the agar).

2. Allow the agar solution to cool to about 45°C and then mix one part to one part double strength medium also at 45°C. Maintain the temperature by keeping in the waterbath.

3. Add one part FCS to 10 parts of the agar/medium mix giving a final concentration of agar of 0.5% mass/vol. in medium supplemented with 10% FCS.

4. Pipette 2 ml of this medium into each 35 mm diameter petri dish and allow the agar to set as a base layer (20 minutes at room temperature).

5. Prepare a series of dilutions of the cell line to be cloned in 1 ml volumes of medium (DMEM + 10% FCS) at room temperature. We find 24 well culture dishes are convenient and economical for the dilutions, suggested dilutions being six 6-fold dilutions from a starting cell concentration in the region of 10^5 cells per ml.

6. Working quickly add 1 ml of the 0.5% agar/medium to each dilution, mix and transfer between 0.5 ml and 1.0 ml to the petri dishes containing the agar base layers. It is best to plate only a few dilutions at a time to avoid the agar setting too soon. The same pipette can be used for several dilutions provided the lower cell concentrations are plated first. Allow the top layer to set and then transfer the dishes to a humidified CO_2 37°C incubator.

7. After 5 to 7 days the clones should be large enough (100–200 cells) to be transferred into liquid culture. This is best done by digging out the clone using a pasteur pipette and expelling the clone into a well of a multi well culture dish containing about 0.5 ml of DMEM + 10% FCS. A stereo dissection microscope is useful but not essential.

Individual clones are usually selected using similar assay procedures as for the original fusion culture wells. The positive cultures are expanded and when there are enough cells in a good state of viability aliquots of cells are frozen to ensure the indefinite survival of the culture. Suitably frozen the cells will survive for many years if kept in liquid nitrogen cooled vessels or alternatively the cells may be stored for a more limited period in –70°C freezers (6 months). Cultures in exponential growth phase (cells in stationary phase are not suitable) with a high viability are taken, the cells are spun down and resuspended in cold (+4°C) freezing medium. Aliquots containing approximately 2×10^6 cells are placed in each sterile freezing vial and following this the cells are transferred directly to a –70°C freezer or put into a polystyrene container suspended in the neck of a liquid nitrogen container. After 24 hours the cells can be transferred to liquid nitrogen storage if required. Although microprocessor controlled temperature cell freezing machines are available we have found that their use is not necessary for the freezing and thawing of hybrid myeloma cell lines with good viability.

Protocol for freezing cells

Materials
Freezing mixture 90% FCS 10% DMSO kept cool on ice, a supply of 2 ml freezing ampoules (Sterilin, Cat. No. 506) labelled with the name of the cell line and the date, also kept cool in ice. Sterile centrifuge tubes (universals).

Procedure
1. Spin down the cells from culture for 7–10 minutes at $400 \times g$ (approximately 10 ml of a culture of cells in good condition, growing in logarithmic phase at a cell density of about $2 \times 10^5 - 5 \times 10^5$ cells/ml for each vial to be frozen).

2. Decant off the supernatant (may be kept for assay) and resuspend the cell pellet in cold freezing mixture (1 ml per ampoule to be frozen) and place the cell suspension in a labelled freezing ampoule.

3. As quickly as possible and without allowing the ampoules to warm up above ice temperature transfer them to a $-70°C$ freezer and leave for at least 24 hours. We have found that it is not necessary to use controlled temperature cooling of rat or mouse hybrid myelomas to maintain high recovery of viable cells, although it is possible to place the ampoules inside a polystyrene container to reduce the rate of cooling.

4. After 24 hours the ampoules may be transferred to liquid nitrogen cooled storage vessels for long term storage. (Cells stored at $-70°C$ lose viability over a period of between 6 to 12 months).

Thawing of frozen cells

Materials
Cold medium (DMEM + 10% FCS). Centrifuge tube (universal). A multi well culture dish or a small 25 cm² Culture flask.

Procedure
1. Bring the cells rapidly to $+4°C$ by warming the vial in a $37°C$ water bath until the ice is just melted.

2. Without allowing the medium to warm above $+4°C$ add the cell suspension quickly to 10 ml of cold medium (DMEM + 10% FCS) and spin the cells down for 10 minutes at $400 \times g$ in a cooled centrifuge if possible.

3. Many cell lines can then be immediately transferred to culture flasks (gassed with 5% CO_2) in about 3–5 ml of culture medium (DMEM + 10% FCS). However for optimal recovery of valuable cell lines it is better to make four doubling dilutions of the cell in 1–2 ml culture wells and place in a humidified CO_2 $37°C$ incubator and observe after 24 hours.

It is of course essential for the long term care of hybrid myeloma cultures that the individual hybrids be cloned properly in the first instance (we suggest at least two sequential cloning operations) and that a sufficient number of ampoules be frozen at each stage to ensure the maximum chances of maintaining the culture for an indefinite period. If the hybrid clone is kept in continuous culture for a period of several months it is likely that variants will accumulate as discussed earlier. Thus it is best to clone such cultures periodically or to return to earlier frozen stocks if culture is to be continued.

IDENTIFICATION OF CLONES AND ANALYSIS FOR VARIANTS OF IMMUNOGLOBULIN PRODUCTION

In addition to screening for the specific antibody production by individual clones we have found it useful to record certain additional properties of the antibodies. The isotypes and chain compositions of the secreted antibodies are normally determined. We routinely take samples of cells of the selected clones and grow them overnight in medium containing radioactively labelled lysine. The internally labelled antibody is then analysed by running the supernatant on reducing Laemmli gels followed by autoradiography[41]. Often it is possible to see differences in the mobilites of different chains of the same type (e.g. two light chains) because of their anomalous apparent molecular weights[42]. However where two different chains have the same mobility it is still possible to run the supernatant on iso-electric focussing gels[42,43,44].

Materials
1. Prepare medium containing no L-lysine from the Gibco-Biocult 'Select amine kit' (Gibco Europe, Cat. No. 062-9050) following the manufacturers instructions.
   2. L-[U-^{14}C]lysine monohydrochloride, 250 micro Curies in 5 ml (Amersham UK, England, Cat. No. CFB.69).
   3. Dialysed FCS. Prepare by dialysing against tissue culture grade water and then add back 10 × balanced salt solution 1 part to 9 parts FCS. Filter sterilize.
   4. Sterile 10 ml round bottomed centrifuge tubes or alternatively kidney tubes.

Procedure
1. Incorporation medium is prepared by adding 1 ml of [^{14}C]-Lysine and 0.5 ml of dialyzed FCS to 9 ml of lysine free medium.
   2. Approximately 1×10^6 cells from an exponential culture are centrifuged in the 10 ml tubes at 400 × g for 10 minutes, and are then resuspended in lysine free medium and pelleted at 400 × g again. The cells are then resuspended in 0.2 ml of incorporation medium and are incubated for 15–20 hours at 37°C.
   3. Spin out the cells at 400 × g for 10 minutes and collect the supernatant. The radioactively labelled antibody can then be analysed by gel electrophoresis.

We also determine the isotype of the antibody produced. The classical way of doing this would be to use immunodiffusion techniques using isotype specific antisera[45]. However we have either made or obtained isotype specific mouse monoclonal anti rat immunoglobulins[46,47,48] and have found that the fastest and simplest way to isotype our rat monoclonal antibodies is to couple the mouse monoclonals to human group O red blood cells or to trypsin treated sheep red blood cells and to then use reverse passive haemagglutination. If the supernatants are titred it is also possible to estimate relative concentrations of antibodies, a useful guide when scaling up production of antibody in vitro. It is also possible to stabilize the coupled red cells for long term storage[49]. Alternatively the anti-isotype monoclonal antibodies may be linked to the red cells or labelled with for example radioactive iodine or an enzyme and then used in isotype specific indirect binding assays on the unknown monoclonal antibodies[38,50].

All of these properties of the secreted antibodies are useful in distinguishing the differences between individual clones (possibly obtained from the same original culture well) and in identifying variants of the original clone.

LARGE SCALE PRODUCTION OF ANTIBODY

Large quantities of monoclonal antibodies can either be obtained as cell free supernatant from culture of cells in vitro or alternatively the cells can be passaged in vivo to obtain the antibody as ascitic fluid. Antibody produced by in vitro culture is free from contamination by other rat or mouse immunoglobulins. However the antibody concentration is often less than 100 μg/ml even in spent culture medium and for very large volumes extra culture equipment is needed such as roller culture or spinner culture facilities. Hybrid myeloma cells derived by fusion of a mouse myeloma with spleen cells from an inbred mouse strain or a rat myeloma with spleen cells from an inbred rat strain will readily grow as tumours in the appropriate strain of mouse or rat. Antibody concentrations may be as high as 10–20 mg/ml of ascites. The animals should be primed with pristane in order to facilitate the rapid growth of the cells as ascitic fluid in the peritoneal cavity.

Procedure
The animals should be primed at least 2–3 weeks earlier with pristane (Sigma, tetramethylpentadecane Cat. No. T 7640), 0.5 ml i.p. each mouse or 1.5 ml i.p. each rat. 5×10^6 to 1×10^7 cells in logarithmic growth will rapidly produce ascitic fluid in such animals (5 ml per mouse in approximately 2 weeks or 40 ml per rat in 9–10 days). The animals are then killed and the ascitic fluid drained from the peritoneum. Second generation transplants can be carried out, the ascites from one mouse or rat will provide enough cells to transplant into 20 others. We do not go beyond 2–3 generations to minimize the accumulation of chain loss variants.

The antibody can be concentrated and partially purified from both ascites and culture supernatants by a number of methods. The first step is usually to precipitate the antibody using 50% of saturation of ammonium sulphate, the precipitate is then redissolved and dialyzed into a suitable buffer of choice such as for example phosphate buffered saline. Subsequent purification steps might involve gel filtration, ion-exchange chromatography or affinity chromatography. Details of these methods can be found in general texts[51,52] (see also ch. 3).

SELECTION OF 8-AZAGUANINE DRUG RESISTANCE MARKER

The use of hybrid myelomas with a drug resistance marker for the derivation of hybrid hybridomas making antibodies of dual specificity has recently been described[27]. It may be that workers will wish to construct such hybrid hybridomas using a parental hybrid myeloma with a different specificity. In general it is found that re-establishing the drug resistance marker is usually quite straightforward in hybrids resulting from the use of a myeloma cell line resistant to 8-Azaguanine.

Materials
Medium (DMEM + 5% FCS) and 100 × 8-Azaguanine stock (described earlier). Multi well culture dish. Prepare 1 × 8-Azaguanine medium (DMEM + 5% FCS with 1 part/100 8-Azaguanine stock).

Procedure
1. Establish the cell line in 12 wells of a multi well culture dish.

2. Feed the first 2 wells with medium and the 10 subsequent wells with medium and medium + Azaguanine in various proportions such that the third well is approximately 10% 8-Azaguanine medium and the last well 100% 8-Azaguanine medium.

3. Observe the growth of cells and gradually on subsequent days move cells growing at lower concentration of 8-Azaguanine to a higher concentration.

4. The cells will eventually be growing in full strength 8-Azaguanine when they should be cloned and frozen and a clone selected for cell fusion experiments.

RECORD KEEPING

Embarking on a project to produce hybrid myelomas secreting monoclonal antibodies is likely to involve much time and effort in complex tissue culture and assay procedures. The identification of positive cultures and then expansion of these cultures followed by repeated freezing and cloning generates an exponentially increasing amount of data to be stored. It is essential that the details of isolation of each clone should be easily accessible so that relationships with other clones of a similar or different specificity may be obtained. Also it is necessary to know how many vials of each cell line are frozen and where they are located so that an important hybrid myeloma line is never irrecoverably lost. It is also good policy to always replace a newly frozen vial as the first action after expansion of a culture thawed from frozen stock.

The simplest way of achieving these ends is to systematically name each clone with a unique number. The method usually adopted is to give each fusion a unique name or number followed by a second number indicating each individual culture well of a fusion, e.g. fusion A culture wells 1–96 would be A1, A2, ... A96. When a given well is cloned then each clone is also given a number, e.g. the 24 clones obtained from well 7 would be A7.1, A7.2 ... to A7.24 and so on with recloning.

Using such a systematic naming system it is very easy to keep track of all the information relating to the culture, storage and assay data for a given hybrid myeloma clone. This data can also be very easily transferred onto computer.

TROUBLE SHOOTING

The most common problem is an inability to obtain or sustain the growth of hybrid myeloma cultures. The most likely case is one of the media components or the preparation and treatment of cells for the fusion. A few simple checks may identify the problem.

1. The medium and fetal calf serum should be checked for their ability to support the growth of the myeloma cell line and preferably a hybrid myeloma cell line at low cell densities.

2. The myeloma cell line should die in medium supplemented with HAT but the toxicity of the HAT and HT should also be tested with hybrid myeloma cell lines or cell lines lacking the 8-Azaguanine drug resistance marker which should therefore grow quite happily in medium supplemented with HAT.

3. The toxicity of the PEG can be assessed on the day following the cell fusion and prior to the addition of HAT for selection. Cell growth and division of the myeloma should have occurred and if the cultures contain a high percentage of dead cells then the treatment may have been for too long. An insufficient treatment with PEG will also result in no hybrid growth but in this case there will be little evidence of cell death on the following day.

4. Plating the cells following cell fusion into cultures at various dilutions with and without feeder cells or conditioned media may help to optimize conditions for cell fusion with the reagents in use in a given laboratory.

5. It is important that the parental myeloma cell line be kept in optimal conditions prior to the fusion growing in logarithmic phase. If the cells are allowed to overgrow, i.e. reach stationary phase it may require subsequent culturing in log phase for at least a week for the cells to give optimum fusion efficiencies.

REFERENCES
1. Burnet M 1959 The clonal selection theory of acquired immunity. Vanderbolt University Press, Nashville, USA
2. Pernis B, Chiappino G, Kelus A S, Gell P E H 1965 Cellular localization of immunoglobulins with different allotypic specificities in rabbit lymphoid tissues. Journal of Experimental Medicine 122: 853–876
3. Potter M 1972 Immunoglobulin producing tumours and myeloma proteins in mice. Physiological Reviews 52: 631–719
4. Cohn M 1967 Natural history of the myeloma. Cold Spring Harbor Symposium on Quantitative Biology 32: 211–221
5. Horibata K, Harris A W 1970 Mouse myelomas and lymphomas in culture. Experimental Cell Research 60: 61–63
6. Cotton R G H, Secher D S, Milstein C 1973 Somatic mutation and the origin of antibody diversity: Clonal variability of the immunoglobulin produced by MOPC21 cells in culture. European Journal of Immunology 3: 135–140
7. Secher D S, Cotton R G H, Milstein C 1973 Spontaneous mutation in tissue culture—chemical nature of variant immunoglobulins from mutant clones of MOPC21. FEBS Letters 37: 311–316
8. Secher D S, Milstein C, Adetugbo K 1977 Somatic mutants and antibody diversity. Immunological Reviews 36: 51–71
9. Cotton R G H, Milstein C 1973 Fusion of two immunoglobulin producing cell lines. Nature 244: 42–43
10. Schwaber J, Cohen E P 1974 Pattern of Ig synthesis and assembly in a mouse–human somatic cell hybrid clone. Proceedings of the National Academy of Science 71: 2203–2207
11. Kohler G, Milstein C 1975 Continuous cultures of fused cells secreting antibody of predefined specifity. Nature 256: 495–497
12. Iscove N N, Melchers F 1978 Complete replacement of serum by albumen, transferrin and soybean lipid in cultures of lipopolysaccharide reactive B-lymphocytes. Journal of Experimental Medicine 147: 923–933
13. Iscove N N, Gilbert L J, Weyman C 1980 Complete replacement of serum in primary cultures of erythropoietin dependent red cell precursors (CFU-E) by albumen, transferrin, iron, saturated fatty acids, lecithin, and cholesterol. Experimental Cell Research 126: 121–126
14. Spitz M, Spitz L, Thorpe R, Eugui E 1984 Intrasplenic primary immunization for the production of monoclonal antibodies. Journal of Immunological Methods 70: 39–43
15. Sirvaganian R P, Fox P C, Bereustein E H 1983 Methods of enhancing the frequency of antigen specific hybridomas. Methods in Enzymology 92: 17–25
16. Stahli C, Staehelin T, Miggiano V 1983 Spleen cell analysis and optimal immunization for high frequency production of specific hybridomas. Methods in Enzymology 92: 26–36
17. Clark M, Cobbold S, Hale G, Waldmann H 1983 Advantages of rat monoclonal antibodies. Immunology Today 4: 100–101
18. Hale G, Bright S, Chumbley G, Hoang T, Metcalf D, Munro A, Waldmann H 1983 Removal of T-cells from bone marrow for transplantation: a monoclonal anti-lymphocyte antibody which fixes human complement. Blood 62: 873–882
19. Hale G, Clark M R, Waldmann H 1985 Therapeutic potential of rat monoclonal antibodies: Isotype specificity of antibody-dependent cell-mediated cytotoxicity with human lymphocytes. The Journal of Immunology 134: 3056–3062
20. Kohler G, Howe S C, Milstein C 1976 Fusion between immunoglobulin secreting and non secreting myeloma cell lines. European Journal of Immunology 6: 292–295
21. Kearney J F, Radbruch A, Liesegang B, Rajewsky K 1979 A new mouse myeloma cell line that has lost immunoglobulin expression but permits the construction of antibody-secreting hybrid cell lines. The Journal of Immunology 123: 1548–1550
22. Clark M R, Milstein C 1981 Expression of the spleen cell immunoglobulin phenotype in hybrids with myeloma cell lines. Somatic Cell Genetics 7: 657–666

23. Schulman M, Wilde C D, Kohler G 1978 A better cell line for making hybrid myelomas secreting specific antibodies. Nature 276: 269–271
24. Galfre G, Milstein C, Wright B 1979 Rat × rat hybrid myelomas and a monoclonal anti-Fd portion of mouse IgG. Nature 277: 131–133
25. Galfre G, Milstein C 1981 Preparation of monoclonal antibodies: strategies and procedures. Methods in Enzymology 73: 3–46
26. Bazin H 1982 Production of rat monoclonal antibodies with the LOU rat non secreting IR983F myeloma cell line. In: Peeters H (ed) Protides of the biological fluids. Pergamon Press, Oxford, 29: 615–618
27. Milstein C, Cuello C 1983 Hybrid hybrid myelomas and their use in immunohistochemistry. Nature 305: 537–540
28. Kohler G, Hengartner H, Milstein C 1978 The sequence of immunoglobulin chain losses in mouse (myeloma × B-cell) hybrids. In: Peeters H (ed) Protides of the biological fluids. Pergamon Press, Oxford
29. Cobbold S P, Waldmann H 1984 Therapeutic potential of monovalent monoclonal antibodies. Nature 308: 460–462
30. Gefter M L, Margulies D H, Scharff M D 1977 A simple method for polyethylene glycol-promoted hybridization of mouse myeloma cells. Somatic Cell Genetics 3: 231–233
31. Mercer W E, Baserga R 1982 Techniques for decreasing the toxicity of polyethylene glycol. In: Shay J W (ed) Techniques in somatic cell genetics. Plenum Press, London, 23–33
32. Norwood T H, Ziegler C J 1982 The use of dimethyl sulphoxide in mammalian cell fusion. In: Shay J W (ed) Techniques in somatic cell genetics. Plenum Press, London, 35–44
33. Sharon J, Morrison S L, Kabat E A 1980 Formation of hybrid myeloma clones in soft agarose; effect of pH and of medium. Somatic Cell Genetics 6: 435–441
34. Szybalski W, Szybalska E H, Ragni G 1962 Genetic studies with human cell lines. National Cancer Institute Monographs 7: 75–89
35. Littlefield J W 1964 Selection of hybrids of fibroblasts in vitro and their presumed recombinants. Science 145: 709–711
36. Hoang T, Gilmore D, Metcalf D, Cobbold S, Watt S, Clark M, Furth M, Waldmann H 1983 Separation of hemopoietic cells from adult mouse marrow by use of monoclonal antibodies. Blood 61: 580–588
37. Watt S M, Metcalf D, Gilmore D J, Stenning G M, Clark M R, Waldmann H 1983 Selective isolation of murine erythropoietin-responsive progenitor cells (CFU-E) with monoclonal antibodies. Molecular Biology and Medicine 1: 95–115
38. Aqel N M, Clark M R, Cobbold S P, Waldmann H 1984 Immunohistochemical screening in the selection of monoclonal antibodies: the use of isotype-specific antiglobulins. Journal of Immunological Methods 69: 207–214
39. Davis J M, Pennington J E, Kubler A M, Conscience J F 1982 A simple, single step technique for selecting and cloning hybridomas for the production of monoclonal antibodies. Journal of Immunological Methods 50: 161–171
40. Sharon J, Morrison S L, Kabat E A 1979 Detection of specific hybridoma clones by replica immunoabsorption of their secreted antibodies. Proceedings of the National Academy of Science 76: 1429–1433
41. Laemmli U K 1970 Cleavage of structural proteins during the assembly of the head of bacteriophage T4. Nature 227: 680–685
42. Kohler G, Milstein C 1976 Derivation of specific antibody-producing tissue culture and tumor cell lines by cell fusion. European Journal of Immunology 6: 511–519
43. Phillips J M, Dresser D W 1973 Isoelectric spectra of different classes of anti erythrocyte antibodies. European Journal of Immunology 3: 524–527
44. Zeigler A, Kohler G 1976 Resolving power of isotachophoresis and isoelectric focussing for immunoglobulins. FEBS Letters 71: 142–146
45. Johnson A, Thorpe R 1982 Immunochemistry in practice. Blackwell Scientific Publications, Oxford
46. Gutman G A 1982 Rat kappa chain allotypes. IV. Monoclonals to distinct RI-1b specificities. Hybridoma 1: 133–138
47. Lanier L L, Gutman G A, Lewis D E, Griswold S T, Warner N L 1982 Monoclonal antibodies against rat immunoglobulin kappa chains. Hybridoma 1: 125–131
48. Springer T A, Bhattacharya A, Cardoza J T, Sanchez-Madrid F 1982 Monoclonal antibodies specific for rat IgG1, IgG2a, and IgG2b subclasses, and kappa chain monotypic and allotypic determinants: reagents for use with rat monoclonal antibodies. Hybridoma 1: 257–272
49. Cranage M P, Gurner B W, Coombs R R A 1983 Gluteraldehyde stabilisation of antibody-linked erythrocytes for use in reverse passive and related haemagglutination assays. Journal of Immunological Methods 64: 7–16

50. Clark M R, Cobbold S P, Waldmann H, Coombs R R A 1984 Detection of monoclonal antibodies against cell surface antigens: the use of antiglobulins coupled to red blood cells. Journal of Immunological Methods 66: 81–87
51. Hudson L, Hay F C 1980 Practical immunology. Blackwell Scientific Publications, London
52. Weir D M (ed) 1973 Handbook of experimental immunology. Blackwell Scientific Publications, London

2

Detection of monoclonal antibodies

Andrew J. McMichael Peter C. L. Beverley

INTRODUCTION

A crucial step in the production of monoclonal antibodies by hybridomas is that of screening culture supernatants for the presence of the desired antibody. Ideally the technique used should fulfill three criteria, accuracy, speed and economy. A common situation is that between 200 and 300 samples have to be tested and the decision as to which colonies to grow and clone must be made before these cultures overgrow. The number of cultures to be maintained must be reduced drastically to keep the work load manageable. Thus, accuracy is necessary to make a definitive assessment of the value of each colony in a single step. Speed is vital to ensure that the result is available before the colonies need further attention. Economy of effort is important if very large numbers of samples are to be checked. Speed and economy may have to be sacrificed however in situations where the antibody can only be detected by complicated bioassays.

The techniques of detection are all dependent on antibody binding to antigen. Because the monoclonal antibody is initially present only in minute quantities, most techniques rely on the use of a second reagent for detection. These include the use of second antibodies, which can be radio-isotope, fluorochrome or enzyme-labelled and the use of second reagents to immunoprecipitate antigen, to aggregate, or lyse cells. If functional assays are used for detection, the antibody is usually tested directly.

The techniques described in this chapter are all based on methods that are currently in use in our laboratories. The emphasis is on practical instructions rather than theory and we have not given a detailed bibliography.

BINDING ASSAYS

Indirect binding assays are the most widely used methods for screening hybridoma cultures. Some general points are common to all techniques. The antigen may be either cellular, particulate (e.g. virus), soluble or fixed. The main requirement is that the antigen can be separated from the antibody, so that it can be washed and then exposed to the second reagent. This is simply achieved when the antigen can be centrifuged, e.g. cells. It is also simple when the antigen is fixed to a solid support such as sepharose beads or a plastic surface. If the antigen is small and soluble, e.g. a hapten group, it is possible to precipitate the monoclonal antibody by using ammonium sulphate (Farr assay)[1] or a precipitating second antibody. Described below are some of the more commonly used methods for radioimmunoassay, fluorescence assay and enzyme linked immunoassay.

RADIO BINDING ASSAYS

Direct labelling of a monoclonal antibody by incubation of the hybridoma with ^{14}C,[3]H or ^{35}S labelled amino acids is possible but impracticable for screening large numbers of separate cultures. Similarly, iodination of antibody requires relatively large amounts and purification of the immunoglobulin from the other proteins in the culture supernatant. Indirect radio binding assays are therefore used for screening hybridomas and only these will be described. The assay described below is based on methods devised by A. Williams and co-workers and a more detailed discussion can be found in their papers[2,3].

Antigen

The antigen must be attached to a solid phase or precipitable by centrifugation. Cells are ideal and can be used live or fixed. Cultured cells must be viable as dead material tends to bind radiolabelled antibody non-specifically. However, the cells can be fixed by treatment with glutaraldehyde or formalin (see Table 2.1) and stored frozen. This procedure is valuable when fresh cells are not constantly available, e.g. leukaemic cells. It should be noted however that antigens are denatured by this procedure and some antigenic epitopes will be lost.

Protein antigens and viruses can be immobilized on solid supports such as sepharose beads. A very simple method is to fix them to 96 U-well polyvinyl chloride plates (Flow laboratories, Irvine, Scotland). This material is negatively charged and by incubating with the protein or virus in protein free phosphate buffered saline at pH 7.4 (PBS), sufficient material adheres to make the assays possible. If insufficient antigen sticks, a higher pH should be tried, e.g. bicarbonate buffer pH 9.0 (1.59g Na_2CO_3, 2.93g $NaHCO_3$ in 1 litre). Protein antigens are made up to 50–500 μg/ml in buffer, (although lower concentrations can be used if the supply of antigen is limited) and 50 μl is dispensed into each well for assay and incubated at 4°C for at least 1 hour. At the end of this time the solution is removed, (it can be saved and recycled) and the protein binding sites in the wells are saturated by filling the wells to the brim with PBS containing 0.5% bovine serum albumin (0.5% BSA-PBS) and leaving for a further hour at 4°C. The wells are then washed thrice with PBS-0.1%BSA using a pipette or syringe and the plate is then ready for assay.

Table 2.1 Glutaraldehyde fixation of cells

1. Wash cells free of protein in PBS (3 centrifugations at 500 g)
2. Resuspend at 10^7 per ml in PBS containing 0.25% (v/v) glutaraldehyde
3. Leave 5 minutes at room temperature
4. Add one tenth of the volume of PBS containing 10% (mass/vol.) bovine serum albumin (BSA)
5. Centrifuge at 500 g for 10 minutes
6. Wash cell three times in PBS-0.5% BSA
7. Resuspend cells at $1–4 \times 10^7$ per ml and store at –20°C. Thaw immediately before use

Antibody

The quality of the second reagent is important. Good anti-mouse immunoglobulin can be purchased from companies such as Dako, (Mercia-Brocades, UK), Meloy (Springfield, Virginia, USA), Miles (Stoke Poges, UK) and this material can be iodinated. It is important to obtain affinity column purified antibody that reacts with all murine immunoglobulin isotypes. Although backgrounds are lower if the F(ab')$_2$ fragment is used, this is not essential. For a single fusion experiment extending over 4 to 6 weeks 25 μg of second antibody, labelled with 1mCi of ^{125}I, should be sufficient. If the second antibody cannot be purchased, or there is a requirement for a large supply, this reagent can be made, although it may take 2 months to do. The method is described at the end of this chapter.

Iodination

Although labelled second antibody can be purchased (Amersham, UK), the half life of ^{125}iodine is 60 days and it is more economical to label one's own reagent[4]. Antibody, 25 μg in 100 μl of PBS in the absence of any added protein, is pipetted into a glass tube, followed by 1mCi of carrier free ^{125}I (Amersham or New England Nuclear). 25 μl of chloramine T (Sigma, Poole) 1.0 mg/ml dissolved in PBS are added. After one minute, 100 μl of a saturated solution of tyrosine (Sigma, Poole) in PBS is added. After a further 2 minutes 100 μl of 10% BSA in PBS is added and solution applied to a 5 ml Sephadex G25 (Pharmacia, Cambridge, UK) column, which has been equilibrated with 0.1% BSA-PBS. After being allowed to sink into the gel, 1 ml of 0.1% BSA-PBS is added and the fraction collected. This procedure is repeated to give five fractions of 1 ml. Each aliquot is counted and the hottest two fractions, normally two and three, pooled. The radiolabelled antibody so obtained should be tested in a standard system before screening a hybridoma fusion. As a guide, we obtain 25 000 counts per minute (cpm) when using 50 μl of rabbit anti-mouse Ig, prepared as above, and diluted 1 in 200, on 10^6 human peripheral blood lymphocytes (pbl) which have been incubated with a saturating concentration of a monoclonal antibody specific for monomorphic HLA Class I antigen, such as W6/32 (Seralab, Crawley Down, UK). In this same assay the low control, pbl incubated with PBS and then labelled antibody, is less than 1000 cpm.

The assay

Cells. Cells are suspended in 0.5% BSA-PBS at $1–4 \times 10^7$ per ml. 25 μl aliquots are dispensed into 3 cm plastic tubes, and the tissue culture supernatant, 25 μl, is added. Tubes are incubated for one hour at 4°C and then washed by the addition of 1.5 ml 0.1%BSA-PBS and spun at 500 g for 5 minutes. Supernatant is removed and the cells resuspended by vortexing. A further 1.5 ml of 0.1%BSA-PBS is added and the procedure repeated. To the pellet is added 50 μl of 1 in 200 ^{125}I labelled anti-mouse immunoglobulin (RAM) (62.5 ng/ml). After a further incubation for one hour at 4°C the cells are washed and counted. It is not necessary to transfer cells to clean tubes before counting unless counts are only marginally above the background, part of which represents non specific binding of the labelled antibody to the plastic.

Plate assay Wells are coated with 50 μl of antigen and then saturated with at least 100 μl of 0.5% BSA as described above. After emptying 50 μl of monoclonal antibody is added to each well and the plate incubated for one hour at 4°C. Wells are then washed using 0.1% BSA-PBS with a syringe or pipette and 50 μl of ^{125}I RAM added. After a further hour, wells are washed three times and then cut out for counting. In our assay a good monoclonal culture supernatant will give 5000 cpm against a background of less than 500 cpm.

ENZYME LINKED ASSAYS

Enzyme linked assays are similar in principle to radiobinding methods. For screening an indirect method is invariably used in which an appropriate enzyme is covalently coupled to anti-mouse or rat immunoglobulin antibody. Binding of anti-immunoglobulin is detected by conversion of enzyme substrate to a coloured reaction product or precipitate. The most commonly used enzymes are horseradish peroxidase and intestinal alkaline phosphatase which are cheap and robust. Coupling of either of these to antibody is relatively simple (Table 2.2) but usually not necessary since commercially available conjugates are of good quality (Dako, Miles, Mercia Brocades, UK).

Enzyme linked assays have the advantage that the use of radioactive isotopes is avoided and that conjugates are stable for long periods. Antibody-peroxidase conjugates have been used in an indirect binding assay to detect antibodies binding to the surface of viable cells and sensitivity is similar to that of immunofluorescent and radiolabel methods[6]. A problem of the use of peroxidase and phosphatase is that some cell types have endogenous enzyme activity so that it may be necessary to treat cells to block the endogenous enzyme. While methods for this are available[6,7] the procedures may alter antigenicity so that treated cells are less reliable as screening material. An alternative which avoids this problem is to use a substrate not metabolised by mammalian enzymes. Bacterial β galactosidase can be coupled to anti-immunoglobulins[8] and used with 4-methyl-umbelliferyl-galactoside[9] the fluorogenic substrate. Other substrates for this enzyme which allow measurement of a colour reaction or form a precipitate will allow its more widespread use for screening antibodies to cells in suspension or on tissue sections[10]. In the meantime peroxidase and phosphatase remain the mainstay of present methods.

Peroxidase assay using fixed target cells

This method utilizes target cells crosslinked to polyvinyl plates (Cooke No. 220-24) with glutaraldehyde to obviate the multiple centrifugations necessary if cells in suspension are used. Detailed descriptions of this type of method have been published by others[7,11].

Cells are washed three times in phosphate-buffered saline and resuspended to 2×10^7/ml in PBS. 50 μl of cell suspension are dispensed into the wells of round bottomed polyvinyl plates and the plates centrifuged at $100 \times g$ for 5 min. The plates are then gently immersed in a large beaker of 0.25% glutaraldehyde in PBS at 4°C. After 5 minutes the plate is removed and glutaraldehyde removed by flicking out the supernatant. The plate is then washed by immersion in three successive beakers of PBS flicking out excess PBS between each. Remaining non-specific binding sites on the plastic are then blocked by adding 200 μl per well of PBS containing 1% bovine serum albumin and 0.1% sodium azide for 1 hour. Plates can be stored at 4°C without changing the buffer for several weeks.

Table 2.2 Preparation of antibody-peroxidase conjugates[5]

1. Dissolve 5 mg horseradish peroxidase (HPRO) (Sigma) in 1 ml of 0.3 M sodium bicarbonate pH 8.1.
2. Add 0.1 ml 1% FDNB★ in absolute alcohol. Stir gently for 1 hour at room temperature.
3. Add 1 ml 0.05 M $NaIO_4$ in distilled water. Mix gently for 30 minutes.
4. Add 1 ml 0.16 M ethylene glycol in distilled water. Mix gently for 1 hr.
5. Dialyse extensively at 4°C against 0.01 M sodium carbonate buffer pH 9.5.
6. Add 5 mg IgG in 1 ml carbonate buffer and mix gently for 2–3 hours at room temperature.
7. Add 5 mg $NaBH_3$ and leave overnight at 4°C.
8. Dialyse against PBS.
9. Separate conjugate from free HPRO by Sephadex G-100 chromatography. An 85 × 1.5 cm column of Sephadex is equilibrated in PBS and the sample applied. Optical density at 280 and 403 nm of the fractions is monitored and conjugate containing fractions (the first peak) are pooled. Conjugate can be stored at –20°C in the presence of 1% BSA.

★FDNB,2,4-Dinitro-1-fluorobenzene

The assay is performed as follows. The PBS-BSA is flicked out and 50 μl of hybridoma supernatant added. Controls containing antibodies known to bind to the target cells and negative supernatants should be included. After one hour incubation the supernatant is flicked out and the plate washed three times by adding 200 μl of PBS-BSA and flicking it out. 50 μl of an appropriate dilution of peroxidase conjugated anti-mouse Ig are added and the plates left for a further 1 hour before washing three times. 100 μl of freshly made up substrate solution is then added. Substrate consists of 40 mg ortho-phenylenediamine (Sigma) dissolved in 100 ml of phosphate-citrate buffer pH 5.0, (24.3 ml 0.1M citric acid, 25.7 ml 0.2M sodium hydrogen phosphate, 50 ml distilled water) to which is added immediately before use 40 μl of 30% hydrogen peroxide. The reaction is stopped after 30 minutes at room temperature by addition of 50 μl of 5M sulphuric acid. Colour can be read visually or 100 μl of supernatant transferred to flat bottomed microplates (e.g. Dynatech) for reading of optical density at 492 nm using a Titertek Multiskan ELISA reader (Flow Laboratories).

Assay for cellular antigens in Terasaki plates
The peroxidase method described above has been adapted for use in Terasaki plates (Falcon 3034). The major advantage being the small numbers of cells and supernatant required for the assay so that 100 μl of supernatant could be tested on several different target cells[11].

The plates are immersed in a solution of 0.1 mg/ml poly-L-lysine in PBS (PLL Sigma) for 30 minutes at room temperature and then washed twice in PBS. After shaking out the PBS 10 μl of a suspension containing 5 × 10⁴ cells is added using a Hamilton dispenser. After 30 minutes at room temperature the cells are fixed by addition to the plate of 15 ml of 0.025% glutaraldehyde in PBS. After 10 minutes the fixative is tipped off and the plate washed 3 times with PBS followed by addition of 15 ml PBS containing 1% BSA and 0.1% sodium azide. Plates can be stored at 4°C.

After removing the PBS-BSA by tipping and then flicking the plate 5 μl of test sample is added to each well and the plate then incubated at room temperature for 1 hour. After 3 washes in which the plate is flooded with PBS-BSA the liquid is tipped off and residue removed by flicking, 5 μl of peroxidase conjugated anti-mouse Ig are added. After a further 1 hour at room temperature and 3 washes 10 μl of substrate is added to each well and plates maintained at room temperature until a strong colour develops in positive control wells. Results can be recorded visually or by polaroid photography. Alternatively, 10 μl of supernatant can be transferred to 96 well micro elisa plates containing 100 μl 1N sulphuric acid per well and the optical density recorded using a plate reader.

This method can also be used to examine the binding of antibody at the single cell level with minor modification[7].

Assay for soluble antigens
Many soluble antigens bind readily to plastic microtitre plates and the method for preparing plates has already been described (see radiobinding assay section). While plate binding assays are most frequently used for assaying antibody to purified proteins we have adapted this method for assaying antibodies to cellular antigens. For the latter, target cells are washed twice in PBS pelleted by centrifugation and resuspended in bicarbonate buffer pH9 (1.59g $NaCO_3$, 2.95g $NaHCO_3$/litre) at 2×10^7 cells/ml. The cells are then sonicated on ice for 30 seconds and diluted to 2×10^6 cell equivalents/ml. One hundred μl aliquots are dispensed into flat bottomed micro-elisa plates. The plates are left at 4°C overnight or can be stored at 4°C for up to 4 weeks (in this case 0.2 g/l of NaN_3 should be added to the bicarbonate buffer). Before use the wells are washed 3 times with PBS containing 0.05% Tween 20 and then incubated with PBS-1%BSA.

For both soluble antigens and cell lysates the assay is carried out in similar fashion[12]. The PBS-BSA is flicked out of the wells and test supernatants added and incubated for 1 hour at room temperature. After 3 washes with PBS-Tween, 100 μl of peroxidase conjugated anti-mouse Ig is added and left for a further hour. The wells are again washed three times with PBS-Tween and 100 μl substrate added. The reaction is stopped after 10 minutes by addition of 50 μl of 5M sulphuric acid and optical density at 492 nm read using an ELISA plate reader.

In all three assays described, phosphatase coupled anti-immunoglobulin can be substituted for peroxidase (Table 2.3). In this case after incubation with the anti-immunoglobulin and washing, phosphatase substrate is added. This consists of 1 g/l p-nitrophenylphosphate (Sigma) in 0.05M bicarbonate buffer containing 10^4M $MgCl_2$ at pH 9.8. The reaction is stopped by addition of 3M NaOH and absorbance read at 400 nm[13].

Table 2.3 Preparation of antibody-phosphatase conjugates[13]

---

1. Add 2 mg of immunoglobulin in 1 ml PBS to 5 mg of enzyme (Calf intestinal alkaline phosphatase Type VII ammonium sulphate suspension, Sigma). Dialyse the mixture against PBS at 4°C.
2. Add 25% glutaraldehyde to give a final concentration of 0.2%. Incubate 1–2 hr at room temperature.
3. Dialyse overnight against several changes of PBS then against 0.05 M Tris buffer pH 8. Add BSA to final 1% concentration and NaN_3 to 0.02%. Store at 4°C. Conjugates prepared in this way can usually be diluted 1:500 or more for use.

Tissue section screening
A useful technique, which has recently been introduced, is to screen hybridoma supernatants by immunoperoxidase or alkaline phosphatase staining of frozen sections of a tissue[14]. For lymphoid antigens, frozen cryostat tonsil sections are convenient and can be prepared quite readily in advance by standard methods. 50 μl

of culture supernatant is added to the slide. After 30 minutes at room temperature, the slide is washed in 0.05 M Tris HCl buffered 0.15M NaCl at pH 7.6.(TBS). Then freshly prepared peroxidase coupled rabbit immunoglobulin anti-mouse immunoglobulin (Dako, Mercia-Brocades) diluted 1 in 200 in 5% human AB serum (to block Fc and cross reactive binding to the human cells) is added. While the slide is incubating for 30 minutes at room temperature, the substrate is made up. Diamino benzidine (Sigma, Poole, UK) (CARE-carcinogenic) 6 mg is dissolved in 10 ml of TBS and 30 μl of 10% by volume H_2O_2 is added just before use. This mixture is added to the section after the second antibody has been washed off, and the slide is incubated for 8–15 minutes. The slide is then washed and dipped into haematoxylin. After 15 seconds the slide is washed thoroughly in tap water and dipped in acid alcohol (2% conc. HCl/98% ethanol). It is then treated successively with one minute washes of 70%, 90%, 100%, ethanol, followed by xylene twice, after which it is mounted in DPX.

This technique which takes less than 2 hours is very useful. Positives and negatives can be distinguished by naked eye and microscopy can distinguish between antibody specific for subpopulations of cells, e.g. T-cells, B-cells or epithelial cells. More details are given in Chapter 6.

FLUORESCENCE ASSAYS

Antigen

Cells or cryostat tissue sections are appropriate. Subcellular particles can also be used.

Labelled antibody. Good fluorescein or rhodamine labelled anti-mouse immunoglobulin reagents are available commercially (e.g. Meloy, Miles). Antibodies should be made up in 0.5% BSA-PBS in the presence of 0.02% sodium azide, to prevent capping. Cross reactivity with human immunoglobulin should be blocked by diluting in 5% human serum. (If other species are being studied the appropriate normal serum should be used).

The assay

The technique for staining cells is very similar to that described above for the enzyme linked assays. Cells, 1×10^6/ml in 0.5% BSA-PBS are incubated with 25–50 μl of culture supernatant. After 1 hour at 4°C cells are washed twice in 0.1% BSA-PBS and then second antibody is added. After 1 hour at 4°C cells are washed again and may then be read. Cells can be fixed at this stage by adding 1% formalin in PBS-1% Fetal Calf Serum (FCS). After this procedure fluorescence does not decline significantly in four weeks though for screening hybridomas the result would be needed much earlier.

Fluorescent labelled cells can also be read by a fluorescence activated cell sorter. The staining procedure is exactly as above and details of the procedure are given in Chapter 9. The advantage of this method for screening is that reactivity with subpopulations can be readily detected. It is particularly valuable for detecting antibodies that bind to rare cell populations in mixtures such as peripheral blood mononuclear cells or bone marrow.

COMPLEMENT MEDIATED CYTOTOXICITY

Introduction

In theory complement mediated cytotoxicity should be a sensitive technique for screening monoclonal antibodies to cell surface antigens. In our experience however, there are serious problems. The first is that IgG_1 antibody, which may constitute 50% of the hybrid myeloma monoclonal antibodies, does not fix complement. Secondly rabbit complement which seems to work best with mouse antibodies can be non specifically cytotoxic to the target cells used, particularly cultured cell lines. The complement (rabbit serum stored at $-70°C$ and thawed immediately before use) must therefore be screened carefully prior to use. We have found that each monoclonal antibody has an optimum concentration of complement with which it is active and at the screening stage therefore problems arise and three to four concentrations of the rabbit serum may have to be used. Reading large numbers of cytotoxicity reactions rapidly requires some skill and is best carried out where the test is performed routinely, e.g. tissue typing labs. The Chromium 51 release assay is easier for non experts and this is described.

^{51}Chromium release assay

Cells are prepared for labelling with ^{51}Cr by resuspending in a tissue culture medium such as RPMI 1640 (Gibco-Europe, Paisley, Scotland) at approximately 10^7 cells/ml. As only small numbers of cells are needed in the assay, this would normally mean less than 0.5 ml total volume. Sodium ^{51}chromate, 100–300 μCi (Amersham) is added and the cells incubated for one hour at $37°C$ after which cells are washed twice in medium containing 10% Fetal Calf Serum FCS or PBS-0.5%BSA. The cells are then made up to 2×10^5/ml and 50 μl aliquots dispensed into round bottomed 96 well microtitre trays. 50 μl of tissue culture supernatant is added and cells and antibody incubated at room temperature for one hour. An equal volume of (100 μl) rabbit complement is then added. Normally a dilution of the serum to 1 in 4 is suitable but this must be determined for each batch of serum before the experiments and as indicated above more than one concentration may be needed. After incubation for another hour at $20°C$, the plate is centrifuged at 1000 rpm for 5 minutes and 100 μl of supernatant pipetted off for counting. Positive and negative controls are essential; the former can be a previously obtained or purchased monoclonal antibody or 2% Triton X-100 (or other detergent); the latter should be cells incubated in medium instead of tissue culture supernatant. The percent positive lysis is calculated by the formula: E-M/H-M × 100 when E is experimental counts per minute, M is medium control cpm and H is high control cpm.

IMMUNOPRECIPITATION

This technique has been used for screening, but about 200 μl of high titre supernatant is needed. It is difficult unless previous expertise in the technique has been acquired. It is probably best therefore to use an alternative screening method first and then immunoprecipitate with selected monoclonal antibodies. A strategy that can be used is to mix 10–20 supernatants, concentrating 5–10 times in an Amicon B15 concentrator to return each to a suitable concentration, and then immunoprecipitating. If a positive result is obtained then each contributing antibody to the group will have to be retested in smaller groups and then individually. The following outline can be used as a guide for using this method.

Labelling of target antigen

Soluble protein antigens can be labelled directly by iodination using the method described above for anti-immunoglobulins. Cell antigens can be labelled internally by culture with radiolabelled amino acids or externally with ^{125}iodine using the lactoperoxidase technique[15].

Internal labelling is most conveniently achieved by the use of ^{35}S-methionine (Amersham or New England Nuclear). For small scale labelling 5×10^6 healthy cells are resuspended in 2 ml of methionine free RPMI-1640 medium (Gibco-Biocult, Paisley, Scotland) containing 10% Fetal Calf Serum (FCS). The cells are incubated at 37°C for 1 hour and then 100 μCi ^{35}S-methionine is added and the incubation continued overnight. The cells are then centrifuged, washed once with PBS and lysed by adding 1 ml of a detergent buffer such as: 50 mmol Tris, 5 mmolMgCl$_2$, 0.5% NP40 containing 0.1M phenylmethylsulphonyl fluoride (PMSF). The last is unstable and should be made up just before use. After 15 minutes at 4°C the tube is centrifuged fast in a microfuge for 10 minutes. The supernatant, which includes plasma membrane proteins can then be stored frozen at –70°C. This method gives sufficient labelled lysate to make up to four precipitations, the labelling can be scaled up to give as much material as is necessary.

Cell surface labelling with ^{125}Iodine must be carried out in a suitable safety hood to protect the operator. 10^7 viable cells are washed free of serum and resuspended in 200 μl of PBS. Dead cells should be avoided as this will result in labelling of cytoplasmic proteins. To these are added at room temperature, 200 μl of lactoperoxidase, (Sigma, Poole, UK) freshly made up at 1 mg/ml in PBS. Iodine-125 (Amersham) 1 mCi, is then added, followed by 50 μl of 30% by volume H$_2$O$_2$. The reaction mixture should immediately start bubbling as oxygen is released. After 5 minutes a further 50 μl of H$_2$O$_2$ are added. Ten minutes later 20 ml of PBS containing 1 mM Tyrosine are added and the cells are centrifuged down. Supernatant is disposed of carefully, as the procedure is inefficient and despite the addition of tyrosine some of the iodine is still free. The cells are then washed a further two times in PBS and lysed with 0.5% Nonidet P40 (NP40, Sigma). After incubation for 30 minutes at 4°C the nuclei are centrifuged down at 600 × g for 5 minutes, and the soluble membranes pipetted off. This fraction can then be passed over a 5 ml Sephadex G-25 column (Pharmacia) equilibrated with medium plus detergent or dialysed overnight against PBS-detergent. The collected labelled peak of material should then be stored in the presence of a neutral carrier protein such as 0.5% BSA in PBS containing NaN$_3$ (0.02%). Only around 1–2% of added iodine is recoverable in protein.

Precipitation

Before precipitation it is advisable to clear non-specifically sticky labelled proteins from the lysate (1 ml) by incubation first with normal mouse serum, 5 μl, for 1 hour followed by 100 μl 10% formalin fixed Staphylococcus A (Cowan strain I) organisms[16] (Calbiochem). The latter should be washed three times in buffer containing 50 mmol Tris, 150 mmol NaCl, 5 mmol EDTA, 0.5% NP40 before use. After 1 hours incubation with the Staphylococcus A the tube is centrifuged in a microfuge and the supernatant used for the immunoprecipitation.

The antigen and monoclonal antibody are mixed. For most antigens 200 μl of high titre culture supernatant is normally adequate to precipitate antigen from 5×10^6 cells. After 1 hour at 4°C 100 μl of 10% formalin fixed staphylococcus A organisms are added. It should be noted that IgG_{2a} and $_{2b}$ bind better to Staphylococcus A than IgG_1. For screening purposes therefore, when the isotype of the monoclonal antibody is unknown, 5 μl of rabbit anti-mouse immunoglobulin (Miles-Yeda, Stoke Poges, UK) should be added after the monoclonal antibody and at least 1 hour before the Staphylococci. The tube should be centrifuged 15 minutes after addition of the latter and the pellet washed three times in buffer containing 50 mmol Tris, 150 mmol NaCl, 5 mmol EDTA, 0.5% NP40. Labelled antigen can then be eluted from the Staphylococcal A-immune complex by boiling in 60 mmol Tris, 0.2% sodium dodecyl sulphate, 50 mmol dithiothreitol, 10% glycerol, pH 6.8, for 5 minutes. The sample is then centrifuged and the supernatant loaded onto a polyacrylamide gel[17].

OTHER ASSAY METHODS

Agglutination

A single monoclonal antibody will cause not agglutination unless it binds to repeating antigenic epitopes. In the presence of a second antibody however it is possible to use this technique. As with complement mediated lysis, the concentration of the second antibody is critical and the optimum may vary for different monoclonal antibodies at different concentrations, as occurs in the screening step. Therefore, although simple in theory the technique requires some skill to make it work. As with many of the techniques it is advisable to work it out with a previously made or purchased monoclonal antibody beforehand.

Western blotting

An alternative to immunoprecipitation is to run an SDS-polyacrylamide gel of a whole cell lysate or antigen mixture, blot onto nitrocellulose and then detect antibodies by incubating with supernatants followed by a radiolabelled second antibody and autoradiography. Unfortunately many antigens are denatured by the SDS-polyacrylamide gel process. However, for some antigens such as HLA Class II, the method does work, under non reducing conditions. The technique may also be valuable when one is deliberately looking for antibodies that bind to denatured separated chains, for instance if searching for reagents to use to detect products of cell free messenger RNA translation. The method is described by Burnette[18].

Functional techniques

A classical virological diagnostic assay is haemagglutination and its inhibition by antibodies is well known. These tests work well with monoclonal antibodies and are simple to perform. Laboratories wishing to use these techniques are likely to be expert in them already. Similarly, enzyme assays can be inhibited by monoclonal antibodies that bind to appropriate epitopes on the enzyme. Again laboratories experienced in these techniques should have no trouble in adapting them for screening although it should be pointed out that binding assays would detect a greater range of monoclonal antibodies.

More complex functional assays can be used for screening. One example was the production of an anti-interferon monoclonal antibody by Secher et al[19]. Antibody was mixed with interferon which was then assayed for inhibition of viral replication. Another complex assay that has been used is the inhibition of lysis of lymphoid cells by cytotoxic T lymphocytes. In these experiments 4 hour chromium release assays were blocked by adding hybridoma culture supernatant at the same time as the effector cells. Several antibodies were detected which inhibited lysis and two new antigens, LFA-1 and LFA-3, were first identified in this manner[20]. It should be noted however in this system that inhibition is only achieved when antibodies were present in amounts sufficient to saturate the effector cell population. This may prove a problem for screening hybridomas in the early stages.

It is not feasible to give details of all the possible functional assays that could be used. Laboratories will only consider these techniques if they are already expert in the assay to be inhibited. In early screening, the antibody concentration may be suboptimal and it may therefore be necessary to follow up any cultures whose supernatant gives small effects on the assay.

PREPARATION OF RABBIT ANTI-MOUSE IMMUNOGLOBULIN

For many of the techniques described above, anti-mouse immunoglobulin is needed. Although good preparations are available from commercial sources the following description should help those who wish to prepare their own.

PURIFICATION OF MOUSE IMMUNOGLOBULIN

To 10 ml of normal mouse serum at 4°C add, 10 ml of ice cold saturated ammonium sulphate, slowly with stirring. A white precipitate forms immediately. Let the mixture stand for at least one hour at 4°C. Resuspend the precipitate in 5 ml 0.025 M Tris-HCl, 0.1 M NaCl, 0.02%NaN$_3$ pH 7.5 and dialyse overnight against the same buffer, 2 × 500 ml, at 4°C.

Prepare a column of diethylaminoethyl (DEAE) sepharose (Pharmacia, Cambridge) such that bed volume is 2 times sample volume, and equilibrate with 0.025 M Tris, 0.1 M NaCl, 3 mmol NaN$_3$, pH 7.5. Apply dialysed sample to DEAE sepharose column and elute in 1 ml fractions with the above buffer. Monitor OD$_{280}$ 1 cm for each sample and pool the peak of protein. Measure OD$_{280}$ of the pool and calculate immunoglobulin concentration, assuming OD$_{280}$ of 1.2 is equivalent to 1.0 mg/ml IgG.

Immunization of rabbit

Prepare 1 mg immunoglobulin in 1 ml of buffer (PBS) and form an emulsion with Freunds Complete Adjuvant (FCA) by passing back and forth into a glass syringe. Immunize at least two rabbits by intramuscular injection of 0.5 mg antigen into each thigh muscle. After 3 weeks repeat using, for each animal 1 mg in incomplete Freunds Adjuvant (IFCA) by intradermal injection into multiple sites on the back. After 2 further weeks, bleed and test antibody activity by carrying out a precipitation assay in an Ouchterlony plate (1% agar in PBS)[8]. In the centre well place antigen (1 mg/ml) and twofold dilutions of the antiserum in the outer wells. Leave overnight at 4°C and then observe for lines of precipitation. A good serum should give lines out to at least a 1 in 8 dilution.

If the antiserum is low titre, reimmunize with 1 mg/ml IgG in IFCA and rebleed. Repeat as necessary. When a good titre has been obtained collect a large volume of rabbit serum by bleeding 50 ml blood at 2-weekly intervals, boosting with antigen every month, or bleeding the animal out.

Purification of rabbit anti-mouse immunoglobulin

Mouse immunoglobulin, 10 mg in 2 ml, is dialysed for 18 hours against 0.1 M $NaHCO_3$, 0.5 M NaCl, pH 8.3 (coupling buffer). Cyanogen bromide activated sepharose 4B (Pharmacia, Cambridge) is swollen in 1 mmol HCl, for 30 minutes and then washed in the same buffer on a scintered glass funnel. The beads, 3 ml, are then washed with coupling buffer (300 ml) and mixed with immunoglobulin (10 mg) in the coupling buffer. This mixture is rotated in a tube gently for 2 hours at 20°C and beads are then washed on a scintered glass funnel with 0.2 M glycine pH 8.5 (300 ml). The beads are then mixed gently in the glycine buffer to neutralise remaining reactive groups, for one hour, after which the beads are packed into a 5 ml syringe column and nonspecifically bound protein desorbed with three washing cycles of 0.1 M sodium acetate, 0.05 M NaCl with acetate buffer pH 4.5, followed by coupling buffer, pH 8.3. Beads can then be stored in 10 mmol Tris, pH 8.0 containing 0.02% sodium azide.

Rabbit antiserum to be applied to the column should be centrifuged at $10\,000 \times g$ to remove aggregates. 10 ml of the rabbit antiserum can then be applied to the column, allowed to bind for one hour at 4°C and then washed with 10 mmol Tris pH 8.0 until no protein is detectable (OD_{280}) in the washings. 50 mmol diethylamine, pH 11.5 is then applied and 1 ml aliquots collected. Each is immediately brought back to neutral pH by addition of 100 μl of 1 M Tris HCl pH 3.5. The OD_{280} of each fraction is measured and the eluted antibody pooled. When no further protein comes off the column it should be washed in a large volume of 10 mmol Tris pH 8.0. It may then be used again for further cycles.

The antibody activity of the eluted antibody is first checked in an Ouchterlony plate as above. It should then be iodinated and tested in binding assays using standard monoclonal antibodies with standard target cells.

CONCLUSIONS

The most popular screening techniques for detecting monoclonal antibodies have been described here. The list is by no means exhaustive and undoubtedly many more procedures will be devised. Much depends on the ingenuity of the investigators, particularly when it is not possible to use the simpler methods. It is obvious but sometimes forgotten however, that there is no point in constructing a complex screening assay when a simple one will do.

REFERENCES

1. Farr R S 1958 A quantitative immunochemical measure of the primary interaction between I BSA and antibody. Journal of Infectious Disease 103: 239–262
2. Jensenius J C, Williams A F 1974 The binding of anti immunoglobulin antibodies to rat thymocytes and thoracic duct lymphocytes. European Journal of Immunology 4: 91–97
3. Morris R J, Williams A F 1975 Antigens on mouse and rat lymphocytes recognised by rabbit anti serum against rat brain: the quantitative analysis of a xenogeneic antiserum. European Journal of Immunology 5: 274–281
4. Greenwood F C, Hunter W N, Glover J S 1963 The preparation of ^{131}I labelled human growth hormone of high specific radioactivity. Biochemical Journal 89: 114–123
5. Nakane P K, Kawasi A 1974 Peroxidase labelled antibody. A new method of conjugation. Journal of Histochemistry and Cytochemistry 12: 1064–1071
6. Posner M R, Antonio D, Griffin J, Schlossman S F, Lazarus H 1982 An enzyme-linked immunosorbent assay (ELISA) for the detection of monoclonal antibodies to cell surface antigens on viable cells. Journal of Immunological Methods 48: 23–30
7. Lansorp P M, Astaldi G C B, Oosterhof F, Janssen M C, Zeijelmaker W P 1980 Immunoperoxidase procedures to detect monoclonal antibodies against cell surface antigens. Quantitation of binding and staining of individual cells. Journal of Immunological Methods 39: 393–401
8. Deelder A M, De Water R A A comparative study on the preparation of immunoglobulin-galactsidase conjugates. Journal of Histochemistry and Cytochemistry 29: 1273–1280
9. Galjaard H, Hoogeveen H, Keijzer W, De Wit-Verbeek E W, Vlek-Woot 1982 The use of quantitative cytochemical analysis in rapid prenatal detection of somatic cell genetic studies of metabolic diseases. Histochemical Journal 76: 153–161
10. Bondi A, Chieregatti G, Eusebi V, Fulcheri E, Bussolati G 1982 The use of β-galactoside as a tracer in immunochemistry. Histochemistry 76: 153–159
11. Heusser C H, Stocker J W, Gisler R H 1981 Methods for binding cells to plastic: application to solid-phase radioimmunoassays for cell surface antigens. Methods in Enzymology 73B: 406–418
12. Zanders E D, Smith C M, Callard R E 1981 A micromethod for the induction assay of specific in vitro antibody responses by human lymphocytes. Journal of Immunological Methods 40: 33–39
13. Voller A, Bidwell D E, Bartlett A 1976 Enzyme immunoassays in diagnostic medicine. Bulletin of the World Health Organisation 53: 3418–3426
14. Naiem M, Gerdes J, Abdulaziz Z, Sunderland C A, Allington M J, Stein H, Mason D Y 1982 The value of immunohistological screening in the production of monoclonal antibodies. Journal of Immunological Methods 50: 145–160
15. Marchalonis J J, Cone R E, Santer V 1971 Enzymatic iodination: A probe for cell surface proteins of normal and neoplastic lymphocytes. Biochemical Journal 124: 991–927
16. Kessler S W 1975 Rapid isolation of antigens from cells with a staphylococcal protein A antibody absorbent: Parameters of the interaction of antibody:antigen complexes with protein A. Journal of Immunology 115: 1617–1624
17. Laemmli U K 1970 Cleavage of the structural proteins during the assembly of the head of the bacteriophage T4. Nature 227: 680–685
18. Burnette W N 1981 'Western blotting'. Electrophoretic transfer of proteins from sodium dodecyl sulphate polyacrylamide gels to unmodified nitrocellulose and radiographic detection with antibody and radioiodinated protein A. Annals of Biochemistry 112: 195–205
19. Secher D S, Burke D C 1980 A monoclonal antibody for large-scale purification of human llucocyte interferon. Nature 285: 446–450
20. Davignon D, Martz E, Reynolds T, Kurtzinger K, Springer T A 1981 Monoclonal antibody to a novel lymphocyte function associated antigen (LFA-1): Mechanism of blockade of T lymphocyte mediated killing effects on other T and B lymphocyte functions. Journal of Immunology 127: 590–595

3
Monoclonal antibodies and immunochemistry

Rosemarie Dalchau John W. Fabre

INTRODUCTION

Antibodies produced by monoclonal hybridomas have many outstanding advantages over conventional antisera in the field of immunochemistry. Not only is exquisite monospecificity inherent in the technique of their production, but the specific antibody is available in concentrations several orders of magnitude greater than in conventional sera, resulting in preparations with extremely high specific activities. In addition, it is possible to introduce stable internal labels into the antibody molecules by culturing the hybridoma cells with radiolabelled amino acids, a possibility not available with conventional sera. These advantages have made certain experimental techniques much simpler and more reliable, and, perhaps more importantly, have allowed the development of powerful experimental approaches not possible with conventional antibodies.

In this chapter, we shall review firstly the immunochemistry of monoclonal antibodies, i.e., the determination of their immunoglobulin class, purification from ascites, and so on, as this is likely to be of general value to those working with monoclonal antibodies. The second part of the chapter will deal with the experimental use of monoclonal antibodies in the field of immunochemistry, concentrating especially on the use of monoclonal antibody affinity columns.

IMMUNOCHEMISTRY OF MONOCLONAL ANTIBODIES

DETERMINATION OF CLASS AND SUBCLASS

It is often useful to know the class and subclass of immunoglobulin to which a monoclonal antibody belongs. Occasionally, it might be so important as to be included very early in the assessment of a fusion, soon after cloning or even before cloning of a fusion well. For example, IgM antibodies usually do not behave well as immunoadsorbents, so that if the aim is to produce monoclonal antibodies for this purpose, it is of value to reject IgM secreting clones at an early stage. Other applications have specific subclass requirements, and certain manipulations (e.g. preparation of $F(ab')_2$) vary depending on the subclass of the monoclonal antibody. Over and above that, even if it is not immediately of importance to know the class and subclass of a monoclonal antibody it is a fundamental characteristic of the antibody and one which may affect its use in the future.

A number of approaches give clues as to the class and subclass of immunoglobulin. For example, the elution pH from protein A columns[1] and the presence or absence of complement fixation can suggest particular subclasses. The IgM class of a monoclonal antibody is suggested by elution of the antibody activity in the void volume of G-200 gel filtration columns, or by showing a 70 000 Mr heavy chain on SDS gels by internal labelling techniques[2]. However, the use of conventional antisera specific for the various immunoglobulin classes and subclasses for Ouchterlony or other techniques is the most widely used and specific approach, and is the one to be favoured. The advent of rat monoclonal antibodies specific for mouse immunoglobulin classes and subclasses should provide new and reliable methods in future.

Double immunodiffusion

Ouchterlony plates. This is perhaps the easiest approach, especially since the advent of low cost, reliable kits from commercial suppliers (e.g. Miles Laboratories). In each test, the mouse monoclonal antibody is assayed for reactivity with antisera specific for IgM, IgG_1, IgG_{2a}, IgG_{2b}, IgG_3 and IgA. The principle of the Ouchterlony test will be well known to all readers, and involves simply the addition to a well in an agar plate of the monoclonal antibody under study, and the addition to nearby wells of the class and subclass specific antisera. Diffusion of these reagents in the agar results in the formation of a precipitin line where the concentration of antigen and antibody are optimal.

It is essential in Ouchterlony analysis to use culture supernatants and not immune ascites, as the latter will obviously be contaminated with normal mouse immunoglobulins. It is also important to note that it is sometimes necessary to concentrate (e.g. 10 fold) the culture supernatant under test, as the formation of the precipitin line is dependent on the correct ratios of antigen and antibody concentrations. Too high or too low a concentration of monoclonal antibody will result in failure of the precipitin line to form.

Rat monoclonal antibodies to mouse immunoglobulin classes and subclasses are unlikely rapidly to replace conventional sera in Ouchterlony tests, as conventional sera are usually better in precipitin reactions.

Serological assays

There are many possible permutations and combinations of assays involving the interaction of labelled anti-immunoglobulin sera, class and subclass specific sera and monoclonal antibodies for the determination of the immunoglobulin class and subclass of the monoclonal antibody.

Radioimmunoassay on PVC plates

As an example of the sorts of assays possible, we shall describe briefly one recently reported radio-immunoassay involving PVC plates as the solid phase[3]. This assay has the advantage of simplicity, and, in addition, several thousand assays can be performed per ml of commercially available class and subclass specific antiserum. Thus if an experiment requires the determination of class and subclass on very numerous occasions, this assay has advantages in terms of cost.

We have not yet had any experience of this assay, but the steps as described by the authors[3] are:

incubate 1 in 100 dilution of the immunoglobulin fractions of commercially available class and subclass specific antisera (e.g. prepared in rabbit) in wells of flexible PVC plate;

remove antisera (for re-use) and block remaining sites with bovine serum albumin (BSA);

remove BSA and wash plate;

add hybridoma culture supernatant;

remove culture supernatant, and wash the plate;

add radiolabelled anti-mouse immunoglobulin, which does not distinguish between classes and subclasses;

wash the plate, and count the radioactivity per well.

Enzyme—rather than radio-labelled anti-mouse immunoglobulin sera can of course be used in the last incubation.

The use of antigen-bound monoclonal antibody

If the monoclonal antibody can be bound to a solid or particulate phase by way of its antigen combining site (e.g. anti leucocyte antibodies to leucocytes), class and subclass could be determined where contaminating immunoglobulins were present (unless of course there is any likelihood of the contaminating immunoglobulins also binding to the target). We have attempted this type of assay using erythrocytes and leucocytes as the particulate phase, in a triple sandwich involving mouse monoclonal antibody, rabbit anti-mouse class and subclass-specific immunoglobulin sera and ^{125}I labelled, affinity purified goat anti-rabbit F(ab')$_2$. However, the commercially available class and subclass specific antisera were not specific enough in this assay, and assay backgrounds were high. The use of rat monoclonal antibodies to mouse immunoglobulin classes and subclasses will very likely provide the desired specificity in the second layer of this test. In that case, however, the rat monoclonal antibody would have to be labelled (e.g. internally) to make the third layer unnecessary, or the third layer would have to consist of an anti-rat immunoglobulin reagent from which the substantial amount of antibody cross-reacting with mouse immunoglobulin had been removed.

PURIFICATION OF MONOCLONAL ANTIBODIES

Monoclonal antibodies in culture supernatants form an excellent preparation for many purposes, e.g. serological assays, immunohistology. Purification and concentration of the monoclonal antibody from the culture fluid is necessary only for special purposes. The advent of protein-free culture media[4] should provide relatively pure antibody in culture supernatants.

On the other hand, monoclonal antibodies present in the form of ascites are generally not ideal for use without some form of purification to remove contaminants such as the oily solutions used to induce and promote ascites formation. The monoclonal antibody in the ascites will already be in a concentrated form, so that concentration of the antibody is not usually an important consideration when choosing the approach for purification.

It is probably worth mentioning in the context of purification that unless the parent myeloma secretes neither heavy nor light chains, the hybridoma products will very likely consist of scrambled light and heavy chains of myeloma and lymphocyte origin, only a proportion of which will be bivalent specific antibody of interest to the experimenter.

Our routine is to raise large volumes (e.g. 100 to 200 ml) of ascites, and to perform a large scale single purification using ion exchange chromatography. However, the immunoglobulin class of the monoclonal antibody, and the degree of purification required, will dictate which technique, or which combination of techniques, is appropriate. Before applying any purification procedure to ascites, it is advisable to centrifuge it (e.g. 20 000 g for 20 minutes) to pellet particulate matter, and to enable removal of the fatty material which floats to the top. It is very important, after any purification procedure, to check the purified preparation in relation to the starting material, and to estimate the yield. Given the high titre of immune ascites, it is not difficult to recover only 1% or less of the original monoclonal antibody, but still to have a high titre preparation.

It is worth bearing in mind that snap-freezing preparations (e.g. in liquid nitrogen) is likely to result in less denaturation of antibody than simply placing solutions at $-20°C$. In the latter case, pure water crystals form, resulting in local high concentrations of protein and salts. After snap-freezing, preparations can be stored in ordinary freezers.

Salt fractionation

Immunoglobulins may be precipitated by adding salts such as $(NH_4)_2SO_4$ or Na_2SO_4. Our preference is for Na_2SO_4, which is added slowly and with constant stirring at room temperature to give 16–18% mass/vol. The precipitates formed are pelleted by centrifugation at 20 000 g for 20 minutes, and resuspended in distilled H_2O. The precipitation is usually repeated once or twice. The final precipitate is resuspended in an appropriate buffer and dialysed to remove Na_2SO_4. The starting ascites, the supernatant(s) after centrifugation and the reconstituted precipitate should all be titrated to determine the yield of antibody activity. The supernatant(s) after centrifugation should not be discarded until this has been performed since it is possible that some monoclonal antibodies will behave atypically.

This purification step may be used on its own or as a preliminary to further purifications. It can of course serve as a concentrating as well as a purifying step.

A variant of salt fractionation is precipitation of IgM by dialysis against distilled water. This is probably not a wise step to use, however, as denaturation might occur.

Ion exchange chromatography

This is a very useful approach as it can deal easily with large volumes and gives a substantial purification in a single step. It can also serve as a concentrating step if antibody preparations are dilute. Our approach is to thaw and pool all of the individual aliquots of a particular batch of immune ascites, and to centrifuge the pool at 20 000 g for 20 minutes at 4°C. The clarified ascites is then dialysed against 50 volumes of 0.05 M Tris, 0.01 M NaCl, 0.02% NaN_3, pH 8.6 at 4°C over 24 hours with one change of buffer, and passed through a column of DEAE CL 6B (Pharmacia,

Uppsala, Sweden) equilibrated in the same buffer. We use approximately 1.5 ml gel for every 1.0 ml ascites to be purified. The column is washed with one column volume of the buffer and eluted with a linear gradient from 10–300 mmol NaCl (500 ml total buffer for a 50 ml column). Fractions are collected and monitored by optical density at 280 nm. Individual peaks may then be pooled and each titrated for antibody activity, together with a sample of the starting ascites so that yield can be estimated. Alternatively, each fraction can be assayed (e.g. at a 1 in 1000 dilution if immune ascites is being purified) for antibody activity, and fractions with specific antibody are pooled. This latter approach probably does not usually increase the purity of the preparation obtained. In our hands, using immune ascites, >90% of the antibody activity is recovered in approximately 20–30% of the starting protein, and the purified preparation consists of reasonably pure immunoglobulin. The antibody concentration in the purified preparation is usually much the same as in the initial ascites.

The column should not be discarded until the assays for antibody activity have been performed because of the possibility that a monoclonal antibody might behave atypically. If the antibody is retained on the column at the end of the salt gradient, the gradient can be increased (e.g. to 500 mmol NaCl) or a pH change can be used for elution.

Gel filtration

Gel filtration on G-200 or S-300 (Pharmacia, Uppsala, Sweden) is a simple purification step, and is particularly useful for IgM antibodies which will elute ahead of the IgG peak. Samples will be diluted approximately 5-fold after gel filtration but this is not usually a problem. For purification of small volumes of unfractionated immune ascites available commercially, gel filtration has a good deal to commend it, as it is quick, simple, and there is virtually no possibility of loss of the antibody.

For processing of large volumes of ascites, gel filtration has the disadvantage that only relatively small samples can be processed at any one time. For good resolution, the sample volume should not be greater than 5% of the column volume, and this is only 25 ml for a 500 ml column.

Fractions from the column can be monitored for OD at 280 nm, and peaks pooled for assay, or individual fractions can be assayed for antibody activity, as described under ion-exchange chromatography.

Protein A affinity chromatography

This is a useful technique for IgG monoclonal antibodies, particularly when higher degrees of purity are required. IgG_1, IgG_{2a} and IgG_{2b} immunoglobulins can be eluted sequentially from protein A columns using pH steps, increasing the degree of purity obtained[1].

Protein A can be purchased already coupled to beads, and columns can be constructed using plastic or glass syringes, but small disposable columns available commercially are preferable (Econo-Columns, Bio-Rad Ltd, Watford, Herts). The capacities of these gels is generally 6–10 mg of immunoglobulin per ml of gel, and they can of course be re-used, but one should perhaps be wary of re-using the same column for antibodies of different specificities. Unless very large columns are constructed, only 5 ml or so of ascites can be processed at any one time, and this is sometimes a disadvantage.

Preparative iso-electric focussing

This is rarely used, since the very high degree of purity possible with this approach is rarely needed. However, the purification of immunoglobulins according to their pI offers the possibility of approaching 100% purity of the specific monoclonal antibody under study. A preliminary purification step will have been performed (e.g. ion-exchange chromatography), and after iso-electric focussing a gel filtration should be used to remove the ampholytes (mol. weight approx 10 000) used to generate the pH gradient.

A number of firms market equipment for preparative iso-electro focussing. The flat bed approach, with which we have had limited experience, is probably preferable to column techniques.

PREPARATION OF Fab AND F(ab')$_2$

Most of the work on the production of immunoglobulin fragments has been done with rabbit and human IgG. Relatively little has been published on mouse immunoglobulins, but this obviously will change with the widespread use of mouse monoclonal antibodies.

Preparation of F(ab')$_2$

The classical technique for preparing F(ab')$_2$ from rabbit IgG (i.e., digestion at pH 4.5 for 20 hours at 37°C at enzyme/substrate ratios of approximately 2% w/w) works well with the rabbit IgG, and reasonably well with human IgG, but very poorly with the IgG of most other species (e.g. mouse, rat, dog, goat). With all of these 'difficult' species, we found that lowering the pH of the digestion to 4.0 or 4.1, i.e. closer to the pH optimum for pepsin, resulted in the production in good yield of F(ab')$_2$ which could be purified by subsequent G-200 gel filtration.

As regards mouse monoclonal antibodies, one recent and detailed review[5] suggests that mouse IgG$_2$ monoclonal antibodies are susceptible to pepsin degradation, but IgG$_1$ monoclonal antibodies are not. In these experiments, the immunoglobulin fraction of monoclonal antibodies was digested at pH 4.8, for 48 hours at 37°C at an enzyme/substrate ratio of 10% w/w. Mason & Williams[6], however, report excellent pepsin degradation and good yields of F(ab')$_2$ with several mouse IgG$_1$ monoclonal antibodies. Their conditions of digestion involved pH of 4.0 and enzyme/substrate ratios of 2% for 20 hours at 37°C. It seems likely, therefore, that IgG$_1$ monoclonal antibodies are relatively resistant to pepsin, but this can be overcome by carrying out the degradation at a pH closer to the pH optimum for pepsin. A satisfactory approach would therefore seem to be to determine the class and subclass of the monoclonal antibody under study, and to perform degradations of IgG$_2$ antibodies at pH 4.5 and IgG$_1$ antibodies at 4.0. It is nevertheless essential to bear in mind that individual monoclonal antibodies might differ substantially in their susceptibility to degradation, and that modifications might be required in specific cases. Moreover, we have no information on pepsin degradation of IgG$_3$ or the other classes of mouse immunoglobulins.

A suitable protocol would be to prepare the immunoglobulin fraction of the immune ascites by salt precipitation, and/or ion-exchange chromatography as described in the preceding section. The immunoglobulin concentration can be roughly estimated by measuring the optical density at 280 nm, and assuming an extinction of 1.4 for a 1 mg/ml solution (and a 1 cm light path). We aim for immunoglobulin concentrations of 5 mg to 10 mg/ml, but have degraded preparations around 1 mg/ml without any problems. The immunoglobulin preparation is dialysed against the digestion buffer, which consists of 0.1 M Na acetate adjusted to pH of 4.5, 4.0, or other appropriate pH with glacial acetic acid. The amount of immunoglobulin to be degraded is calculated, and 2% or 4% of this amount of pepsin is weighed out, dissolved in a small volume of the digestion buffer, and added to the immunoglobulin. In our experience, this generally results in a slight cloudiness of the solution, but this is no cause for concern. The mixture is then incubated with constant stirring or shaking at 37°C for 20 hours. At the end of the digestion, the reaction mixture is lightly centrifuged (e.g. 1000 g for 15 minutes) and any precipitate discarded. The reaction is then stopped by raising the pH to 7.5 with 2 M Tris buffer, which irreversibly inactivates the pepsin. $F(ab')_2$ can then be purified from this preparation by G-200 or S-200 gel filtration.

As IgG and $F(ab')_2$ do overlap to some degree on G-200 gel filtration, a preliminary separation of any undigested IgG can be performed as described by Parham et al[5] by dialysing the digest against 5 mmol Tris HCl, pH 7.5 and passing it down a DEAE ion exchange column equilibrated in the same buffer. $F(ab')_2$ and any F(ab) pass through the column, and IgG is retained. The same effect can be achieved by passing the reaction mixture through a protein A column. However, this preliminary step is not really necessary, and it is easier simply to discard the front of the $F(ab')_2$ peak.

An alternative to the use of low pH pepsin degradation of IgG_1 monoclonal is suggested by Parham et al[5] and involves digestion with preactivated papain (in the absence of free cysteine). If papain digestion of IgG_1 is performed in the presence of free cysteine, $F(ab')_2$, Fab and Fc are produced as a result of incomplete reduction of disulphide bonds in the hinge region. Papain is preactivated by incubation in 3 mmol EDTA, 50 mmol cysteine, in 0.1 M Na acetate pH 5.5 for 30 minutes at 37°C. The activated papain is separated from cysteine by desalting on small G25 gel filtration columns (e.g. PD-10, Pharmacia, Uppsala, Sweden) previously equilibrated in 3 mmol EDTA, 0.1 M Na acetate pH 5.5. Papain elutes in the void volume, and can be followed by OD at 280 nm, and by its yellow colour. Activation is carried out just before use, although it can be stored frozen for small periods (e.g. 1 day or less). Typical conditions[5] involve IgG_1 monoclonal antibody at 10 mg/ml incubated for 18 hours at 37°C with 0.5 mg/ml of preactivated papain in 3 mmol EDTA, 0.1 M Na acetate, pH 5.5. A further aliquot of 0.5 mg/ml of activated papain (frozen in the interim) is added after 9 hours. At the end of the incubation, papain is inactivated by adding 30 mmol iodoacetamide. The suggested approach for purification of $F(ab')_2$ from this reaction mixture involves preliminary removal of undigested IgG and of Fc by DEAE ion exchange chromatography as described above, followed by gel filtration. It is suggested that small scale pilot experiments be performed in the first instance. In these experiments, only an aliquot of the reaction mixture is inactivated at 18 hours, the rest being frozen. This aliquot is analysed by PAGE in SDS for production of F(ab')$_2$. If sufficient digestion has occurred, the reaction mixture is thawed and inactivated with iodoacetamide. If not, the reaction can be continued.

F(ab')$_2$ preparations should be checked for purity by SDS gels using reduced and non-reduced samples. IgG migrates at an Mr of 150 K non-reduced, and 50 K and 25 K reduced. F(ab')$_2$ migrates at 100 K non-reduced, and as a single 25 K band when reduced. Therefore, any contamination of the F(ab')$_2$ preparation with IgG is immediately obvious.

Preparation of Fab

A simple approach is to prepare Fab from F(ab')$_2$ by reduction with 10 mM cysteine for 1 hour at 37°C. The reaction is stopped and free sulphydrils alkylated by incubating with 30 mmol iodoacetamide for 1 hour at room temperature. Fab is separated from unreduced F(ab')$_2$ by G-200 gel filtration. The aim with this approach is reduction of the inter-heavy chain disulphide bonds, without affecting the heavy–light chain disulphide bonds. Parham et al[5] comment that bifunctional thiols such as dithiothreitol, are not as selective for the inter-heavy chain disulphide as cysteine and β2-mercaptoethanol, so that reducing agents such as dithiothreitol should not be used.

The more usual approach to Fab preparation is papain digestion of immunoglobulin in the presence of free cysteine, with separation of Fab from Fc fragments by ion exchange chromatography. For example, the method originally used by Porter on rabbit immunoglobulin[7] involves digestion of IgG at an enzyme substrate ratio of 1% w/w in phosphate buffer of pH 7.0 with 10 mmol cysteine and 2 mmol EDTA for 16 hours at 37°C. We are not aware of a systematic study of papain digestion on mouse immunoglobulin subclasses, but Parham et al[5] report that with mouse IgG$_1$ monoclonal antibodies, the above conditions (except for the use of 50 mM rather than 10 mmol cysteine) give complete degradation of the IgG$_1$ resulting in a mixture of F(ab')$_2$, Fab and Fc. The Fc can be removed by DEAE ion exchange chromatography as described above (or with protein A columns) and the F(ab')$_2$ separated from Fab on G-200 gel filtration. How well this works with the IgG$_{2a}$, IgG$_{2b}$ and IgG$_3$ subclasses and with the other classes of mouse immunoglobulin, we do not know.

MONOCLONAL ANTIBODIES AS REAGENTS FOR IMMUNOCHEMISTRY

Immunochemistry can be defined as the utilisation of antibodies for determining the structure and biochemical characteristics of molecules (the chemistry of the antibody molecules themselves is not relevant to the present discussion). Monoclonal antibodies have made possible monospecific reagents of very high specific activity to virtually any molecule of interest, bringing the possibility of using immunochemical techniques to almost every laboratory.

The major function of the antibody in immunochemistry is the selective removal for subsequent analysis of the target antigen from complex mixtures, and this can be done in the liquid phase (immunoprecipitation techniques) or with the antibody bound to a solid phase, (e.g. monoclonal antibody affinity chromatography, various techniques with antibody immobilized on plates). Alternatively, antibody can be used to identify the target molecule during biochemical separation procedures of complex mixtures, and thereby give information on the biochemical nature of the molecule (e.g. Western blots after SDS PAGE, inhibition assays after gel filtration, or ion-exchange chromatography). Other immunochemical uses of monoclonal antibodies include, for example, serological definition of the topography of a molecule by competitive inhibition studies; looking for clues as to the biochemical nature of the antigenic determinant (and therefore of the molecule bearing the determinant) by exposure of the molecule to various specific degradations (e.g. proteinases, glycosidases) and looking for loss of antigenic activity. Of these and other uses in immunochemistry, monoclonal antibodies have had the greatest impact on two areas: antibody affinity chromatography and the ability readily to distinguish distinct antigenic sites on complex molecules. Both of these areas were, if not quite impossible, then at least extremely difficult, in the days before monoclonal antibodies.

In this chapter, we shall concentrate on the use of monoclonal antibody affinity chromatography both for bulk purification of target molecules, as well as the use of small columns for a variety of purposes. The use of monoclonal antibody covalently bound to beads for small scale solid phase 'immunoprecipitations', and some other areas, will also be discussed.

MONOCLONAL ANTIBODY AFFINITY CHROMATOGRAPHY

This involves the use in columns of beads to which monoclonal antibodies have been bound.

Major experimental uses

Large-scale purification of target antigens
A pure preparation of the target molecule is a prerequisite for any substantial studies on structure, and, in addition, it offers great potential for studies of function.

Our experience has been with membrane glycoproteins, and here 1 mg of pure antigen provides enough reagent for extensive structural studies. As well as the simple determination of amino acid and carbohydrate composition, more detailed studies on the nature of the oligosaccharide chains can be performed[8]. It is possible nowadays to take advantage of modern techniques for amino acid sequencing for N terminal and (after preparation of fragments) internal sequences. These can be used to construct genetic probes for c DNA and genomic libraries, and the full amino acid sequence of the protein, and the nucleotide sequence of the structural gene, can be determined. The technology to follow this path is now more-or-less established as a routine.

Small columns for use with radiolabelled antigens
Small (e.g. 0.5–1 ml) columns can be used to separate target antigens from radiolabelled mixtures for subsequent analysis. For example, the Mr of a molecule can be determined by passing ^{3}H or ^{125}I labelled, detergent solubilized membranes

through a column, eluting the molecule and analysing it on SDS gels. Detection can be by gel-slicing techniques[9] or autoradiography. The incorporation of phosphate, various sugars or other moieties can be tested for in this way, by culturing target cells with radiolabelled metabolites.

We are currently testing the use of small quantities (e.g. 50–100 μl) of beads for binding the labelled molecule, with the beads being washed in a test-tube rather than in columns. If it proves generally applicable, this will be a faster technique than the use of small columns but is not as versatile.

Small columns for determining molecular relationships of antigenic determinants and for functional studies

If a few ml of the target tissue or cell suspension is solubilized, passed through a small affinity column, and the bound antigen eluted, the following reagents are generated:

complex mixture

complex mixture specifically depleted of target antigen

enriched target antigen.

These three reagents form a powerful experimental tool. Serological analysis of the reagents with different monoclonal antibodies will rapidly establish if they are directed at the same molecule. More complex molecular relationships of different antigenic determinants can also be demonstrated. For example, we were able to demonstrate[9] that two monoclonal antibodies showing very different patterns of reactivity among leucocytes were nevertheless directed at different determinants on the **same** molecule. The complexity arose because one of the determinants was present on all the molecules under study, while the other determinant was present on only **some** of these molecules. Molecular heterogeneity in families of molecules can readily be demonstrated in this way.

The three reagents also form a powerful combination for studies of function, e.g. enzyme activity.

The use of small columns for specifically immobilizing the target molecule

A small column, saturated with the target molecule, might be a useful method for studying molecular interactions.

Preparation of the monoclonal antibody affinity column

The covalent coupling of antibodies to beads is extremely simple nowadays because of the availability of many commercially prepared pre-activated gels. Cyanogen bromide activated gels (e.g. from Pharmacia, Uppsala, Sweden) are most commonly used, and these link the protein to Sepharose beads via primary NH_2 groups. The columns are stable for many years, and, with care, can be re-used many times.

The aim is to produce high capacity columns, so immune ascites must of course be used, and a preliminary simple purification procedure to remove as many contaminating proteins as possible is strongly advisable. We use ion-exchange chromatography as outlined in a previous section and usually prepare 15–20 ml of gel. We couple 10 mg of protein per ml of gel, which is at the upper limit of the recommended rate of coupling. Protein content of the purified ascites is best measured precisely[10] but with purified ascites, one may assume an extinction over 1 cm at 280 nm of 1.4 for a 1 mg/ml solution, in which case the protein content is calculated as mg/ml. In the latter case, because of potential inaccuracies in the measurement, it is best to couple at 5 mg protein/ml gel.

On the day before coupling the appropriate amount of antibody is thawed and dialysed against 0.1 M $NaHCO_3$, 0.5 M HCl pH 8.5 (the coupling buffer). This serves two purposes, the first being to bring the pH of the preparation up to the range where coupling is most efficient, and the second to remove any Tris from the preparation since the NH_2 groups of the Tris will compete with the protein for reactive groups on the gel beads. The concentration of protein in the ascites we have coupled has been in the range of 1 to 5 mg/ml.

On the day of coupling the desired amount of CNBr activated Sepharose 4B (supplied as a freeze-dried powder) is weighed out (1 g of freeze dried powder swells to 3.5 ml gel). The gel is swollen for 15 minutes in approximately 100 ml of 1 mmol HCl, pH 3.0, and then washed with 200 ml 1 mmol HCl per g dry gel on a scintered glass filter, porosity G3, on a Buchner flask. The pH of the gel is then brought up to 8.5 by washing the gel in the coupling buffer (100–200 ml). It is very important to check that this pH has been achieved by measuring the pH of the last few ml of buffer that have passed through the gel. The gel is then sucked dry and transferred to a suitable tube. The pH of the dialysed antibody is checked to be 8.5 and it is added to the gel. The gel and antibody are then mixed by end-over-end rotation for 2 hours at room temperature.

At the end of the incubation, the mixture is transferred to the scintered glass funnel and sucked dry. The optical density of the recovered fluid is measured at 280 nm to check the efficiency of the coupling. Usually approximately 90% of the protein is bound to the gel. The gel is then washed with several hundred ml of coupling buffer before blocking the remaining active groups of the gel by incubating in 1 M ethanolamine at pH 8.0 for 2 hours, preferably in a tube as for the coupling. At the end of the incubation the gel is sucked dry and again washed with several hundred ml of coupling buffer. Any non-covalently adsorbed protein is then removed from the gel by subjecting it to 3 cycles of alternating low pH (0.1 M Na acetate 1 M NaCl, 0.02% NaN_3 pH 4.0) and high pH (0.025 M Tris, 1 M NaCl, 0.02% NaN_3 pH 8.2). The pH of the buffer coming through the gel must be measured and the next wash should not be started until the appropriate pH has been attained. Finally the gel is washed in Tris buffered saline (0.025 M Tris, 0.15 M NaCl, 0.02% NaN_3 pH 7.4 at 4°C) and stored at 4°C in this buffer in an airtight container. The OD at 280 nm of all buffers that pass through the gel are measured against the appropriate blanks to check that most of the initial OD has bound to the gel.

Solubilization of antigen

Introduction
The molecules of interest must obviously be in aqueous solution to allow the use of affinity chromatography. If the molecules are naturally water soluble, this simplifies considerably the experimental approach. If they are not approaches must be devised for the preparation in good yield of stable aqueous solutions. Our experience has been with the use of detergents for solubilizing membrane glycoproteins, and this is likely to be the area of interest to most readers. We have not studied membrane glycolipids,

nor non-membrane proteins such as are present in ribosomes, microfilaments, virions, etc.

The use of detergents involves in the first instance finding a detergent that solubilizes the target molecule in good yield, and this is by and large a matter of trial and error. However, we have found the weakly anionic detergent Na deoxycholate, and the non-ionic detergent Brij (a 2:1 mixture of Brij 99: Brij 96) to be most satisfactory. In many published studies, the non-ionic detergent NP-40 is used without any knowledge as to its efficiency in solubilizing the target molecule of interest, and in our experience using quantitative studies on yields, NP-40 appears to be rather a poor detergent.

The definition of solubility is an operational one, a molecule being considered soluble in a detergent if it remains in the supernatant after ultracentrifugation (e.g. 80 000 g for 75 minutes). When this occurs, it is assumed that each molecule is associated with a single detergent micelle, which is probably true if a sufficiently high ratio (2 to 1) of detergent micelles to protein molecules is used.

Choice of detergent

Sodium deoxycholate has proved to be a very useful detergent. It is extremely efficient at solubilizing membranes and also has the advantage that it has a small micelle size (approximately 1000 to 10 000 daltons depending on the ionic strength of the medium)[11] so that the size of the molecule plus detergent is usually not much larger than the molecule alone. This latter point is an advantage if one wishes to submit the solubilized membrane to gel filtration, which separates on the basis of molecular size, as differences between molecules are not so blurred as when the detergent micelle has a molecular weight of approximately 100 000 daltons, which is usually the case with the non-ionic detergents. Sodium deoxycholate has, however, a number of disadvantages. Firstly, it will lyse the nuclear membrane as well as the external cell membrane, whereas the non-ionic detergents leave the nuclei intact. For this reason, deoxycholate usually results in viscous solutions when the usual cell suspensions and homogenates are used. Secondly, solutions of deoxycholate will gel if the pH of the solution falls much below 8 or if the ionic strength of the solution is too high and in particular if it contains divalent cations. Thirdly, being ionic, separation procedures depending on charge (e.g. ion-exchange chromatography, iso-electric focussing) cannot be used on membranes solubilized in deoxycholate.

The non-ionic detergents are not such efficient solubilizers as deoxycholate, but the Brij detergents are very good and appear to be the best of the group in this respect. A 2:1 mixture of Brij 99/Brij 96 is our non-ionic detergent of choice as it remains in solution at 4°C, whereas solutions of Brij 96 tend to come out of solution after several hours at 4°C.

We use the non-ionic detergents directly as supplied, but the deoxycholate is used after one crystallization, to remove impurities, which vary from batch to batch. This is done as follows (A F Williams, personal communication). Approximately 150 g of sodium deoxycholate (Sigma, London, UK) is dissolved in 1.2 litres of a 4:1 mixture of acetone and water, in a water bath at 75°C. The acetone/water mixture boils at 63°C, and to avoid inhaling the fumes this should be done in a fume cupboard. The solution is filtered while hot through filter paper using pre-warmed Buchner funnel and flask. It is then allowed to cool slowly and is left overnight at 4°C. The crystalline precipitate is removed by filtering through filter paper and washed with some cold acetone/water mixture. The crystals are allowed to dry in a fume cupboard overnight, and the drying process completed by placing them under vacuum with $CaCl_2$ overnight. The result should be a white crystalline powder.

Choice of protocol for solubilization

Direct solubilization in non-ionic detergents. Membrane antigens can be directly solubilized by non-ionic detergents, particularly Brij, but this is entirely unpredictable. Our protocol for solubilization is to take homogenate at 25% solid tissue (approximately 10 mg of homogenate protein ml^{-1}) or cells at 5×10^8 ml^{-1} in 0.01 M Tris, 0.15 M NaCl, 0.02% Na azide pH 7.3 at 4°C and add an equal volume of 10% mass/vol. of the non-ionic detergent in the same buffer. The mixture is incubated for 1 hour on ice with constant stirring and then centrifuged for 15 minutes at 1500 g at 4°C to remove nuclei. The supernatant is then ultracentrifuged at 80 000 g for 75 minutes at 4°C.

Direct solubilization in deoxycholate. This is possible wherever there are no or few nuclei in the sample to be solubilized, e.g. platelets, erythrocyte membranes. Otherwise, the nuclei will be disrupted, and a viscous solution produced. The samples to be solubilized are suspended in 0.01 M Tris, 0.02% Na azide pH 8.4, and incubated with an equal volume of 4% deoxycholate in the above buffer for 1 hour on ice. The sample is then ultracentrifuged at 80 000 g for 75 minutes at 4°C. Direct solubilization in deoxycholate of brain homogenates (particularly if they have been frozen and re-washed after homogenisation) is possible but gelling does occur occasionally[12].

Solubilization by use of a non-ionic detergent followed by deoxycholate. Some non-ionic detergents, particularly Tween 40[13] will not usually solubilize the molecule under study, but will result in the formation of membrane fragments which require ultracentrifugation for sedimentation. The protocol is precisely as for direct solubilization with non-ionic detergents, except that 4% Tween 40 detergent is usually used. The membrane-containing ultracentrifuge pellet is resuspended in 0.01 M Tris, 0.02% Na azide, pH 8.4 at 4°C, usually to the original volume of cell or homogenate suspension. After resuspension with a pipette, it is wise to use a ground-glass homogenizer as the small pellet will frequently be difficult to disrupt. An equal volume of 4% deoxycholate in the same buffer is then added, incubated for 1 hour on ice with constant stirring, and then the mixture ultracentrifuged at 80 000 g for 75 minutes at 4°C. The antigen should then be in the supernatant. The above procedure works well with single cell suspensions, but does not appear to be effective with tissue homogenates.

Assays in the presence of detergents

While testing for a suitable detergent, and subsequently during purification procedures, the concentration of antigen in various fractions should be assayed (e.g. by quantitative binding assays[14] to allow the calculation of yields of antigenic activity. If the target is susceptible to detergent lysis, and this will frequently be the case, the target must be protected or a non-lysable system chosen. Possible solutions to this problem are as follows:

The use of targets 'fixed' by agents such as glutaraldehyde. The simplest procedure is to fix the target cell, homogenate or whatever else is in use with a reagent such as glutaraldehyde[15]. The target suspension is washed in protein-free medium three times, and then resuspended to 2×10^8 cells ml^{-1} or 2–4 mg of homogenate protein ml^{-1}. An equal volume of 0.25% glutaraldehyde in the same buffer is then added, mixed, and incubated for 5 minutes at room temperature. The reaction is stopped by adding excess protein (e.g. 1/10 volume of 10% bovine serum albumin (BSA) or undiluted serum) and the targets washed immediately three times by centrifugation in protein-containing media. After fixation, the cells may be stored frozen in aliquots, in protein-containing buffers.

Glutaraldehyde-fixed targets are usually resistant to freezing, non-physiological salt concentrations, detergents, and almost any other insult, but two important things should be noted. Firstly, even after fixation, detergent interference is occasionally a problem, so appropriate detergent controls must be included in all assays even though fixed targets are used. In some cases, 10% BSA will be necessary in the assay system even with fixed targets (see next section). Secondly, even mild fixations as described above will denature some antigenic determinants so that preliminary antibody titrations against fixed and fresh targets must be performed to check for denaturation. Although partial denaturation usually occurs, this does not preclude the use of the fixed targets in assays.

The use of protein in the assay system. Living cells or other detergent-susceptible targets may be used if high concentrations of protein are included in the reaction mixture[16]. A final concentration of 10% BSA in the mixture is what we aim for in the first instance, but up to 30% may be necessary, depending on the particular detergents in use and their concentrations. BSA may be introduced by using 20–30% BSA for (i) resuspension of target cells; (ii) dilution of the antibody; or (iii) dilution of the antigen.

The use of plate assays. Many detergent solubilized molecules will bind to flexible PVC plates (e.g. Flow Laboratories, Irvine, Scotland), and their presence may be detected by adding monoclonal antibody and then labelled anti-mouse immunoglobulin antibodies. This approach cannot be used while the molecule under study is a minor component of a complex mixture, because of competition for binding to the plate. However, once the molecule is reasonably pure (e.g. as it is eluted from the affinity column) it can usually be readily bound to PVC plates.

If immunoglobulin is non-specifically eluted along with antigen from the affinity column (as does happen occasionally), it will bind to the plate and result in false positives, but this latter difficulty can be easily detected by including a control that omits incubation with the monoclonal antibody.

We have used plate assays in two ways. Our main use has been simply to detect the presence of antigen in fractions during chromatographic purification (e.g. Fig. 3.1). For this test, 50 μl of the soluble antigen are added to wells and incubated for 3 hours or overnight at 4°C. The solution is removed from the plate with a pipette and 200 μl of 5% BSA are added to each well to saturate protein binding sites. After incubation for one hour, this is removed and the wells are washed three times in 0.5% BSA/PBS. 50 μl of the monoclonal antibody are added at dilutions sufficient to saturate the antigen, and incubated for 1 hour. The plates are washed 3 times, and 50 μl of ^{125}I labelled, affinity purified anti-immunoglobulin is added (approximately 300 000 cpm). After a further 1 hour's incubation, the wells are washed 3 times, cut

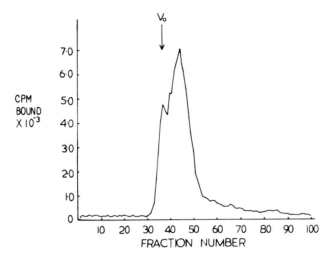

Fig. 3.1 Use of a plate assay in the presence of detergent to monitor purification of antigen by gel filtration. Monoclonal affinity column purified F8-11-13 antigen was submitted to Sepharose CL 6B gel filtration chromatography and 50 μl of each fraction placed in polyvinyl plates. Antigen containing fractions were detected by adding F8-11-13 monoclonal antibody and then ^{125}I labelled rabbit anti-mouse immunoglobulin to each well.

out, and placed into counting tubes to measure radioactivity. This is a very useful and rapid assay for antigen, but it is not quantitative. Another way to use plate assays is precisely as one would use any other target. For example, after quantitative absorption analysis, residual antibody can be detected by incubation in antigen coated wells[8].

Potential difficulties with detergent solubilization
Ideally, a detergent should give perhaps 20% or better yield of soluble antigen from the starting material.

A suitable solubilization is given in Figure 3.2.

The potential difficulties with solubilization are as follows:

the antigen is solubilized not at all or in low yields by the detergents selected

the antigenic determinant under study is denatured by the detergent

the monoclonal antibody is of too low affinity to react with soluble, monomeric antigen

the concentration of antigen in the tissue to be solubilized is too low to allow quantitative detection after the dilutions and losses involved in solubilization

the target cells, even if fixed with glutaraldehyde, require further protection from detergent with BSA

the monoclonal antibody is denatured by the detergent.

Inhibition of proteolysis
It is essential in most experiments to retain the molecule under study in its original form. The proteolytic enzymes present in the tissues can cause considerable problems in this respect and it will usually be vital to take great care to avoid proteolysis.

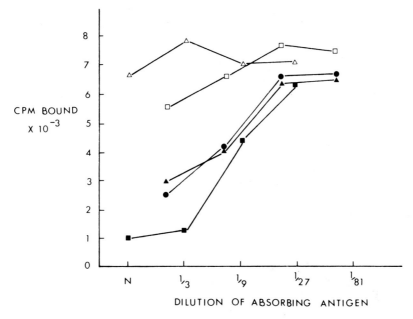

Fig. 3.2 Testing a detergent for adequacy of solubilization by quantitative absorption analysis. Aliquots of F10-44-2 monoclonal antibody[25] at 1 in 15 000 dilution were absorbed with tripling dilutions of samples taken at different stages of solubilization and tested for residual antibody activity by an indirect radiolabel binding assay using glutaraldehyde fixed spleen cells at 5×10^7/ml. Spleen homogenate, ■———■; spleen homogenate plus 4% Brij 99/96 after 1 hour incubation, ●———●; supernatant of Brij incubated spleen homogenate after low speed centrifugation to remove nuclei, ▲———▲; ultracentrifuge pellet, □———□; 2% Brij 99/96 control, △———△

All of the following precautions should be taken routinely:
1. Keep all solutions on ice or at 4°C at all times.
2. Perform all procedures in the minimum time possible, particularly in the early stages before substantial purification.
3. Avoid acidic pH's, where acid proteases will be most active.
4. Avoid the presence of divalent cations, since some proteases require them for activity, and use 5 mmol EDTA in all solutions.
5. Use 2.5 mmol iodoacetamide (IAA) in all solutions.
6. Use 2 mmol phenyl methyl sulphonyl fluoride (PMSF) in all solutions.

The PMSF and IAA each inactivate a different class of proteases. IAA is readily soluble in water, and can be used without difficulty. PMSF is poorly soluble in water, but is much more readily soluble in detergents. It is also very toxic. Problems with proteolysis occur mainly after addition of detergents, so that the PMSF may be dissolved to 4 mmol in the detergent prior to addition to the tissue. Both IAA and PMSF must be prepared fresh immediately before use.

Affinity chromatography with monoclonal antibody columns

Introduction and design of pilot experiments
Once the antigen has been solubilized in good yield and the affinity column prepared,

there are still some obstacles to be negotiated. For this reason, it is advisable to perform pilot experiments to pin-point potential difficulties, and these experiments are best performed with small columns. We routinely use 0.7 ml of gel in disposable plastic columns (Econo-columns; Bio Rad, Watford, Herts). The column is washed with 5 ml of buffer without detergent and then with 5 ml of buffer with 0.5% detergent to equilibrate the column. This is done simply by applying the washing solution to the top of the column with a Pasteur pipette, and takes only a few minutes. The column is then pre-eluted to remove any proteins that can be removed from the column by the eluting procedure chosen. One may use either low pH (e.g. 1 M propionic acid, pH 2.6) or high pH (e.g. 0.05 M diethylamine, pH 11.5) solutions in 0.5% detergent for elution, although obviously only the high pH solution is appropriate for systems with deoxycholate. 2 or 3 ml of the eluting solution are passed through the column, after which it is brought quickly back to the starting pH by passing through buffer with 0.5% detergent. It is useful to use pH paper to check quickly that the column is back to a reasonable pH. The column is now ready for use.

We apply a few ml, usually 4 ml, of antigen solution to the column at the rate of 2 ml per h. A useful system which we have devised for use with small volumes of detergent solution (and in particular for radiolabelled solutions) is given in Figure 3.3. The solution is forced out of the plastic syringe used as a reservoir by pumping air at a controlled rate into the syringe. This system is doubly useful since, by reversing the flow of air, the sample can be sucked into the syringe at the beginning of the experiment.

After 1 or 1.5 ml of sample has passed through the column, a 1 ml sample is collected as the 'depleted' fraction. After all the sample has passed through the column, it is washed with 0.5% detergent in the appropriate buffer. The first 1 ml of wash is applied at the same rate as sample application, so that the antigen solution in the column will not be wasted by being rapidly washed through. Then 10–20 ml of detergent solution is applied by pipette to wash the column and this can be done quite rapidly. The column is then eluted by low or high pH, or other appropriate solution in 0.5% detergent, by applying 6×0.5 ml aliquots of the eluting solution and collecting each as a separate fraction. Each fraction should be neutralized immediately if a pH change is used to effect elution. With the 0.05 M diethylamine, pH 11.5 buffer, the use of solid glycine in the collecting tube is a useful method, since in saturated glycine the pH is brought rapidly down to approximately 8. If 1 M propionic acid is used for elution the sample after collection can be neutralized with 2 M Tris, but this can be quite a delicate procedure, and perhaps less concentrated Tris solutions should be used with these small fractions. All else being equal, we routinely use high pH elution in the first instance. Once the eluting solution has been applied, the column should be brought back to a more physiological pH by washing with, e.g. 0.15 M NaCl, 0.02% N azide, 0.025 M Tris, pH 7.4 at 4°C. Note that where deoxycholate is used, it is essential that it be washed out of the column with the low salt, pH 8.4 buffer before the Tris/saline buffer just mentioned is applied.

The starting detergent solution, the depleted samples and the first 4 elution fractions are then tested by quantitative techniques for the amount of antigen present. In the majority of cases the picture seen is similar to that given in Figure 3.4 for bulk purification from larger columns, showing complete depletion of antigen from the applied sample, and its recovery in good yield in the eluted fractions. The

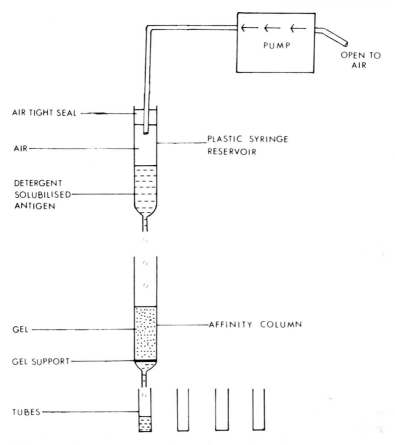

Fig. 3.3 Experimental system for work with small affinity columns, especially when using radiolabelled antigens

antigen will usually be concentrated on elution, and the degree of concentration will depend mainly on the ratio of the volume of the applied and eluted samples.

Potential problems with affinity columns
Most affinity columns prepared with IgG monoclonal antibodies will function well. Our experience and that of others is that IgM monoclonal antibodies generally do not behave well as immunoadsorbents, but there are exceptions. When problems do arise, it is sometimes useful to investigate the situation before discarding a system as valueless. The problems that might arise are as follows:

1. The antigen passes unretarded through the columns either because the antibody is of too low affinity to function effectively, or the antibody is denatured by the coupling procedure. It is also possible that the concentration of specific antibody in the coupled ascites is too low.

2. The antigen is retained on the column but antigen activity cannot be detected in the eluted fractions. This can be the result either of the antigen remaining bound to the column in spite of the elution procedure used[17] or the antigen being eluted from the column in a denatured form.

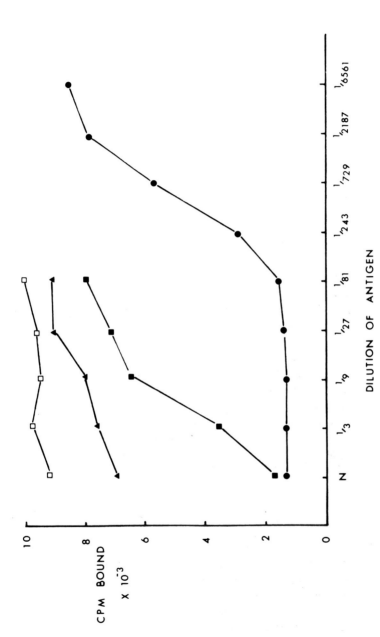

Fig. 3.4 Purification of antigen by monoclonal antibody affinity chromatography monitored by quantitative absorption analysis. Aliquots of F10-44-2 monoclonal antibody[25] at a 1 in 15 000 dilution were absorbed with tripling dilutions of samples and assayed by an indirect radiolabel binding assay using glutaraldehyde fixed spleen cells. Brij 99/96 solubilized spleen homogenate before ■——■ and after ▲——▲ passage through an F10-44-2 monoclonal antibody affinity column; high pH eluate of the column, ●——● ; and 2% Brij 99/96 control, □——□ . 600 ml of solubilized antigen was passed through the column and the elution volume was 10 ml.

3. Very occasionally, with some monoclonal antibodies, large amounts of immunoglobulin are eluted from the column, and this can substantially complicate the picture.

Bulk purification of molecules

Introduction. A monoclonal antibody affinity column offers the opportunity in one step to purify a membrane molecule one hundred to several hundred fold in good yield in relation to total tissue protein. In addition to this high factor of purification, a specific affinity step has theoretical advantages over conventional biochemical techniques, since the purification does not depend on any biochemical characteristics of the molecule. (The usual biochemical procedures purify groups of molecules with similar characteristics). It can be applied to very large volumes of antigen containing material, and serves as a concentrating as well as a purifying step. An example of bulk purification of a lymphocyte membrane molecule is given in Figure 3.4.

Practical aspects of chromatography. Once the preliminary work has been completed, bulk purification is essentially a scaling up of the procedures outlined in the section on pilot experiments. We generally use columns (Econo-columns, Bio Rad) containing 8–10 ml of gel, and apply 200–500 ml of soluble antigen at 10–20 ml per hour, using a pump. The soluble material is first passed through a 10 ml column of Sepharose 4B (in series with the affinity column) to remove any material which might adhere non-specifically to the affinity column. The solution that has passed through the column is collected into 10 ml fractions. It is vital at this and at all subsequent stages to use disposable plastic or thoroughly cleansed glassware to avoid introducing contaminants into the purified solution. All steps are carried out at 4°C in the presence of proteolytic inhibitors.

After the sample has passed through, the column is washed with at least 100 ml of 0.5% detergent in the appropriate buffer, at 10–20 ml per hour using a pump. Fractions are collected and the optical density at 280 nm is measured. When the optical density is zero, or has stabilized close to zero, the column is eluted as described in a preceding section using approximately 5 column volumes of eluting solution. This can be done quite quickly by hand-pipetting, and 5 ml fractions are collected. The fractions are neutralized (if pH change has been used for elution) and the first 5 or 6 eluted fractions, the starting solution, and every 5th or 10th of the depleted fractions (to check when and if the column has been saturated) are analysed for antigen activity. If a plate assay is possible for detecting antigen, it can be particularly useful for detecting the eluted antigen.

The antigen-containing fractions are pooled, and we routinely apply them to a gel filtration column for two reasons. Not only does it serve as an extra purification step, but it effectively 'desalts' the antigen, removing the eluting and neutralizing substances (e.g. diethylamine, glycine). Concentration of the antigen prior to gel filtration is usually not necessary, as up to 25 ml can be loaded on to a 500 ml column for gel filtration. (We use Sephacryl S-300 or Sepharose CL 6B (Pharmacia, Uppsala, Sweden)). The gel filtration column should of course be equilibrated in 0.5% detergent in the appropriate buffer, and care must be taken that the antigen concentration in the sample is sufficiently high to be detected after a 5-fold or so dilution as a result of the gel filtration. We test all or alternate fractions for their content of antigen, and antigen containing fractions are pooled, sometimes after checking each fraction for purity on SDS gels. We find it useful at this stage to concentrate the sample 4 or 5 fold by positive pressure filtration (Amicon, Woking, Surrey) and then, because the detergent might be concentrated along with the antigen, to dialyse the sample against 0.5% detergent in the appropriate buffer. We then divide it into aliquots which are stored at –80°C.

Concentration of antigen. It is usually necessary to know the concentration of antigen in the sample, and this for our work means protein estimations. The usual technique for measuring proteins are modifications of the much-quoted paper by Lowry et al.[10] In the context of the present discussion it is vital to note that detergents will frequently form precipitates and interfere with the colour reaction, but this can usually be overcome by including 1% SDS in the alkaline copper reagent. The standard curve must contain the same concentration of detergent as that in the sample. If these precautions are taken, reasonable certainty can be attached to protein measurements.

Checks of purity. The purity of the sample should be checked, and SDS gels are now almost universally used for this purpose for protein antigens. It should be stressed that 'purity' is a relative and not an absolute term, and, moreover, that it is uncommon for the material eluted from a monoclonal antibody affinity column to give a single band on SDS gels. For the SDS gels we aim to load 10 μg of protein for each sample, and perform the electrophoresis on slab gels. If the molecular weight of the molecule under study is unknown, both high (e.g. 12%) and low (e.g. 6%) percentage acrylamide gels should be used, so that both low and high molecular weight regions can be surveyed. At the termination of electrophoresis, the gels are usually stained for protein (e.g. Coomassie blue or silver stains) but stains for carbohydrate (e.g. periodic acid-Schiff reaction) can be useful for heavily glycosylated proteins.

If there is difficulty in obtaining the antigen in a form concentrated enough to load approximately 10 μg of protein on the gels, it can be precipitated by use of acetone or trichloroacetic acid. However, we have found it very useful simply to freeze-dry the sample and then resuspend it in loading buffer. If the antigen is in low salt and in 0.5% detergent, 300 to 400 μl can be freeze-dried and resuspended in 100 μl of loading buffer without difficulty. Apart from simplicity, freeze-drying does not have the potential problem of selective precipitation, which might occur with the above-mentioned reagents.

It is vital to note that it is not a simple thing to relate a band on a gel to the target molecule of the monoclonal antibody. If the molecular weight is known it may be clear that the antigen has been successfully purified but if not, it is unwise to conclude that a particular band represents the antigen, even if there is only a single band on the gels. In the absence of other corroborative evidence, the point should be proved either by performing Western Blots (discussed in a subsequent section) or by assaying for antigen from the gel itself[3]. A good example of how errors can arise is in relation to monoclonal antibodies to β2 microglobulin (mol.wt.12 000). These will purify HLA ABC antigens from cell membranes, and when analysed on, e.g. 6% acrylamide gels, the β2 microglobulin will migrate with the dye while a major band will be seen at the 45 000 Mr position. The monoclonal antibody however, is clearly not directed at this band.

If there are several bands on the gel, additional purification procedures might be necessary depending on the use to which the sample will be put. It is sometimes useful to pass the sample through gel filtration a second time, and the information obtained from the first gel filtration can be used to choose the most appropriate gel for the second run. Additional purification procedures can be used. We have used both lectin affinity and ion-exchange chromatography for final purification of Brij solubilized antigen. Preparative isoelectric focussing is also possible, but clearly both ion-exchange and iso-electric focussing techniques can be used only with non-ionic detergents. A number of other approaches are possible[18] but these additional techniques are not as yet widely in use.

Small affinity columns for molecular weight estimations on SDS gels

The use of small affinity columns with systems previously tested as described in the previous sections has several advantages over the conventional immunoprecipitation technique for molecular weight estimation, particularly as there is no problem with regard to antibody or antigen excess for the precipitation step. In addition, samples that are specifically depleted of antigen after passage through the column are available, and these frequently provide useful corroborative evidence for the Mr estimation[8,9,12]. Because the amount of antigen eluted is small, its detection requires the use of radiolabels, followed by gel slicing techniques or autoradiography.

Cell surface molecules can be labelled by a number of techniques. Because at least the majority of proteins on the outer surface of cell membranes are glycosylated, they can be labelled with ^{3}H by way of the terminal sialic acids of their oligosaccharide chains, using sodium periodate and NaB^{3}H$_4$[19]. This technique is useful only if the molecule under study is heavily glycosylated, but it is an especially attractive system when it works, because of its selectivity. The more usual approach is to iodinate the protein with ^{125}I, and here the iodogen method is very useful[20]. It is a better technique than lactoperoxidase catalysed iodination, in that iodination seems to be restricted much more to cell surface proteins. Proteins solubilized in detergent solutions can also be iodinated using either the chloramine T or iodogen methods, but this is usually of value only if the solubilized material has been substantially purified prior to iodination. With cultured cells and cell lines, one can introduce labelled amino acids, sugars or other metabolites biosynthetically. It should also be noted that labelling with ^{3}H and ^{125}I can easily be applied to tissue homogenates[12].

We aim to label a minimum of 2×10^8 lymphocytes by the ^{3}H method or 2×10^7 with ^{125}I. With lymphocytes, generally 10^6 cpm are incorporated per 10^8 cells using the ^{3}H label, and 5×10^6 cpm per 10^7 cells using iodogen for ^{125}I labelling. Because of the long half-life of ^{3}H (12 years) quite large numbers of cells can be labelled, and the soluble, labelled membranes stored frozen. After the cells have been labelled and washed, we resuspend ^{3}H labelled lymphocytes to $1-2 \times 10^8$ ml^{-1}, and ^{125}I labelled lymphocytes to approximately 2×10^7 ml^{-1}, for subsequent solubilization. After addition of detergents, we proceed as rapidly as possible in the presence of proteolytic inhibitors carefully maintaining the solutions at 0°C to 4°C at all times.

For the chromatography, the volume of sample loaded should be approximately 2 ml. We aim to load approximately 10^6 cpm with ^{3}H labelled samples and 3 to 5×10^7 cpm with ^{125}I, although the amount loaded will vary with the system under study, and the more loaded, probably the better. Elution of the antigen may be performed as outlined in a preceding section, but for analyses on SDS gels we find that it is better to remove the washed gel from the column in a small amount of 0.5% detergent solution, sediment the beads by centrifuging at 400 g for 5 minutes in a glass tube, and then to add approximately 0.5 ml of 2% SDS in 0.25 M Tris, pH 6.8. This is then placed in a boiling water bath for 5 minutes with shaking; the sample is centrifuged again at 400 g for 5 minutes and the supernatant recovered.

For analysis by PAGE in SDS, we use 3 mm thick slab gels. With ^{3}H labelled samples, we aim to analyse the sample before application to the affinity column, the depleted sample and the eluted material. With ^{125}I labelled samples, only the eluted material is analysed. For ^{3}H labelled samples we aim to load 50 000 to 100 000 cpm for the starting and depleted samples, and 10 000 to 20 000 cpm for the eluted material. With ^{125}I labelling of cell surfaces, we tend to load 10 000 to 20 000 cpm for the eluted material. If the samples are too dilute to allow a suitable number of counts to be loaded, protein-bound radioactivity may be precipitated from a larger volume using acetone or trichloroacetic acid or, more simply the sample can be freeze-dried and resuspended in the appropriate volume of loading buffer.

OTHER USES OF MONOCLONAL ANTIBODIES FOR IMMUNOCHEMISTRY

Monoclonal antibodies can be used in a variety of ways to give clues to the structure of the target molecule. Three of the more useful approaches will be discussed briefly here.

Monoclonal antibody coupled beads for solid phase immunoprecipitation

Beads to which monoclonal antibodies have been covalently coupled may be used for solid phase immunoprecipitation in test tubes, as an alternative to their use in small affinity columns. We have had only little experience with this approach, but there are reports in which it has been used successfully[21]. As variations on this theme, monoclonal antibody is first allowed to interact with radiolabelled soluble antigen, and is then removed from solution with beads to which anti-immunoglobulin antibodies[22] or protein A have been coupled. Staphylococci have also been used to adsorb the immunoglobulin[23]. These approaches have the advantage of speed as compared to the use of small columns, but they are not as versatile. When compared to liquid phase immunoprecipitations, however, there are fewer potential problems with poorly controlled variables.

A suspension containing 50 or 100 μl of 50% beads to which monoclonal antibody has been coupled is transferred to a glass test tube, and centrifuged at 400 g for 5 minutes. The supernatant is removed, and the beads resuspended in approximately 500 μl of detergent solubilized extract of radiolabelled membranes. This is incubated for 1 hour on ice in the presence of proteolytic inhibitors, with shaking every 15 minutes. The beads are then washed three times in 0.5% detergent in the appropriate buffer. The beads are finally resuspended in 200 μl of 2% SDS and placed on a boiling water bath for 5 minutes. The beads are then centrifuged again, and the supernatant removed for analysis in SDS gels as described previously.

Liquid phase immunoprecipitation

This approach appears to be losing popularity as techniques involving the use of beads to which monoclonal antibodies, protein A or anti-immunoglbulin sera have been coupled gain more widespread acceptance. The principle is simple: the monoclonal antibody is mixed with a detergent extract of a radiolabelled preparation, allowing the antibody to interact with the target molecule. The mouse immunoglobulin, including the radiolabelled antigen in the complexes, is then precipitated with an anti-mouse immunoglobulin serum and the precipitate is analysed on SDS gels. The major problem with liquid phase immunoprecipitation is that care must be taken to avoid antigen or antibody excess for the precipitation step, i.e. the amount of mouse immunoglobulin in the preparation used to form monoclonal antibody/antigen complexes must be taken into account when adding the precipitating anti-immunoglobulin sera. We have in our work invariably used monoclonal antibody coupled to beads, and therefore cannot offer any experience with liquid phase immunoprecipitation.

Monoclonal antibodies as markers for individual components of complex mixtures, with particular reference to Western blots

The most widespread approach to obtaining biochemical information as regards the target molecule of a monoclonal antibody is the use of solid or liquid phase immunoprecipitations of radiolabelled material, followed by analysis on SDS gels to give the Mr of the target molecule. A recently described alternative is the use of 'Western' blots[24]. Here, the complex solution containing the target molecule is submitted to SDS polyacrylamide gel electrophoresis, and the separated proteins are then transferred electrophoretically to nitrocellulose paper so that an exact image of the SDS gel is reproduced on the paper. The position of the target molecule on the nitrocellulose paper can then be determined, usually be incubating the paper with monoclonal antibody, followed by an incubation with radiolabelled or peroxidase labelled anti-mouse immunoglobulin antibodies.

The advantage of this approach is that the band on the gel is directly identified as the target of the monoclonal antibody, so that the potential errors inherent in ascribing bands on gels as the targets of monoclonal antibodies are overcome. Moreover, where molecular structures consist of two or more polypeptide chains, it is sometimes possible to identify with which polypeptide the monoclonal antibody interacts.

There are, however, potential problems. Some antigenic determinants will be denatured when the native molecule is exposed to SDS, even without boiling. Because of this possibility, samples are usually analysed unreduced and without boiling in SDS before electrophoresis, and this in our experience results in loss of resolution and blurring of bands. Because the determinant under study might be resistant to these procedures (e.g. if it is a carbohydrate determinant) it is useful to analyse a boiled and reduced sample as well as the non-boiled, non-reduced sample. A special example of denaturation is where non-covalently associated polypeptides are important for the structure of the complex. For instance, when $\beta 2$ microglobulin is dissociated from the HLA-ABC heavy chain, the conformational changes in the heavy chain result in the loss of many determinants present on the native molecule[5].

Western blots are in fact a special case of identifying the target molecule **after** biochemical separation of complex mixtures. One can also, for example, submit the sample to gel filtration and follow antigenic activity so as to obtain an idea of size. One should remember here, however, that the Stokes' radius of membrane glycoproteins as measured by gel filtration is very much higher than that for globular proteins of corresponding molecular weight. Whether this is a result of the shape of the molecule, or their aggregation, is not certain.

REFERENCES

1. Hudson L, Hay F C (eds) 1980 Practical immunology, 2nd edn. Blackwell Scientific Publications, Oxford, p 223
2. Kohler G, Milstein C 1975 Continuous culture of fused cells secreting antibody of predefined specificity. Nature 256: 495–497
3. Storch M-J, Lohmann-Matthew M-L 1984 A new and rapid method for immunoglobulin class and subclass determination of mouse monoclonal antibodies using a solid phase immunorediometric assay. Journal of Immunological Methods (In press)
4. Cleveland W L, Wood I, Erlanger B F 1983 Routine large scale production of monoclonal antibodies in a protein-free culture medium. Journal of Immunological Methods 56: 221–234
5. Parham P, Androlewicz M J, Brodsky F M, Holmes N J, Ways J P 1982 Monoclonal antibodies: purification, fragmentation and application to structural and functional studies of class 1 MHC antigens. Journal of Immunological Methods 53: 133–173
6. Mason D W, Williams A F 1980 The kinetics of antibody binding to membrane antigens in solution and at the cell surface. Biochemical Journal 187: 1–20
7. Porter R R 1959 The hydrolysis of rabbit gamma globulin and antibodies with crystalline papain. Biochemical Journal 73: 119–126
8. Lakin K H, Allen A K, Fabre J W 1983 Purification and preliminary biochemical characterisation of the human and rat forms of the central nervous system specific molecule, F3-87-8. Journal of Neurochemistry 41: 385–394
9. Dalchau R, Fabre J W 1981 Identification with a monoclonal antibody of a predominantly B lymphocyte specific determinant of the human leucocyte common antigen: evidence for structural and possible functional diversity of the leucocyte common molecule. Journal of Experimental Medicine 153: 753–765
10. Lowry H, Rosebrough N J, Farr A, Randall R J 1951 Protein measurement with the Folin reagent. Journal of Biological Chemistry 193: 265–275
11. Tanford C, Reynolds J A 1976 Characterisation of membrane proteins in detergent solutions. Biochimica et Biophysica Acta 457: 133–170
12. Lakin K H, Fabre J W 1981 Identification with a monoclonal antibody of a phylogenetically conserved, brain-specific determinant on a 130 000 molecular weight glycoprotein of human brain. Journal of Neurochemistry 37: 1170–1178
13. Standring R, Williams A F 1978 Glycoproteins and antigens of membranes prepared from rat thymocytes after lysis by shearing or with the detergent Tween 40. Biochimica et Biophysica Acta 508: 85–96
14. Morris R J, Williams A F 1975 Antigens on mouse and rat lymphocytes recognized by rabbit antiserum to rat brain: the quantitative analysis of a xenogeneic serum. European Journal of Immunology 5: 274–281
15. Williams A F 1973 Assays for cellular antigens in the presence of detergents. European Journal of Immunology 3: 626–632
16. Springer R A, Strominger J L, Mann D 1974 Partial purification of detergent soluble HL-A antigen and its cleavage by papain. Proceedings of the National Academy of Sciences (USA) 71: 1539–1543
17. Dalchau R, Kirkley J, Fabre J W 1980 Monoclonal antibody to a human leucocyte specific membrane glycoprotein probably homologous to the leucocyte common antigen of the rat. European Journal of Immunology 10: 737–744
18. Hoffmann-Ostenhof O, Breitenbach M, Koller F, Kraft D, Scheiner O (eds) 1978 Affinity chromatography. Pergamon Press, Oxford
19. Gahmberg C G, Andersson L C 1977 Selective radioactive labelling of cell surface sialoglycoproteins by periodate-tritiated borohydride. Journal of Biological Chemistry 252: 5888–5894
20. Hudson L, Hay F C (eds) 1980 Practical immunology, 2nd edn. Blackwell Scientific Publications, Oxford, p 241
21. Meuer S C, Acuto O, Hussey R E, Hodgdon J C, Fitzgerald K A, Schlossman S F, Reinherz E L 1983 Evidence for the T3 associates 90K heterodimer as the T cell antigen receptor. Nature 303: 808–810

22. Howard J C, Butcher G W, Galfre G, Milstein C P 1979 Monoclonal antibodies as tools to analyse the serological and genetic complexities of major transplantation antigens. Immunological Reviews 47: 139–174

23. Morishima Y, Kobayashi M, Yang S Y, Collins N H, Hoffman M K, Dupont B 1982 Functionally different T lymphocyte subpopulations determined by their sensitivity to complement dependent cell lysis with the monoclonal antibody 4A. Journal of Immunology 129: 1091–1098

24. Towbin H, Staehelin T, Gordon J 1976 Electrophoretic transfer of proteins from polyacrylamide gels to nitrocellulose sheets: Procedure and some applications. Proceedings of the National Academy of Sciences 76: 4350–4354

25. Dalchau R, Kirkley J, Fabre J W 1980 Monoclonal antibody to a human brain-granulocyte-T lymphocyte antigen probably homologous to the W3/13 antigen of the rat. European Journal of Immunology 10: 745–749

4

The production of human monoclonal antibodies

Paul A. W. Edwards Michael J. O'Hare

INTRODUCTION

This chapter is concerned primarily with the production of human monoclonal antibodies by construction of human-human hybridomas although two alternative strategies—the use of Epstein-Barr (EB) virus transformation and hybridization of human lymphocytes with mouse myelomas—will also be considered briefly. We discuss why human monoclonal antibodies are useful, how they can be made in principle and in practice, the difficulties and pitfalls that can be encountered, and some prospects for the future. We will assume that the reader is already familiar with the production of monoclonal antibodies and therefore the general principles of hybridoma technology (see elsewhere in this volume and references[1-3]).

It is now possible to make human–human hybridomas routinely but it would be wrong to give the impression that it is as easy as making rodent hybridomas; there is now so much enthusiasm for making human monoclonal antibodies that the emphasis in this chapter is on caution. We would advise anybody contemplating making human–human hybridomas first to ask carefully why they are making human rather than rodent hybridomas; secondly, how they are going to make them; and thirdly whether the hybridomas they will be able to make will be satisfactory for their ultimate purpose and whether they will be obtainable with a reasonable amount of effort.

WHY MAKE HUMAN MONOCLONAL ANTIBODIES?

Two main reasons are usually given for wanting to make human hybridomas: (1) to capture and 'immortalize' particular human immune responses; and (2) to make human antibodies for therapeutic purposes. Examples under the first heading include (a) antibodies to human polymorphic antigens such as blood groups and histocompatibility antigens; (b) human immune responses in disease such as putative responses to tumours; (c) auto-immune responses, for example in systemic lupus erythematosus, rheumatoid arthritis or autoimmune endocrine syndromes. In addition it has been suggested or implied that the human immune system may make different antibodies to a particular antigenic challenge than a rodent, and there might be situations where the specifically human immune response was interesting.

All these reasons are, on closer inspection, subject to some reservations.

60

The case for making rodent monoclonal antibodies at the present time or waiting for improved techniques

The concept that human antibodies will recognize antigens in qualitatively different ways from rodent antibodies is in general naive. It should be possible to obtain rodent antibodies that bind to a particular distinctive structure recognized by a human antibody provided enough hybrids are generated and screened. **At the present time** cell lines producing human monoclonal antibodies are far more difficult to make than rodent cell lines producing rodent antibodies and they are often less satisfactory, as discussed below. Also, it is not usually possible to immunise humans optimally. An important reason for the success of rodent fusions is that an animal is hyperimmunised and boosted for fusion, and hybridization is remarkably selective for B-cells responsive to, and hence stimulated by, the antigen boost.[4]

Thus in practice the greater suitability of human antibodies has to be balanced against the far greater practical problems, at present, of making human rather than rodent monoclonal antibodies.

Monoclonal antibodies to human polymorphisms can often be raised without difficulty using rodent systems. A number of mouse antibodies have been made to HLA types.[5]

Mouse antibodies to some human blood groups have been made and at least one appears suitable for routine blood grouping use.[6] However, conventional serology suggests that antibodies to rhesus antigens would be difficult to raise in non-human species. Human monoclonal antibodies have been made to rhesus D by using lymphocytes from volunteers who have been immunised for production of anti-D serum.[7]

Although a number of laboratories, including our own, have fused human lymphocytes from tumours and from lymph nodes draining tumours to probe possible anti-tumour responses, little has yet been achieved, as discussed below.

Cell lines producing human auto-antibodies have been made[8,9,10] but other laboratories have failed in spite of many attempts. If the antigen recognized by an autoimmune antibody is known, rodent monoclonal antibodies can often be made (e.g. anti-DNA antibodies[11] and anti-blood group antigen I[12]) so there has to be a specific reason for needing the human antibodies. On the other hand, if the antigen is not known it may be difficult to devise a relevant screening assay for identifying the human monoclonal.

Are human monoclonal antibodies needed for therapy?

It cannot be assumed that human antibodies are **necessary** for therapy and it can be argued that at present rodent antibodies are more suitable for developing therapeutic applications, for example in studying the targetting of antibodies to particular antigens in vivo. The conventional argument is that the antibody response to injected rodent antibody in a patient[13,14,15] will be stronger than the antibody response to injected human immunoglobulin. However, part of the immune response to an injected monoclonal immunoglobulin is the so-called anti-idiotype response, the response to the unique binding site of the antibody. A patient may mount an anti-idiotype response which would be weak and perhaps slow to develop but might eventually be almost as much a problem as a response to injected rodent monoclonal immunoglobulin. An alternative approach is to give a large ($>$100 mg) single dose of mouse monoclonal antibody to swamp the anti-mouse immune response for several days[13] or to work out techniques for developing immunological tolerance to injected mouse immunoglobulin in man. In any case where antibodies conjugated to toxins or drugs are to be used, there will be an antibody response to the toxin or drug, regardless of the species of the immunoglobulin to which it is attached.

Secondly, because of the limitations of current human hybridoma systems that will be discussed below (such as the production of mixed antibody molecules by hybrids), it may be that antibody-producing hybrids generated now will not be suitable for therapeutic use, and effort put in now will only have to be duplicated later when the technology has been improved.

Thirdly, unlike mouse monoclonal antibodies, human monoclonal antibodies cannot be produced cheaply in bulk in the form of ascites fluid and this is an important practical, financial consideration.

Attempts to make human monoclonal antibodies to tumours
A number of laboratories[16,17,18,19,20,21,22] have set out to make hybrids using lymphocytes from lymph nodes taken from patients with tumours or using lymphocytes isolated from the tumours themselves, with the general aims (1) to study the immune response, if any, to the tumours (2) to obtain antibodies to tumour-related or tumour-specific antigens for therapy. The results have so far been disappointing from both points of view. Most of the antibodies made this way react with cytoplasmic antigens[16,19,20] so that they are no use for targetting to tumour cells in vivo. Typically, the yield of antibodies that bind to cell surface antigens is less than 1% of hybrids[19,20] (we have screened about 200 hybrids for antibody binding to cell surface antigens without success) and the specificities have almost all been inappropriate for targetting. The antibodies, whether to cytoplasmic or surface antigens, have not been tumour-specific in any obvious way. Some of them may show a limited tissue specificity[16,18] but the best characterized antibodies[19,20] show restricted and bizarre specificities and look as though they might be to polymorphisms. Before we can interpret these antibodies as examples of an anti-tumour rather than normal response (or for that matter validate putative autoimmune antibodies[9]) they must be compared with antibodies from hybrids made with lymphocytes from normal tissues or normal lymph nodes, a significant number of which also react with cytoplasmic antigens.[19] Also, few hybrids have been characterized because of the low yields of hybrids with present methods (see below). As an example Houghton et al[20] obtained only 16 wells producing antibody to cell surface antigens from a total of about 10^9 lymphocytes fused, and only one cloned hybrid was finally isolated.

At present, far more antibodies to human tumour cell surfaces can be made using rodent hybridomas. Many antibodies have already been made that are suitable for the development of therapeutic methods, and a number of rodent monoclonal antibodies have already been injected into patients with tumours.[13,14,23] For the time being, mouse monoclonal antibodies are more convenient tools for exploring the technical problems facing this field and studying antigen expression by tumours and normal tissues. Perhaps antigens suitable for targetting will be identified using rodent monoclonal antibodies, and then eventually human monoclonal antibodies will be raised to them using in vitro immunization methods[24,25,26,27,28]

Conclusion: Human versus rodent monoclonal antibodies

At present making human monoclonal antibodies is so much more difficult than making rodent monoclonal antibodies, that for many applications it is more profitable to make rodent antibodies. Human antibodies are, of course, preferable or absolutely necessary for certain applications such as studying putative immune responses to tumours in humans; the choice is then whether to wait for or develop improved technology, or to accept the difficulty.

AVAILABLE METHODS FOR GENERATING HUMAN MONOCLONAL ANTIBODIES

Despite these caveats the attractions of human monoclonals has led to the development of a number of systems.

Human monoclonal antibodies can be generated from:

human × mouse hybridomas, fusing human lymphocytes with a mouse myeloma cell line

human lymphoblastoid lines obtained by direct transformation of lymphocytes with EB virus

human × human hybridomas, fusing human lymphocytes with a human B-cell line (myeloma, lymphoma or lymphoblastoid)

We will consider the first two alternatives briefly before giving a detailed account of human × human hybridisations.

Fusions with mouse myelomas

A number of workers have successfully fused human lymphocytes with mouse myeloma cell lines such as NSI.[10,20,29,29-31]

Such hybrids were expected to be unstable because, like most human × mouse hybrid cells, they lose human chromosomes. They were, however, expected to produce high levels of immunoglobulin and to be generated in large numbers because of the efficient fusion characteristics of NSI. In practice a small proportion of the hybrids obtained are very stable secretors of human immunoglobulin after careful repeated cloning, possibly because of the tendency of such heterohybridomas to preferentially retain certain human chromosomes.[32] However, the large number of unstable clones in which human Ig secretion is lost tends to balance out the high number obtained initially. Surprisingly, secretion levels do not seem to be higher in general than those obtained by fusion with human lymphoblastoid lines[19].

Overall experience[17,19,20] suggests that the final yield of useful hybrids is comparable to or is lower than the yield of human–human hybrids in current systems (which will probably be improved upon), and that meticulous cloning is required to maintain the stable lines that do emerge. One advantage of this approach, however, is that non-secretor mouse myelomas are available, e.g. NSO[1] and X63-Ag8.653[33] which have lost all ability to produce their own immunoglobulin chains. True non-secretor human B-cell lines suitable for fusion are not yet available.

Transformation by EB virus

Making human lymphoblastoid lines by direct transformation with EB-virus has been somewhat neglected, partly because it was thought that the yields of immunoglobulin would be low. Human B lymphocytes can be transformed by EB virus into lymphoblastoid cell lines that continuously secrete immunoglobulin. The lines are usually diploid or nearly so (although near-tetraploid variants sometimes arise spontaneously) and characteristically carry the EB-virus nuclear antigen (EBNA).[34]

Lymphocytes are infected, with (mycoplasma-free) culture supernatant from a cell line that produces large amounts of virus, usually the B95–8 marmoset line.[35]

The lymphocytes proliferate and begin polyclonal immunoglobulin secretion, typically producing of the order of 1 μg/ml immunoglobulin.[34,36] Clones are then selected and recloned until a stable line is established. Only a very small number of cells in the initial polyclonal strain can be cloned and will be good stable secretors of antibody and some of the lines die out after some weeks or months in culture. Some appear to lose antibody production even after repeated cloning, though whether this is due to instability or inadequate cloning is debatable. To make the task of cloning out these lines easier, most successful laboratories have first isolated lymphocytes capable of producing antibody to the antigen of interest by a procedure such as rosetting out the lymphocytes with antigen-coated or antigen-bearing erythrocytes.[7,37] A further refinement is to grow the transformants as clones from the outset by plating, directly after infection with virus, in a large number of small wells on a feeder layer at low plating densities (10^2–10^3/well).[7,38]

It may also be possible to stabilize promising lines or enhance their secretion of immunoglobulin by hybridising them with a suitable stock myeloma or lymphoblastoid line.[39]

For further technical details of EBV-virus transformation see[7,37,38,40]

Recently, several stable lines have been reported, notably a line producing 5-20 μg/ml antibody to the hapten NNP[41] one making anti-influenza virus at 10–20 μg/ml[27,7] and an anti-rhesus D line producing around 20 μg/ml[7]. These are among the best reported and cannot be considered typical; compare the line of Steinitz & Tamir[40] which produces 1-2 μg/ml of rheumatoid factor antibody. Just how frequently stable high-secretors can be made will only emerge with time.

It is difficult to compare published success rates for transformation using EB virus with human–human hybridoma results, especially as estimates of transformation frequencies are for initial transformation, not for establishment of permanent high-secreting lines.[36] It may be valid to consider how many stable transformants are obtained by infecting a certain number of selected B lymphocytes. Crawford et al,[7] characterised one stable, cloned, high-secreting transformant from 10^5 rosetted lymphocytes infected; Winger et al,[38] obtained around 1 antibody-secreting transformant per 10^3/to 10^4 antigen-binding lymphocytes but their secretion levels, long-term stability and ability to clone were not generally tested. This is equal to or better than current rates for fusion with B-cell lines, and might mean a superior recovery of producing lines, but note that hybridisations have generally been with unselected lymphocytes including T-cells.

The EB virus transformation method has disadvantages: the requirement for careful and repeated cloning and the problems of handling the virus. On the other hand, the absence of irrelevant immunoglobulin chains belonging to a fusion partner is an advantage at present.

Conclusion

In summary, fusion with non-secretor mouse myelomas and transformation by EB virus have not yet been completely superseded by human–human hybridization as ways of making human monoclonal antibodies. We expect all three methods to be used for the present. But making human–human hybrids is probably easier and it should become the method of choice when better human lines for fusion are developed (see below).

HUMAN × HUMAN HYBRIDOMAS: CHOOSING A SYSTEM

DESIRABLE PROPERTIES OF A PARENT CELL LINE FOR PRODUCING HUMAN × HUMAN HYBRIDOMAS

The desirable qualities of a cell line for human fusions are listed in Table 4.1. None of these are trivial, all have been or are real problems.

First, and certainly not least, the line should be human! We know of at least three laboratories that have generated hybrids with lines supposed to be derivatives of the RPMI 8226 myeloma, and have subsequently found them to be non-human by karyotyping.[42] (see also p 78).

The yardstick for measuring the performance of human hybridoma systems should be the mouse system based on lines such as NSO[1] and P3-X63-Ag8 .653[33] both derived originally from the P3 myeloma. The comparable ideal human fusion partner would give one stable secreting hybrid per 10^5 immunized lymphocytes or better, double in 24 h or less, give hybrids that secrete stably of the order of 10 μg/ml or more immunoglobulin in culture, and be easy to clone. It would also probably be HAT-sensitive, so that hybrids can be selected in HAT medium, or else it has to be suitable for some equally convenient selection method (see below). The line should also be a true chain-loss variant.

Chain-loss variants and the mixed molecule problem

A chain loss variant is a line that has lost the ability to specify immunoglobulin chains. Such variants are usually derived from a high-secreting line that therefore has the cellular machinery for a high-secreting state. Such **non**-producers should not be confused with **low**-secretors that are merely lines that produce very small amounts of their immunoglobulin chains. Low-secretors can be expected either to give low-secreting hybrids or in high-secreting hybrids to show reactivation of synthesis of the parent B-cell lines' immunoglobulin chains, and so be no better than hybrids made with a normally-secreting line (though exactly what happens in practice is not yet known for all lines). For example, the parent B-cell line developed in this laboratory, LICR-LON-HMy2,[43] is a rather low secretor of IgG, but its high-secreting hybrids produce high levels of HMy2's characteristic IgG together with new immunoglobulin from the fused lymphocyte.

It is important to realise that the production by hybrids of immunoglobulin chains specified by the immortal B-cell parent is not merely a problem of contamination of the lymphocyte-specified immunoglobulin. Mixed molecules are secreted, made up of more or less random combinations of the various chains synthesised, so that in a

Table 4.1 Desirable properties of a human fusion partner*

Characteristic	Remarks
Qualities of the ideal line	
High fusion frequency	Measurements can be unreliable
Non-producer (NOT low secretor)	True chain loss variants desirable
High secretion in hybrids	Measurements are not standardized and vary widely
Stable secretion in hybrids	Difficult to measure on large scale
Rapid growth <24 h doubling time	
Readily clonable	Conditions may be critical, e.g. serum batch
Convenient selection system	Preferably HAT-sensitive
Quality control on existing lines	
Human	Test karyotype, LDH isoenzymes, and/or HLA type
Authentic origin	Lines may become contaminated with other lines or lose fusibility due to inappropriate maintenance
Stable to reversion in selection system	Plate in HAT with lymphocytes without PEG treatment. Beware viable non-dividing cells that divide after removal of HAT
Mycoplasma	Test by fluorescent staining. Contamination prevents fusion
Clonable	Use feeder layers and particularly test Fetal Calf Serum

hybrid between two IgG-producing cells only one molecule in **16** of the secreted immunoglobulins will have all four chains specified by the lymphocyte fusion partner, unless preferential association occurs.[44] Only one molecule in 16 will then have two fully active binding sites for antigen: in other words up to 15/16 of the antibody secreted may have little or no activity. Hybrids produced with the present generation of human B-cell fusion partners must be expected to suffer from this problem.

CRITERIA FOR CHARACTERIZING HYBRIDS

One of the pitfalls of human hybridoma production is the generation of cells that masquerade as hybrids. Lymphoblastoid lines can arise spontaneously from donors of lymphocytes carrying EB virus, and virus could be produced by a lymphoblastoid parent line or its hybrids. These lines may produce immunoglobulin transiently or stably. The parent cell line may give HPRT⁺ revertants, (see p 76) aminopterin-resistant HPRT⁻ variants, or a small number of cells that persist in HAT medium for days or even weeks. The lymphocytes used will often proliferate for some days, perhaps mounting a mixed lymphocyte response to the immortal cell parent line.

In developing a human fusion method or setting it up in a new laboratory, it is important to establish that human hybrids are really being made. Subsequently this becomes less important, because once cell lines are being generated that stably produce new immunoglobulin, that is perhaps the only endpoint that matters.

The principal methods for identifying hybrids are:

karyotype or DNA analysis by flow cytometry

immunoglobulin secretion: assay for chain types

immunoglobulin secretion: analysis by electrophoresis and isoelectric focussing

HLA typing

DNA analysis

Probably the best way to screen the products of a fusion for hybrids, and incidentally, to see how polyclonal the hybrids are, is to measure their DNA content on a flow cytometer or fluorescence-activated cell sorter (Fig. 4.1).[18]

The fluorescent DNA stain propidium iodide can be used: cells are fixed and permeabilized, incubated with RNAase and stained.[45] Samples can be stored after fixation. They can be analysed faster than one a minute. Relatively cheap analytical flow cytometers are available: a full fluorescence-activated cell sorter is not required. Hybrids will usually have DNA content per cell between 1.3 and 2 times the parent line, each clonal hybrid having a distinct peak value (Fig. 4.1). The parent line should always be run as a control together with some diploid cells such as lymphocytes. A near-tetraploid variant of our parent B-cell line LICR-LON-HMy2 has arisen in at least one stock from the originally pseudodiploid line.[43] It is clearly HMy2 as it has the same marker chromosomes (Fig. 4.2), HLA type, and light chain by isoelectric focussing, and it gives hybrids with hypertetraploid karyotypes.[46]

Revertants, aminopterin-resistant variants, stimulated lymphocytes and most EB-virus transformants, will be distinguished by this approach. Note, however, that for complete confirmation of a successful hybrid, DNA analysis should be performed after cloning.

Karyotyping

Karyotyping is an acceptable alternative to DNA analysis but is enormously more laborious. If suitable marker chromosomes have been identified in the parent B-cell line (Fig. 4.2) true hybrids can be distinguished from (probably rare) lymphoblastoid tetraploid transformants. The presence of a few tetraploid cells among a basically diploid stock is not of itself evidence that a hybrid line has been generated, although occasional hybrids may have a near-diploid mode.

Assays for types of immunoglobulin chain secreted

Probably the next most convenient test is for the production of immunoglobulin chains not produced by the parent cell line. This has, however, limited value as proof that hybrids are being made. A satisfactory method is to coat plastic wells with anti-human polyclonal antibody, then incubate sequentially with: the unknown sample of human immunoglobulin; a mouse monoclonal antibody that binds specifically to a particular human immunoglobulin chain; finally iodinated or enzyme-conjugated polyclonal anti-mouse antibody.[47]

When a fusion is plated the lymphocytes will inevitably produce some

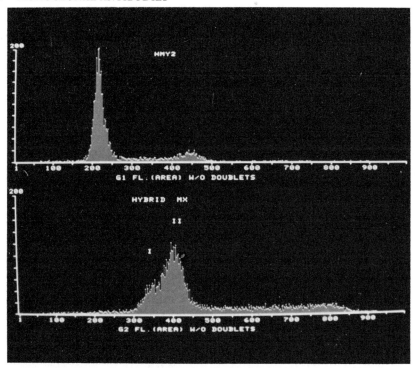

Fig. 4.1 Histograms of DNA content of parent cell line HMy2 (above) and uncloned hybrid MX (below), obtained by fluorescent staining of the DNA and analysis in a flow cytometer. x axis: DNA fluorescence (arbitrary scale), y axis: number of cells. The channel numbers containing the peak of fluorescence were 214 for HMy2 and 400 for the hybrid MX. Note the shoulder (marked I, channel number 350) on the peak (marked II) for the hybrid, suggesting two hybrid populations are present in this uncloned sample.

immunoglobulin and after immunization this may be specific and considerable amounts may be produced if the lymphocytes are stimulated to short-term growth. Thus production of new immunoglobulin chains at an early stage can be misleading.

After repeated feeding or subculture, there is still the problem that lymphoblastoid transformants may be producing immunoglobulin. Finally, a parent cell line that produces low levels of immunoglobulin, may give hybrids that produce high levels of the parent cell line's immunoglobulin chains. So for example a parent cell line such as WI-L2-HF$_2$ (Table 4.2) that has surface IgM and secretes low levels of IgG might be able to give hybrids that produce these immunoglobulins in abundance. In these cases an assay for substantial levels of both γ and μ would probably detect hybrids but they might not necessarily be making new (i.e. lymphocyte specified) immunoglobulins. The assay can also be applied to cloned hybrids to demonstrate secretion of immunoglobulin chains from both the B-cell line and the lymphocyte fused.[43]

Electrophoresis and iso-electric focussing of immunoglobulins
More revealing, but much more difficult and laborious is the analysis of immunoglobulin secretion by SDS/polyacrylamide gel electrophoresis and iso-

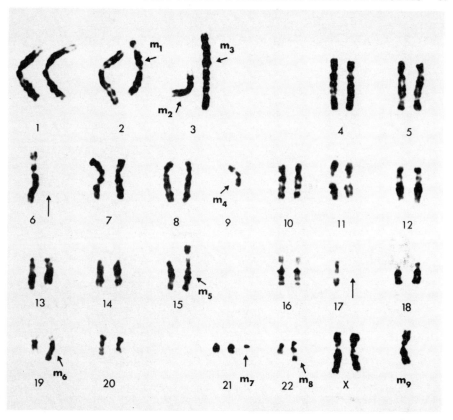

Fig. 4.2 G-banded karyotype of the pseudo-diploid stock of LICR-LON-HMy2. m_1 to m_9 indicate structurally altered chromosomes, due mainly to translocations. The same marker chromosomes are seen in the pseudo-tetraploid variant that arose spontaneously[46].

electric focussing of immunoglobulin that has been radioactively labelled by growing the cells with labelled amino acids (Fig. 4.3). SDS gel electrophoresis provides the same information as chain-specific assays, but is perhaps less liable to artifact. Iso-electric focussing of separated immunoglobulin chains is the most powerful technique, because individual 'mu, gamma, kappa and lambda' chains can be distinguished on the basis of iso-electric point. For example, if a hybrid secretes two kappa chains, one from the B-cell line and one from the lymphocyte, they can be distinguished as two bands, one in the position characteristic of the parent B-cell line's kappa chain (Fig. 4.3). Although a classical approach and definitive proof that an individual cloned hybrid produces immunoglobulins specified by both the cells fused,[43,48] we do not recommend its use except where the quality of information obtained justifies the effort. In particular, hybrids must be cloned before analysis, whereas for example, DNA analysis is performed cell by cell and reveals hybrids even when they are mixed with other hybrids or non-hybrid cells.

HLA typing

HLA typing is also informative but typing cell lines is not as easy as typing lymphocytes. It requires experience and does not always give a clear result. It is,

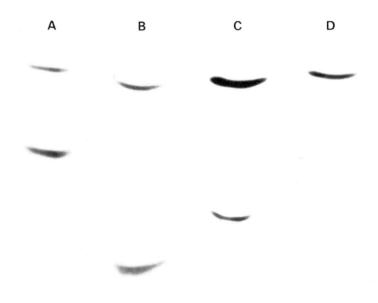

Fig. 4.3 Isoelectric focussing of light chains secreted by parent cell line HMy2 (track D) and various cloned hybrids labelled arbitrarily A, B and C. The common band is the kappa light chain of HMy2, the other bands are new light chains secreted by the hybrids. The cells were grown in the presence of [14C] lysine. The radioactively-labelled, secreted immunoglobulins were concentrated from the culture fluid by immune precipitation and subjected to isoelectric focussing in agarose as described[43]

therefore, probably not useful for many laboratories, even those with access to a routine tissue typing facility. It would be expected that hybrids would express the HLA types of both the immortal parent and the lymphocytes fused, and this has been observed in the construction of human T-cell hybrids for example[49] and some B-hybrids.[8]

Surprisingly, it does not always work this way. We have had a series of hybrids that were made with HMy2 HLA-typed by two laboratories, and essentially they express only the HLA types of HMy2 itself, possibly because lymphoblastoid lines express higher levels of HLA antigens than normal lymphocytes.[34] While this adds to the evidence that the bulk of the cells carry HMy2 genes, and so again shows we are not making transformants, it does not on its own prove that hybrids are being produced. With the development of monoclonal anti-HLA reagents it may one day be possible to screen hybrids for the presence of a particular HLA type that is characteristic of the parent B-cell line (and preferably rare in the general population), perhaps using fluorescence and cytofluorimetry.

Conclusion

In summary, the best method for routine identification of hybrids is measurement of DNA content per cell by cytofluorimetry, but controls must be included.

HUMAN × HUMAN HYBRIDOMA SYSTEMS AVAILABLE

The human × human hybridoma systems that we know to have been used by more than one laboratory are tabulated in Table 4.2. For systems that have only been described in abstracts or very recently, see Kozbor & Roder.[50]

Problems in interpreting the literature

The literature on human hybridomas needs to be read with great caution. Few reports have demonstrated rigorously that true hybrids were being made. A number of reports of human × human hybridomas have appeared which have not been confirmed. In particular, as already mentioned, three laboratories used cell lines supposed to be samples of the human myeloma line RPMI 8226 to develop fusion partners and only later discovered that the samples were of non-human origin.[42]

Note also that some lines have been renamed following cloning or additional selection (see Table 4.2), though their essential characteristics have probably changed very little.

Three difficulties of measuring the relative performance of lines should be noted. Fusion frequency is difficult to measure absolutely because the ability of different samples of lymphocytes to fuse cannot usually be controlled. However, the low fusion frequencies seen with human × human fusion are not just due to poor performance of the lymphocytes, because when lymphocytes have been fused with mouse myelomas in parallel with human B-cell lines,[19,20,59] the mouse myeloma has usually given many more hybrids. Secondly, fusions using lymphoblastoid lines may produce EB-virus transformants, and the proportion of these may vary. Thirdly, levels of immunoglobulin secretion by cultured cells are often quoted but rarely measured in a way that permits accurate comparison. The actual level measured depends on the technique used and the precise conditions of culture, let alone the optimism of the authors. For example, assays with polyclonal antisera calibrated with polyclonal Ig when applied to monoclonal immunoglobulin may give artificially high readings (e.g. in single radial immunodiffusion) or low readings (e.g. in ELISA assays). Assays using target antigen will give very low readings if a hybrid under test produces mixed Ig molecules. In our original characterization of HMy2 we quoted Ig secretion from hybrids at routine passage, knowing that around three-fold higher concentrations of Ig could be achieved, at limiting densities.[43]

Lymphoblastoid lines versus true human myelomas

It was originally thought that lymphoblastoid lines would give hybridomas that produced low levels of immunoglobulins. Results from several laboratories suggest that this was a misconception: it has been shown that when a large number of hybrids that were made with the parent lines HMy2 (lymphoblastoid), NSI (mouse myeloma) and U266 (human myeloma-like) are compared, there is no great difference in the distribution of secretion levels.[19,20] On propagation, it is conceivable that some hybrids made with lymphoblastoid lines may give rise to variants secreting lower levels of Ig: but whether this actually happens remains to be seen. It is, however, said to be difficult to find chain-loss variants of lymphoblastoid lines, so complete loss is not expected.

Another prejudice is that products of lymphoblastoid lines will be inferior to

Table 4.2 Well-established human × human hybridoma systems

Original cell line	Type of line	Reference	Variant used for fusion	Reference	Ig Chains coded or secreted
U266	Myeloma	51	SKO-007	57	λ, ϵ
			FU-266	58	
			'U266' (derived from SKO-007	19, 20	
			U266 (independent HAT-sensitive derivative)	59	
GM1500	Lymphoblastoid	52	GM1500 A1*	60, 8	κ, γ_2
			GM4672*	9	
			KR4*	39	
ARH77	Lymphoblastoid†	53, 43	LICR-LON-HMy2 (also referred to as LICR-2)	43, 46	κ, γ_1
WI-L2	Lymphoblastoid	54, 55	UC729-6	61, 62	κ, μ (and perhaps also $\gamma)^+_+$
			WI-L2-729-HF$_2$	63§§	κ, γ, μ
			H351.1	64	κ, μ (and perhaps also $\gamma)^+_+$
RPMI 8226	Myeloma	56			γ

Quoted secretion level for hybrids $\mu g/ml$**	Comparative studies	References to other users††	HLA type	Karyotype	Remarks
3-11	65		A2, A3, B7, Bw60, Bw6, Cw3[66]	Diploid: mode 44, for markers and details see[66]	Original 266 line and SKO-007 contaminated with mycoplasma
0.3–40**	69, 20				
0.2 (antigen-specific)	59				
ND	20, 59		A2 Aw19 B27, B18 Cw6[8]		Success has been restricted to a few laboratories.
0.3–40** ; 5-25 grown to exhaustion (15)					Some reported 'hybrids' obtained with GM4672 have apparently diploid modal karyotypes 67 so may be transformants.
4, 6					KR4 is a ouabain-resistant derivative of GM1500 A1.
Random‡‡ survey uncloned 1-6, cloned 2-20; 0.3–40**	19, 20, 59	22, 18	A2, A3, B7 (weak) Bw35, Cw3, Cw4[46]	Diploid: mode 43. Some stocks mode 78 details in Fig. 4.2.	The low and high-secretor strains isolated by cloning[43] were lost to mycoplasma. Cloning should be re-attempted.
3-9	59			Diploid: mode 46, 21p+ for details see[61, 62]	Low-secretor line, coding both γ and μ.[63]; not known whether these chains are secreted vigorously by hybrids.
Most polyclonal 5-30 clones 10-20 N.D.	59				
					At least 3 reported derivatives of 'RPMI 8226' were non-human by karotype. Human samples obtainable from ATCC in our hands are slow-growing difficult to clone.

All lines listed are HAT-sensitive. None are true non-producers. For availability see the References and Appendix. For more extensive list of lines see ref.[50]. Note that not all reports prove that true hybrids were made.

*Apparently GM4672 is the same as GM1500A1. It is reported to be negative for EBNA antigen[9] but this seems unlikely as pointed out in ref.[50].

†The ARH-77 line as distributed is lymphoblastoid and distinct from the myeloma originally described.

‡Since 729-HF$_2$ is reported[63] to produce traces of γ also.

§HF$_2$ was derived by Dr R Lundak[63] from W1-L2-729 independently of UC729-6.

**Secretion levels: in comparative studies Cote et al[19] and Houghton et al[20] found that secretion levels (0.3 to 40 μg/ml) were independent of fusion partners for fusions with NSI, U266, GM4672 and HMy2 (referred to as LICR-2).

††Independent reports of fusion not cited elsewhere in the Table.

‡‡corrected from ref.[43] to levels at exhaustion of the medium.

products of myeloma lines because they may contain DNA from the transforming Epstein-Barr virus. Lymphoma lines that are not EB-transformed (such as RH-L4)[65] do not suffer from this problem, but it would be naive to assume that these and the true myeloma lines, particularly from long term culture, are free of comparable transforming viruses. Mouse hybridomas produce retrovirus capable of infecting species other than mouse.[68] In all cases antibody that is to be injected into patients may have to be processed to destroy all contaminating nucleic acid.

The present choice of fusion partner

At present there is no human line that matches up to the specifications laid down in the previous section and Table 4.1. In particular, fusion frequencies are lower than obtained in rodent systems, and fully-authenticated non-producer (non-secretor) lines are not yet available.

There have been three comparative studies reported where different fusion systems were compared[19,20,59] and the results seem consistent with rumours from other laboratories. Taking the lines as listed in Table 4.2: the original derivatives of the myeloma cell line U266, such as SKO-007, were infected by mycoplasma[66] and have not subsequently given hybrids; when freed of mycoplasma[19,20,59,65,66] they gave hybrids, but they were slower growing and fewer than those obtained with the lymphoblastoid LICR-LON-HMy2 and 729 lines.[19,20,59] Similarly U266-derived lines compared unfavourably with RH-L4[65] derived from a histiocytic lymphoma line.

Some samples of the other long-established human myeloma, RPMI 8226, that have been used for fusion, are not human.[42] One (presumably human) derivative of the line has been fused but did not perform well in a comparative study.[59]

There have been some successes with derivatives of the lymphoblastoid line GM1500 (Table 4.2) but only in a few laboratories, and although true hybrids have been made, some supposed hybrids are like EB-virus transformants in that they appear to have near-diploid modal karyotype[67]. Again, this line performed poorly in comparative studies.[20,59]

Our lymphoblastoid line LICR-LON-HMy2 has been used successfully in several independent laboratories[18-20,22,59] and performed well in comparative studies.[19,20,59]

We have documented in detail fusion frequencies, karyotypes, HLA types and secretion patterns of the HMy2 hybrids.[43,46]

Derivatives of the lymphoblastoid lines WI-L2, particularly UC729-6 and WI-L2-729-HF$_2$ (for references see Table 4.2) are also being used in a number of laboratories and performed well in a comparative study.[59] These lines appear to give somewhat higher fusion frequencies than LICR-LON-HMy2, but a lower proportion of the hybrids secreted immunoglobulin[59] and this has been observed independently by Cote & Slater (personal communication). At the risk of being pedantic, it could still be that a substantial number of 'hybrids' produced by the 729 lines are EB-virus transformants. However this may not matter if stable production of new immunoglobulin is achieved. The 729 lines produce only very low levels of IgG and IgM but they should not be thought of as non-secretors—it may be that full secretion of these chains is reactivated in hybrids[63]—as far as we know this remains to be determined. For the present they should be regarded as secretors like the other lines currently available. 729-HF$_2$ has been claimed to give high fusion frequencies,

($\sim$1 in 10^5) i.e. comparable to mouse systems[63], however in a comparative study fusion frequencies with UC729-6 and 729-HF$_2$ were similar.[59] High density platings of 'hybrids' gave growth in a large number of wells but this is reminiscent to us of the apparently polyclonal lymphocyte growth seen in high density platings of LICR-LON-HMy2 fusions in the short term. We have tested a sample of UC729-6 and found it to give apparent fusion frequencies slightly better than LICR-LON-HMy2, as judged by growth in HAT, although we made no attempt to establish the hybrid nature of the growing cells.

Conclusion

In summary, human hybrids can be most reliably made at present with the lines LICR-LON-HMy2 and the 729 lines, UC729-6 and 729-HF$_2$ (for availability, see Appendix). None of these is a truly non-producer line, and all appear to give fusion frequencies an order of magnitude or more lower than obtained in rodent systems.

GENERATION OF PARENTAL B-CELL LINES AND THEIR FUSION WITH HUMAN LYMPHOCYTES

The generation of human hybridomas on a routine basis is still a relatively recent achievement, and techniques are still developing. The current methods do not, therefore, have the status of definitive protocols. Rather than giving a step-by-step method we will use our previously published method for the HMy2 system[43,46] to illustrate what appear to be the critical steps in the procedure, and to comment on the underlying rationale. Other published methods and modifications used successfully by other workers with our HMy2 cell-line will also be considered. We hope by this means to encourage experimentation in certain as yet unexplored areas and to prevent slavish adherence to a protocol that may not yet be optimal.

SELECTION, CHARACTERIZATION AND CULTURE OF PARENTAL B-CELL LINES

Most methods for generating lymphocyte hybrids use HAT-sensitive cell-lines to act as the immortal parent and stem from the general strategies originally devised by Littlefield[69] for hybridization and selection of fibroblast hybrids by enzyme complementation. The principles on which such procedures are based are important because they determine the type of selective medium used to cultivate the fusion products, and this may influence hybrid yield.

The HAT selection method

The enzyme hypoxanthine-guanine phosphoribosyl transferase (HPRT) (EC.2.4.2.8) is specified by a gene located in the terminal band (q27) of the long arm (Xq) of the X-chromosome.[70]

   Present in all tissues it converts both hypoxanthine and guanine to their respective ribonucleotides (i.e. IMP and GMP). Its presence is not essential for cell viability or proliferation as it belongs to a group of enzymes that enable cells to utilize exogenous purines for DNA synthesis by the so-called 'salvage' pathways.[71] The HAT selection method uses enzyme-deficient mutant (usually HPRT⁻) cell lines. Deficiency of such a purine phosphoribosyltransferase in cells renders them sensitive to inhibitors of de novo purine and pyrimidine synthesis. This, and the fact that in tetraploid hybrids two active X-chromosomes are tolerated[72] constitutes the basis of the HAT (*Hypoxanthine-Aminopterin-Thymidine*) selection system.[69,73]

Aminopterin (4-aminofolic acid) and amethopterin (4-amino-10-methylfolic acid, Methotrexate) are folic (pteroylglutamic) acid antagonists that inhibit dihydrofolate reductase and prevent de novo purine synthesis from glutamine[74] as well as conferring an additional requirement for exogenous pyrimidines by inhibiting the tetrahydrofolate-dependent uridine methyl transferase. Addition of both a purine (hypoxanthine) and a pyrimidine (thymidine) is therefore necessary for hybrid survival. Other nucleotides are formed by interconversion and/or uptake and metabolism by other salvage pathway enzymes activities[75] (such as, for example, adenine phosphoribosyl transferase (APRT)).

Generation of enzyme-deficient parental cell lines

Hypoxanthine-guanine phosphoribosyl transferase-deficient lines (HPRT⁻) are, in our experience, the easiest to generate from human myeloma and lymphoblastoid cells, compared with other potentially useful mutants such as adenine phosphoribosyl-transferase (APRT) (EC.2.4.2.7) or thymidine kinase-negative (TK⁻) cells [76]. All enzyme-deficient human cell-lines for B-cell hybridization of which we are aware are HPRT⁻ although APRT⁻[77] and TK⁻ mouse myelomas have been used for fusion.[3]

The relative ease with which HPRT⁻ cells can be obtained in culture (<1 in 10^5)[78] is probably a consequence of the fact that (as an X-linked gene) only one active copy is present in each cell. Translocations and deletions of X-chromosome fragments[79,80] can be associated with loss of HPRT activity. A structural mutation within the gene is probably not, therefore, the only source of HPRT⁻ cells, at least in culture systems. By comparison, the rate of spontaneous mutation to an APRT⁻ phenotype in normal homozygous cells is <1 in 10^8.[81]

Selection with purine analogues

HPRT⁻ cells can be selected for in culture by addition of cytotoxic purine analogues[73] commonly 6-thioguanine (6-TG) or 8-azaguanine (8-AG). HPRT⁺ cells convert them to the corresponding substituted nucleotides, which kill them, primarily by incorporation into DNA in the case of 6-TG, and into RNA with 8-AG.[82]

6-Thioguanine is, in principle, the better choice for selection of HPRT⁻ variants. It is more stable in culture medium[83] and has the higher affinity for HPRT.[84] Purines in culture medium do not, therefore, reduce the selection pressure exerted on HPRT⁺ cells to the same extent as with 8-AG. In practice, however, we have observed that different unselected human lymphoblastoid/myeloma cell lines often exhibit widely differing relative sensitivities to 6-TG and 8-AG, and that 6-TG is not always the most toxic, nor the most effective for selection purposes.

We recommend that selection be commenced on separate cultures of the same line using each analogue at a low concentration (0.05–0.1 μg/ml), gradually increasing the dose two-fold until a concentration of 3–5 μg/ml is tolerated in continuous passage. This is, in our experience, the minimum concentration at which usable levels of HPRT deficiency are obtained. To avoid possible 'leakiness' in the selection system we further select stocks resistant to both purine analogues up to their solubility limits (64 μg/ml with 8-AG and 32 μg/ml for 6-TG). If variants have been selected in 8-AG it is essential to check for 6-TG resistance, because selection in the former does not always result in HPRT⁻ cells, whereas the latter almost invariably does, due to differential utilization of the two purine analogues.[85] The success of such step-wise selection is probably due to the fact that cells can express different levels of HPRT activity;[86,87] survival of a significant proportion of treated cells at any given concentration probably assists continued growth. Stepwise selection regimes are not, however, as successful in our experience when selecting for other enzyme-deficient phenotypes, including thymidine kinase-negative cells with 5-bromodeoxyuridine and adenosine phosphoribosyl transferase-negative cells with 2,6-diaminopurine or 2-fluoroadenine. In such instances the use of mutagens such as ethylmethane sulfonate (EMS), or γ-irradiation may be necessary.

The LICR-LON-HMy cell lines

We successfully applied the above selection methods to 3 human cell-lines, U-266[51], ARH-77[53], and RPMI 8226[56], giving LICR-LON-HMyl, HMy2 and HMy3 respectively.[43,46] LICR-LON-HMy2 (hereinafter called HMy2) has been used successfully in the generation of B-cell hybrids by this, and several other independent laboratories (see Table 4.2).

Characterization of parent B-cell lines

Authentication of human origin of cell line: The human origin of cell lines used for fusion partners must be verified, whatever their source. This can be done readily by karyology and HLA typing, if available, and by enzyme isotyping.[88]

The simplest method is electrophoretic separation of lactate dehydrogenase (LDH) isozymes, staining with chromogenic substrate[89] and comparison with bona fide human LDH from serum or cell lines. The LDH isozyme pattern of HMy2 is illustrated in Figure 4.4, its karyotype in Figure 4.2, and its HLA type is A2, A3, Bw35, B7, Cw3, Cw4.

HPRT-activity: HMy2 possesses less than one per cent of the HPRT levels of unselected ARH-77 stocks, when tested by the method of Albertini & De Mars[87] ¹⁴C-Hypoxanthine is used as a substrate with appropriate cofactors, and the sequentially-formed product of HPRT activity IMP, and inosine (formed from IMP by 5′-nucleotidase) separated by high performance liquid chromatography. Cells must be mycoplasma-free (see below) when tested, because HPRT⁺ micro-organisms can result in a false-positive result when HPRT⁻ cells are infected[90] and the reversible activity of nucleoside phosphorylase (in which mycoplasmas are rich) can simulate HPRT activity by directly converting an excess of hypoxanthine to inosine. Irrespective of the actual levels of HPRT remaining in selected cells (if any) it is the consequent sensitivity to aminopterin (and its stability) that it is the key to its utility as a fusion partner.

Reversion frequency: Some types of 8-AG resistant cells exhibit high spontaneous reversion rates, and can simulate hybrids when using HAT-selection systems. Parental cell lines for fusion, should, therefore, be carefully checked by periodic culture of stocks in hybrid selecting medium. With HMy2 we have found that

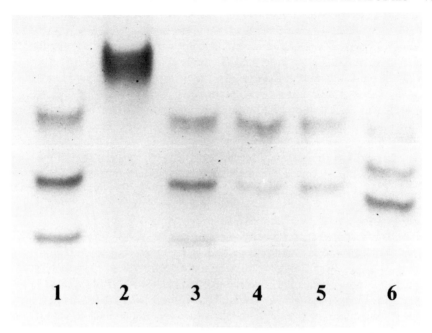

Fig. 4.4 Electrophoretic separation of isoenzymes of LDH (lactate dehydrogenase) to distinguish species of cells. Cells are lysed in hypotonic medium and subjected to electrophoresis in polyacrylamide gel (without SDS) and the gel is stained with a chromogenic substrate[89]. A kit is available from Sigma Chemical Co. (St. Louis, Missouri). Tracks 1 and 3 to 5 are human; track 2 is mouse; track 6 is bovine. Track 1 myeloma cell line U266 (see Table 4.2 for details of cell lines); 2 myeloma NS1; 3 myeloma RPMI 8226; 4 LICR-LON-HMy2; 5 human peripheral blood lymphocytes; 6 Fetal calf serum.

reversion rates are negligible (<1 in 10^8 per generation), and sublines have been cultured for up to 30 consecutive passages at a high split ratio (1:40) without loss of HPRT⁻ phenotype, or detection of revertants. Nevertheless, we routinely repassage them in 8-AG-containing medium at an appropriate concentration (64 μg/ml) once every 6–10 subcultures. Others[65] prefer continual culture in 8-AG or 6-TG containing medium and this may be necessary for some lines. Cells should, however, be passaged in analogue-free medium immediately prior to fusion.

Mycoplasma contamination: All stock cultures of selected lines for fusion must be regularly tested for mycoplasma contamination. Mycoplasmas can enter cultures by operator contamination, from other cultures, from fetal calf serum[91] or from supposedly sterile commercially-prepared defined medium.[92] The antibiotic kanamycin does have some anti-mycoplasmal activity.[93]

Its use for routine culture, as in our original method[43] is, therefore, a two-edged sword. While it may suppress contamination it may encourage emergence of antibiotic resistant forms subsequently difficult to eradicate.

When present in high numbers mycoplasmas can abort the growth of hybrids by depleting the medium of thymidine[90,94] because of their high levels of nucleoside phosphorylase (EC.2.4.2.4). They can also cause chromosome damage, possibly by arginine depletion with some species[95] and glutamine levels may also be significantly reduced. The use of one parental line for human hybridoma production (SKO-007) was originally vitiated by mycoplasma contamination.[66]

Tests for mycoplasma: The simplest, and most reliable methods for detecting mycoplasma contamination are based on staining with DNA-binding fluorescent dyes which show the micro-organisms as bright extranuclear bodies (Fig. 4.5). We originally used 4',6-diamidino-2-phenyindole (DAPI) to stain living cells according to Russell et al.[96] We now prefer to stain smears of methanol: acetic fixed cells, using the fluorescent DNA-binding bisbenzimid dye Hoechst 33258[97] according to Chen.[98]

The sensitivity of this technique can be enhanced by several orders of magnitude by an indirect indicator modification.[99] Cells and medium supernatant to be tested are co-cultivated with a suitable monolayer cell type, free of mycoplasma but susceptible to infection, grown in antibiotic-free medium. Mouse 3T3 fibroblasts (kindly provided by Dr T Harrison) have proved very effective.

Elimination of mycoplasma contamination: Should stocks become contaminated, even at low levels, they should be discarded. If, however, cells are contaminated but cannot be replaced, we recommend that the heat-shock method of Hayflick[100] be used first for attempted eradication. This method has been successfully applied to SKO-007 to yield a mycoplasma-free subline.[66] 42°C for 36 hours has proved a suitable protocol for sublines of HMy2. If this fails then techniques such as clonal growth with macrophage feeders[101] treatment with 5-bromouracil[102] or combination therapy with various antibiotics may be tried. Among the latter, kanamycin, gentamycin, erythromycin, lincomycin and various tetracyclines (including minocyclin) have been reported active[93] as well as tylosin and sodium aureothiomaleate. As a final resort growth in nude mice may be attempted.[103]

HMy2 will grow when inoculated subcutaneously in nu/nu mice (Dr P Thorpe, personal communication).

THE FUSION PROCEDURE

Culture of parental B-cell line

HMy2 and other myeloma/lymphoblastoid lines that we have selected or tested are not particularly fastidious with respect to the defined tissue culture medium used. We use Dulbecco's Eagles medium (DMEM) buffered to 5% CO_2 with bicarbonate and containing 10% fetal calf serum (FCS) plus antibiotics (100 μg/ml penicillin/streptomycin). Iscove's modification of DMEM[104] can also be used. Such 'rich' media tend to permit a somewhat higher limiting density ($<5 \times 10^5$/ml) than media with lower amino-acid and vitamin concentrations, such as the widely used RPMI 1640. In the case of HMy2, the bulk cultures are not exceptionally fastidious with respect to the batch of serum used, although for cloning, and particularly for hybrid growth this is a very significant variable (see below).

A prerequisite for all successful fusions is to ensure that the parental cell line is in optimum condition. It should contain no detectable dead or dying cells ($>98\%$ viability by trypan blue exclusion) and be proliferating at its maximum rate (18–20 hours doubling time in the case of HMy2). The cells should be at mid-point of log-phase growth at a density of 5×10^4–10^5 cells/ml. HMy2 stocks are grown routinely in DMEM with 10 per cent FCS in 75 cm^2 flasks and split 1:40 about every

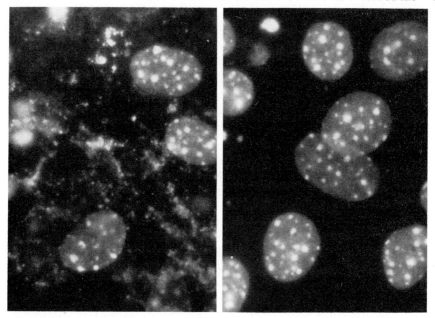

Fig. 4.5 Staining of cells for mycoplasma contamination by using the fluorescent stain for DNA, Hoechst 33258, on an indicator culture of 3T3 mouse fibroblasts. A culture of 3T3 cells exposed to medium from a contaminated cell line (left) shows bright fluorescence outside the nucleus due to staining of the DNA in mycoplasma. Right: control culture, showing fluorescence only inside the nucleus. X780.

5 days. When used for fusion the cultures have their medium volume doubled on each of 2 days prior to fusion, with 100 ml yielding approximately 10^7 cells/flask. The desirability of rapidly proliferating cells is self-evident, although its value may also stem from the fact that mitotic cells are particularly susceptible to fusion with poly(ethyleneglycol).[105] Unlike some other lines for lymphocyte fusion, HMy2 cells tolerate both very low (10^3/ml) and high ($>10^6$/ml) densities without difficulty. While this facilitates routine culture it does not obviate the use of carefully controlled conditions prior to fusion.

Lymphocyte:HMy2 ratios

In our original protocol[43] we fused HMy2 cells with normal lymphocytes at a ratio of 1:10 (10^7 HMy2 plus 10^8 lymphocytes), diluting the fusion products into two polystyrene 48-well culture plates ($\equiv 10^5$ HMy2 per well). Cote et al[19] report, however, significantly better hybrid yields (<1 in 5×10^5 lymphocytes) using a 1:1 ratio with this cell line. Immediately prior to fusion the HMy2 cells and the lymphocytes are separately rinsed once in serum-free, air-buffered L-15 medium. Viable cells are counted with the trypan blue exclusion test, and appropriate aliquots combined and spun down in a round-bottomed 25 ml polystyrene tube and the supernatant removed completely by aspiration.

The fusogen

We have used poly(ethyleneglycol) (PEG)[106] as our fusogen, as have all other published reports of human lymphocyte fusion. A solution of PEG 1500 (50% w/w) is prepared in L-15 medium without serum, and 1 ml added to the combined pellet. The tube is tapped to loosen the pellet, which is gently stirred with the tip of a pipette for 1 minute, following which it is incubated at 37°C for a further 2–4 minutes. The PEG solution is then diluted with 10 ml of warm serum-free L15, slowly (1 ml/min) for the first minute with the remainder added over the next 4 minutes, essentially as described by Galfre et al[107]. Preliminary experiments on the optimum time of exposure to PEG indicated that a total of 3–4 minutes was most appropriate for HMy2. Following dilution of the PEG, the cells are spun down and resuspended in 50 ml of hybrid-selecting medium for plating out in multi-well plates.

As a precaution, we routinely omit the hybrid selective antimetabolite (azaserine or aminopterin) from one well plated from each fusion, checking for vigorous growth of unfused HMy2 cells during the next 3–4 days.

Attempts to improve hybrid yield by centrifuging the combined cell pellet in PEG[108] were inconclusive. We have not examined hybrid yield as a function of the molecular weight of the PEG; other workers with HMy2 (and other human systems) have successfully used PEG 1000–4000 at concentrations from 50–35% (mass/vol.). If the mouse system is anything to go by[3] optima for the timing, temperature, concentration and molecular weight of PEG are probably fairly broad, although the latter two parameters are probably linked. In contrast, control of pH may be more critical. In the mouse system[109] a pH of >8.0 is optimal. We use a PEG solution of pH 8.5, as determined electrometrically; this gives a strawberry-pink colour with the phenol-red indicator in the L15 medium. (It should be noted that neither the electrometric pH nor colour are directly comparable to normal medium because of the high concentrations of polymer present). Selection of a 'good' batch of PEG is reportedly important, as some contain toxic oxidation products[110]; we use batches which give good results with mouse hybridoma systems. However, prolonged storage of PEG solutions, and repeated melting of the solid, are undesirable with solutions becoming progressively more acidic and toxic. Addition of antioxidants[111] such as butylated hydroxytoluene (BHT) is probably not necessary on a routine basis. DMSO enhances fusion frequency with mouse cells[112] and can be included (5% v/v) in PEG solutions for human fusions.

Although there is no evidence that PEG is intrinsically less suited to human systems, alternative fusogens to PEG, such as virus, liposomes, lysolecithin, 8-bromohexane or electrical pulse-induced fusion have yet to be tested systematically with human lymphocyte hybrid systems.

Selection of hybrids

Concentrations of HAT used to select human hybrids have generally conformed to Littlefield's original[69] method, viz 1×10^{-4}M hypoxanthine (14 μg/ml), 4×10^{-7}M aminopterin (0.2 μg/ml) and 1.6×10^{-5}M thymidine (4 μg/ml). Some workers have used reduced concentrations of thymidine (1.6×10^{-6}M) and aminopterin (2×10^{-8}M)[57,65,113] in so-called 'human' HAT medium.

Amino-acid supplementation: Normal levels of glutamine in culture medium (2 mM) are generally adequate for hybrid growth (in the absence of mycoplasma); it is, however, labile and medium must be freshly prepared or separately supplemented. The synthesis of glycine is inhibited by aminopterin and it was also supplemented (3×10^{-6}M) in Littlefield's[69,86] method but levels in media such as Dulbecco's (nearly 1 mmol) are sufficient.

Thymidine toxicity: At high concentrations thymidine will inhibit cell proliferation in culture. This effect can be relieved by adding deoxycytidine[114,115]. Some workers have, therefore, supplemented HAT medium with deoxycytidine (1×10^{-5}M) when generating human lymphocyte hybrids. Foung et al[116] reported a four-fold enhancement of human T-hybrid yield using selective medium without exogenous thymidine but containing deoxycytidine. The B-cell line HMy2, and its hybrids are, however, not affected by 10 times the standard concentration of thymidine (i.e. 1.6×10^{-4}M). Parental T-cell lines seem, however, to be more sensitive (10^{-5}M)[117,115].

HA_z selection medium: Azaserine (6-(1'-methyl-4'-nitro-5'-imidazoly) serine) is an alternative inhibitor of de novo purine synthesis that can be used for hybrid selection. This diazo analogue of glutamine irreversibly inhibits the glutamine dependent amidation of formylglycinamide ribonucleotide (FGAR), thus blocking synthesis of IMP[118]. It does not (unlike aminopterin) inhibit pyrimidine synthesis significantly at concentrations sufficient to block purine synthesis[119]. Hypoxanthine (but not thymidine) is required in the medium (HAz medium). Azaserine was found to yield more mouse hybrids[120].

We obtained our first successful human fusions with an azaserine-containing selective medium, although we retained 1.6×10^{-5}M thymidine for practical convenience and did not add cytidine as fetal calf serum contains such nucleotides. HAT medium is also effective with HMy2[18-20,22,59]. If azaserine is used, it must be added at a higher concentration than aminopterin as it is less stable in culture medium, particularly at acid pHs.[119]

We have determined that 0.4 µg/ml is the minimum concentration at which effective selection is exerted; others have used 1 µg/ml.[120,116]

Amethopterin can be substituted for aminopterin (so-called HOT medium) but we know of no advantages.

Other selection methods: Alternatives to HAT, HOT or HA_z selection with HPRT⁻ (or TK⁻) variants have been devised for preparing lymphocyte hybrids. Apart from other enzyme deficiencies such as APRT⁻ (see above) alternative strategies are available which do not require a mutant parent cell lines. These can, for example, be applied speculatively to new B-cell lines, to see if they will fuse. The general principle is to poison the B-cell line before fusion and rescue it by fusion with an unpoisoned lymphocyte. Diethylpyrocarbonate[121,122] and inhibitors of RNA synthesis (emetine/actinomycin D)[123] have been used. In practice, however, they have not achieved widespread use. The most serious difficulty is getting a reproducible level of poisoning, and they are apparently not applicable to all B-cell lines. The diethylpyrocarbonate method, as originally described by Wright[121], does not, for example, seem to work with HMy2. Furthermore, the extreme lability of this reagent in water makes it difficult to titre the dose reproducibly. The actinomycin D method, by contrast, presents the opposite problem. It is so stable that when it is liberated from dying parental cells in the fusion mixture, it will kill any nascent hybrids, unless it is removed by frequent medium changes (Stimson, personal communication).

Conventional selection systems seem, therefore, to still provide the method of choice for generating human lymphocyte hybrids, with the use of azaserine perhaps marginally preferable on account of its less severe antimetabolic effects, compared with aminopterin.

Growth of hybrids

Time course of HMy2 death: HMy2 cells do not proliferate in HAT (or HAzT) medium formulated as described above; living cells can, however, be detected up to 7–10 days after selection has commenced. If the hybrid-selecting medium is removed too early such residual parental cells can occasionally regrow. We, therefore, retain full-strength selective medium on all hybrid cultures until the colonies have been grown up, cloned and characterized. Such delayed death of the parental B-cell-line has been reported with other human lines for fusion[66], although the UC 729-6 line, by contrast, dies within 3–4 days.

Time course of hybrid growth: We plate out fusion products in 1 ml aliquots in 2 ml wells in 24-well plates at a density of 2×10^5 HMy2 cells/well, and feed the cultures with another 1 ml of full strength selective medium after 7 days, when the plates are sealed with adhesive tape and left undisturbed in the incubator at 37°C with 5% CO_2, 95% air for a further 2 weeks. Hybrid colonies are first detectable at about $2\frac{1}{2}$ weeks with most new colonies appearing over the next 2 weeks; some even emerge as late as 5 weeks post-fusion. Cultures should be refed with fresh selective medium at 4 weeks if no hybrids are yet visible; we discard them after 6 weeks if no growth is evident. This prolonged latency of human hybridomas, also noted by other workers[66] contrasts with rodent systems and places a premium on good sterile techniques. Prolonged maintenance in multi-wells tends to facilitate fungal contamination, and for this reason we include amphotericin B in the medium, despite its somewhat greater toxicity towards mammalian cells compared with some other antibiotics. Under these conditions we have generated several hundred hybrids.[43] The use of certain brands of multi-well plate (e.g. Nunc) tends, in our experience, to limit spread of occasional fungal contamination from well to well, as compared with others of different design, while 24-well plates facilitate phase-contrast observation, compared with the 96-well variety.

The reasons for the delayed growth of human hybridomas are not evident at present. They may relate to thymidine toxicity, they may reflect the relative paucity of purine metabolizing enzymes in typical lymphocyte populations[71] or they may be the consequence of an extended period of chromosomal rearrangement and/or instability. More simply they may denote the fact that optimal conditions for hybrid growth have not yet been established. Hybrids with HMy2 are, on the whole, significantly slower growing than the parent line (doubling times typically 24–56 hours).

Optimum conditions for hybrid growth

The most important parameters that we can presently define as relevant to successful hybrid growth are (a) the batch of fetal calf serum used, and (b) the presence of a suitable feeder layer.

Fetal calf serum. Bulk stock cultures of HMy2 will grow rapidly in most batches of fetal calf serum (FCS), but when cells are cloned by serial dilution cloning efficiencies vary from <1–20%. Preliminary selection of FCS should, therefore, be made by testing at least 4–6 samples and choosing that with the highest cloning efficiency for stock HMy2 cells. With established proved hybrids only about 20–25% of FCS samples are adequate for hybrid propagation and up to 25% of commercial batches we have tested cannot even support their bulk culture let alone clonal growth. When hybrids are available they are, therefore, the best method for selecting suitable serum batches. The requisite serum concentration for culture of fusion products is 10–20%, with 15% a suitable compromise; higher concentrations are undesirable. We use heat-inactivated FCS, (2 hours at 56°C) but have no evidence that this is crucial.

Feeder layers. Fusions should be cultured with a feeder layer. Fusions with HMy2 are plated into 2 ml wells, preseeded with peritoneal macrophages from untreated Balb/c mice at a density of $2–5 \times 10^3$ attached cells/well. Compared with feeder-free cultures a five-fold enhancement in hybrid yield has been noted[43]. Mouse thymocytes, as used for mouse fusions, have proved of little value with HMy2 although they are effective in some other human hybridoma systems.[113] Human foreskin fibroblasts have been employed with UC 729-6[61] and it has recently been reported that human monocytes from peripheral blood are particularly effective.[113] Macrophage feeders aid in clearing cultures of cell debris and facilitate identification of hybrid clones at an early stage. Leukocyte growth factors in the form of supernatants from agglutinin-stimulated tonsil cells have been included in human hybrid-selecting medium[124] although effects on hybrid yield have not been documented. Human endothelial cell culture supernatant (HECS) has been recommended for mouse–human hybrids.[125]

Metabolic cooperation. Metabolic cooperation[126] may, in theory at least, enable limited growth of HPRT⁻ parental stock cells to take place. Such metabolic cooperation has been demonstrated with normal and HPRT⁻ lymphocytes co-cultured in vitro.[127] The use of very dense feeder layers of HPRT⁺ cells for hybrid selection is, therefore, not recommended.

Bulk growth of hybrids. The most crucial stage in the growth of hybrids is their transfer from the original 2 ml multi-well plates to bulk culture. If transferred prematurely with overdilution of hybrid cells then up to 50% may be lost at this stage. We split cultures 1:2 into fresh 2 ml wells with fresh HAT medium without feeders when the well contains about 10^4 cells. If growth is vigorous without feeder cells the cultures can then be transferred into 25 cm² flasks with 5 ml medium; if not then hybrids can sometimes be rescued at this stage by re-adding peritoneal macrophages. With these precautions, we have been able to establish at least 75% of wells with visible hybrids in bulk culture. At this stage (3–5 weeks post-fusion) unstable hybrids do not seem to be a problem.

Morphology of hybrids. As mentioned above, most hybrids grow slower than HMy2. When clonal they show a range of individual morphologies and growth rates, both of which are in our experience stable for at least 6 months or more of continuous subcultivation. In general, they tend to form much larger clumps composed of larger cells than the HMy2 cells (Fig. 4.6), are less adhesive to the culture substratum than HMy2, which attaches loosely at lower densities. Some hybrids do not survive as isolated cells in the absence of feeder layers. Ultrastructurally (Fig. 4.6) hybrids show a similar lymphoblastoid morphology to the parent line.[128]

Cloning of hybrids. Cloning is best attempted with macrophage feeders, in 96-well plates, using a carefully selected FCS batch. Wells are seeded with diluted stocks and

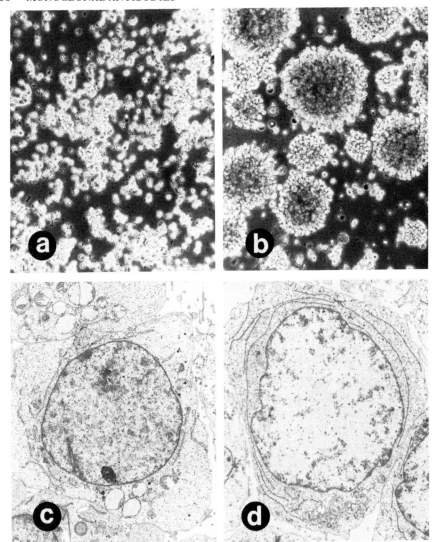

Fig. 4.6 Morphology of parent cell line HMy2 and hybrids. (a) phase contrast (x45) of parent cell line HMy2 (b) phase contrast (x45) of typical hybrid (c) electron micrograph of HMy2 (x2450) (d) electron micrograph (x2450) of hybrid shown in (b).

checked by phase-contrast microscope for the presence of single cells. After a week's culture single growing clones are identified. Clones are transferred to 2 ml wells after 10–14 days. Alternatively, single cells can be isolated. In the method of Sijens et al,[129] drops are dispensed and inspected for the presence of one cell, then transferred to culture wells. We have successfully picked cells manually with a fine (40 μM) micropipette according to Zagury et al[130]; see also Cunningham's method in Dresser[131]. To rely solely on the statistics of serial dilution is not adequate.

Serum-free growth. Although we ourselves have not attempted serum-free or low-serum growth of HMy2 hybrids this is possible using Iscove's modification of

DMEM[104] containing transferrin plus soyabean lipids, with insulin (5 μg/ml) (T Alderson, personal communication). We are not, however, aware of anyone who has successfully generated human hybrids in serum-free medium from scratch.

Freezing of hybrids. We have had no difficulty in freezing and thawing human hybrid cultures, once they have been established in bulk. We transfer them to an air-buffered medium such as Leibovitz's L-15, with 5% (v/v) dimethylsulfoxide and freeze them in the neck of a Union Carbide liquid N_2 container, preferably at a density of $>10^6$ cells/ml. Serum is not necessary in the freezing medium, but may be used with less robust or more dilute hybrid cultures. Thawed cells should be preferably plated onto macrophage feeder layers.

Sources of lymphocytes for fusion

Hybrids have been successfully prepared with human B lymphocytes from spleen,[57] peripheral blood,[60] tonsils and lymph nodes[43] and tumours.[18] We have not observed any differences in yield of hybrids per B-cell although tonsils did give some of our best results. The lymphocytes were simply obtained with centrifugation of the samples on sodium metrizoate-Ficoll solution (1.077 g/l; Lymphoprep). Tonsils were surface-sterilized in 70% ethanol and the lymphocytes expressed by scraping with a scalpel blade into HEPES-buffered McCoy's medium 5A containing penicillin, streptomycin, kanamycin, gentamycin and amphotericin B. (Surface sterilization was omitted with surgical lymph node samples.) Olsson et al[66] have reported lower hybrid yields from PBLs compared with spleen, but did not correct for B-cell content.

The major difference that we have noted was between donors. Hybrid frequencies ranged from 1 hybrid per 10^8 lymphocytes to 1 in 10^6, using standardized methods with the same reagents. This invalidates comparisons between fusions using different lymphocyte preparations. One way to avoid this problem is to use a standardized lymphocyte analogue, such as a frozen stock of CLL cells from a single patient as[59] a means of comparing different human hybridoma systems.

Given these low and variable hybrid yields, can any manipulation of the lymphocytes in vitro enhance and standardize the procedure? Warenuis et al[22] for example, pre-culture with pokeweed (PWM) and report two-fold enhancement of hybrid yield. Our experiments with lymph-node lymphocytes treated in this manner have been inconclusive. Lymphocytes were cultured in RPMI 1640 with 10% FCS and 10^{-5}M mercaptoethanol plus 3 μg/ml PWM for 3–4 days, at which point the total lymphocyte number has been increased two-fold and the cells are at their peak rates of DNA synthesis. We found, however, that these pre-stimulated lymphocytes continued to proliferate in HA_zT selective medium for several days even in the absence of PWM. This resulted in significant overcrowding of the wells and acidification of the medium under our standard conditions (2×10^6 lymphocyte/well) and no dramatic increase in hybrid yield per lymphocyte was obtained using this particular protocol. Different protocols with regard to timing may be more successful, with perhaps fusion attempted at time of peak Ig secretion. Thus Olsson et al[66] using PBLs noted a significant increase in hybrid yield (<1 in 5×10^5) with RH-L4 lymphoma line when lymphocytes were precultured in PWM (2.5 μg/ml) plus HAT for 5–7 days. Kozbor & Roder[124] also report significant enhancement with PBLs and EB (as compared with PBLs plus PWM), recording a five-fold enhancement in TT-specific hybridomas, most of which produced IgM. Overall hybrid yields were still, however, relatively low (3×10^{-6}).

Ouabain-resistant parental B-cell lines

One means of preventing continued polyclonal growth of stimulated wild-type lymphocytes after fusion is to use ouabain-resistant parental B-cell lines. Kozbor et al[39] have prepared a ouabain-resistant mutant of the GM 1500 A1 6TG line, which they have designated KR-4 (see Table 4.2). This lymphoblastoid line enables the HAT-selective medium for hybrids to be supplemented with 5×10^{-6}M ouabain. This kills the wild-type lymphocytes (or EB-transformed lymphoblastoid cell-lines), the aminopterin kills the parental cells, and by complementation only hybrids survive. Such lines have been used to stabilize EB-transformed lines[39] and such hybrids reportedly show enhanced levels of specific Ig secretion in some cases. Similar procedures have been employed with mouse myeloma lines, which are intrinsically more resistant to ouabain than human cells.[132]

We have now derived a comparable cloned, mycoplasma-free ouabain-resistant ($<10^{-5}$M) variant of the HAT-sensitive HMy2 (HMy2OR).

FUTURE DEVELOPMENTS

Present methods for making human monoclonal antibodies are reproducible, but reproducibly produce too few hybrids with satisfactory properties. How can the situation be improved?

Improved fusion partners

When the rodent myelomas particularly the rat Y3 line[133] were developed for fusion, they gradually increased their fusion frequency during long-term passage in spinner culture. It may be that similar treatment of human lines would be successful, although our own attempts with HMy2 have not been, so far. Other human B-cell lines should be tested for fusion frequency, particularly lines that are already non-producers. We isolated high- and low-secretor clones from HMy2.[43] One of the low-secretors seemed to be a non-producer of heavy chains, but the clones were contaminated with mycoplasma and have not been used for fusion. Such cloning could be repeated, perhaps using fluorescence-activated cell sorting to isolate cells with no surface heavy chain, but it seems to be general experience that chain-loss variants of lymphoblastoid lines are very difficult to isolate compared with chain-loss variants of mouse myelomas.

An interesting idea for improving the stability of rodent x human hybrids is being investigated by Kaplan and colleagues.[58] They are developing as fusion partners, HAT-sensitive 'heteromyelomas', hybrids between the mouse myeloma X63-Ag 8.653 and the human myeloma U266. In an attempt to stabilize the heteromyelomas against human chromosome loss the U266 myeloma was first given neomycin-resistance genes by transfection, and the heteromyelomas are maintained in the presence of a neomycin analogue. They hope that these heteromyelomas will retain the excellent characteristics of the mouse myeloma but will have acquired a tendency to form stable hybrids with human cells, and it will be interesting to see if their strategy is successful.

When testing new lines for fusion it is convenient to by-pass the derivation of a HAT-sensitive derivative. Clark et al[122] successfully used the method of Wright described above, in which the cells are treated with metabolic poisons immediately before fusion. Lines that do fuse should, however, then be made HAT-sensitive for routine use.

New fusion methods

It seems unlikely that significant advances will be made by modifying conditions of exposure to PEG. However, only 1 in 10^4 to 10^5 lymphocytes can successfully be fused even in rodent systems and this may in part be because in a cell pellet the chances of forming 1:1 heterokaryons between a myeloma cell and a lymphocyte are very low—most cells will form inappropriate heterokaryons or not fuse at all. A fusion procedure is needed that causes predominantly 1:1 fusion. The antigen-directed fusion method[134] may be a step in the right direction: working with the mouse, myeloma cells were coated with a hapten to encourage fusion with lymphocytes capable of binding that hapten.

Improved lymphocytes

An important advantage of the rodent systems is that animals are hyperimmunized, and in addition they are boosted to give a high proportion of dividing, antibody-secreting cells at fusion. To achieve a parallel situation in the human requires the development of methods for immunising human lymphocytes in vitro in which a response is not only triggered but significant selective proliferation of reactive cells occurs. There seems to have been substantial progress with in vitro immunization techniques recently,[24-26,28] and we can presumably expect future methods to employ T-helper cell clones and various preparations of lymphocyte growth factors. It may eventually be possible to grow normal B-cell clones as human T-cell clones already can be grown with high efficiency.[135]

Alternatives to fusion

Transformation of lymphocytes by SV40 and transfection with DNA have been suggested but seem unlikely to be better than transformation by EB virus. To cut the cost of commercial production of useful human monoclonal antibody it may eventually be worth transferring the genetic information for such an antibody into a bacterial cell by cDNA techniques.

CONCLUSION

The making of human monoclonal antibodies, in contrast to mouse or rat monoclonal antibodies, is still in the development stage. The highest priorities for many workers in the field seem to be the development of better fusion systems, in vitro immunization, and the study of interesting antigens using rodent monoclonal antibodies first.

ACKNOWLEDGEMENTS

We would like to thank in particular, Clare Madin (Smith) for her invaluable assistance in setting up the HMy2 hybridization system and distributing the line. Thanks are also due to Rob Skilton for help with chain-specific assays, Dr M G Ormerod and Andrew Payne for flow cytometry of DNA, Dr P Monaghan for ultrastructural studies, Dr B Reeve for karyotyping HMy2 and Dr K Welsh and Mr W Wakeling for its HLA type and especially Dr Dorothy Crawford for discussions on the EB-transformation system. We gratefully acknowledge numerous colleagues who have given us valuable feedback on the HMy2 system as distributed, and for preprints which have helped in the writing of this chapter, as well as the UC729-6 line from Dr H Handley. We also express our gratitude to Professor A M Neville, without whose suggestion and encouragement we would not have embarked on the development of human hybridoma systems and Mrs C Cassell for typing the manuscript.

APPENDIX

AVAILABILITY OF RECOMMENDED LINES*

LICR-LON-HMy2	Dr M O'Hare, Ludwig Institute for Cancer Research, The Haddow Laboratories, Clifton Avenue, Sutton, Surrey SM2 5PX.
UC729-6	Dr H Handley Director, Cell Distribution, UC San Diego Cancer Center, TO11, University of California of San Diego, La Jolla CA 92093, USA.
WI-L2-729-HF$_2$	Dr R Lundak Techniclone 3301 South Harbor Blvd., Santa Anna, CA 92704, USA.

*Many of the other lines are available from the laboratory of origin, see the appropriate reference.

REFERENCES

1. Galfre G, Milstein C 1981 Preparation of monoclonal antibodies: strategies and procedures. Methods in Enzymology 73: 3–47
2. Edwards P A W 1981 Some properties and applications of monoclonal antibodies. Biochemical Journal 200: 1–10
3. O'Hare M J 1984 Monoclonal antibodies of murine and human origin: their generation, characterisation and use. In: Panayi G, David C (eds) International medical reviews: Clinical Immunogenetics. Butterworths, London

4. Kohler G, Schulman M J 1978 Cellular and molecular restrictions of the lymphocyte fusion. In: Melchers F, Potter M, Warner N L (eds) Lymphocyte hybridomas, Springer-Verlag, Berlin, Heidelberg, New York, pp 143–148

5. Parham P, Androlewicz M J, Brodsky F M, Holmes N J, Ways J P 1982 Monoclonal antibodies: purification, fragmentation and application to structural and functional studies of class I MHC antigens. Journal of Immunological Methods 53: 133–173

6. Voak D, Sacks S, Alderson T, Takei F, Lennox E, Jarvis J, Milstein C, Darnborough J 1980 Monoclonal anti-A from a hybrid-myeloma: evaluation as a blood grouping reagent. Vox Sanguinis 39: 134–140

7. Crawford D H, Harrison J F, Barlow M J, Winger L, Huehns E R 1983 Production of human monoclonal antibody to rhesus D antigen. Lancet: 1, 386–388

8. Eisenbarth G S, Linnenbach A, Jackson R, Scearce R, Croce C M 1982 Human hybridomas secreting anti-islet autoantibodies. Nature 300: 264–267

9. Shoenfeld Y, Hsu-Lin S C, Gabriels J E, Silberstein L E, Furie B C, Furie B, Stollar B D, Schwartz R S 1982 Production of autoantibodies by human–human hybridomas. Journal of Clinical Investigation 70: 205–208

10. Valente W A, Vitti P, Yavin Z, Yavin E, Rotella C M, Grollman E F, Toccafondi R S, Kohn C D 1982 Monoclonal antibodies to the thyrotropin receptor: stimulating and blocking antibodies derived from the lymphocytes of patients with Graves disease. Proceedings of the National Academy of Sciences of the United States of America 79: 6680–6684

11. Andrzejewski Jr C, Stollar B D, Lalor T M, Schwartz R S 1980 Hybridoma autoantibodies to DNA. Journal of Immunology 124: 1499–1502

12. Gooi H C, Uemura K-I, Edwards P A W, Foster C S, Pickering N, Feizi T 1983 Two mouse hybridoma antibodies against human milk-fat globules recognise the I(MA) antigenic determinant β-D-Galp-(1→4)-β-D-GlcpNAc-(1→6). Carbohydrate Research 120: 293–302

13. Sears H F, Atkinson B, Mattis J, Ernst C, Herlyn D, Steplewski Z, Hayry P, Koprowski H 1982 Phase-I clinical trial of monoclonal antibody in treatment of gastrointestinal tumours. Lancet 1: 762–765

14. Miller R A, Levy R 1981 Response of cutaneous T cell lymphoma to therapy with hybridoma monoclonal antibody. Lancet 1: 226–230

15. Levy R, Miller R A 1983 Biological and clinical implications of lymphocyte hybridomas: tumor therapy with monoclonal antibodies. Annual Review of Medicine 34: 107–116

16. Schlom J, Wunderlich D, Teramoto Y A 1980 Generation of human monoclonal antibodies reactive with human mammary carcinoma cells. Proceedings of the National Academy of Sciences of the United States of America 77: 6841–6845

17. Wunderlich D, Teramoto Y A, Alford C, Schlom J 1981 The use of lymphocytes from axillary lymph nodes of mastectomy patients to generate human monoclonal antibodies. European Journal of Cancer and Clinical Oncology 17: 719–730

18. Sikora K, Alderson T, Phillips J, Watson J V 1982 Human hybridomas from malignant gliomas. Lancet: 11–14

19. Cote R J, Morrissey D M, Houghton A N, Beattie Jr E J, Oettgen H F, Old L J 1983 Generation of human monoclonal antibodies reactive with cellular antigens. Proceedings of the National Academy of Sciences of the United States of America 80: 2026–2030

20. Houghton A N, Brooks H, Cote R J, Taormina C, Oettgen H F, Old L J 1983 Detection of cell surface and intracellular antigens by human monoclonal antibodies: hybrid cell lines derived from lymphocytes of patients with malignant melanoma. Journal of Experimental Medicine 158: 53–65

21. Sikora K, Alderson T, Ellis J, Phillips J, Watson J 1983 Human hybridomas from patients with malignant disease. British Journal of Cancer 47: 135–145

22. Warenius H M, Taylor J W, Durack B E, Cross P A 1983 The production of human hybridomas from patients with malignant melanoma. The effect of pre-stimulation of lymphocytes with pokeweed mitogen. European Journal of Cancer and Clinical Oncology 19: 347–355

23. Miller R A, Maloney D G, Warnke R, Levy R 1982 Treatment of B-cell lymphoma with monoclonal anti-idiotype antibody. The New England Journal of Medicine 306: 517–522

24. Callard R E 1979 Specific in vitro antibody response to influenza virus by human blood lymphocytes. Nature 282: 734–736

25. Lane H C, Volkman D J, Whalen G, Fauci A S 1981 In vitro antigen-specific antibody production in man. Journal of Experimental Medicine 154: 1043–1057

26. Misiti J, Waldmann T A 1981 In vitro generation of antigen-specific hemolytic plaque-forming cells from human peripheral blood mononuclear cells. Journal of Experimental Medicine 154: 1069–1084

27. Crawford D H, Callard R E, Muggeridge M I, Mitchell D M, Zanders E D, Beverley P C L 1983 Production of human monoclonal antibody to X31 influenza virus nucleoprotein. Journal of General Virology 64: 697–700

28. Rossio J L, Knost J A, Pickeral S F, Abrams P D Human–human hybridomas producing antigen-specific IgG using in vitro immunized peripheral blood cells as fusion partners. (In press)

29. Schwaber J 1975 Immunoglobulin production by a human–mouse somatic cell hybrid. Experimental Cell Research 93: 343–354

30. Nowinski R, Berglund C, Lane J, Lostrom M, Bernstein I, Young W, Hakomori S 1980 Human monoclonal antibody against Forssman antigen. Science 210: 537–539

31. Gigliotti F, Insel R A 1982 Protective human hybridoma antibody to tetanus toxin. Journal of Clinical Investigation 70: 1306–1309

32. Croce C M, Shander M, Martinis J, Cicurel L, D'Ancona G G, Koprowski H 1980 Preferential retention of human chromosome 14 in mouse × human B cell hybrids. European Journal of Immunology 10: 486–488

33. Kearney J F, Radbruch A, Liesegang B, Rajewsky K 1979 A new mouse myeloma cell line that has lost immunoglobulin expression but permits the construction of antibody-secreting hybrid cell lines. Journal of Immunology 123: 1548–1550

34. Nilsson K 1979 The nature of lymphoid cell lines and their relationship to the virus. In: Epstein M A, Achong B G (eds) The Epstein-Barr virus, Springer-Verlag, Berlin, Heidelberg, New York, pp 225–281

35. Miller G, Lipman M 1973 Release of infectious Epstein-Barr virus by transformed marmoset leukocytes. Proceedings of the National Academy of Sciences of the United States of America 70: 190–194

36. Pope J H 1979 Transformation by the virus in vitro. In: Epstein M A, Achong B G (eds) The Epstein-Barr virus, Springer-Verlag, Berlin, Heidelberg, New York, pp 206–281

37. Kozbor D, Roder J C 1981 Requirements for the establishment of high-titred human monoclonal antibodies against tetanus toxoid using the Epstein-Barr virus technique. Journal of Immunology 127: 1275–1280

38. Winger L, Winger C, Shastry P, Russell A, Longenecker M 1983 Efficient generation in vitro, from human peripheral blood cells, of monoclonal Epstein-Barr virus transformants producing specific antibody to a variety of antigens without prior deliberate immunization. Proceedings of the National Academy of Sciences of the United States of America 80: 4484–4488

39. Kozbor D, Lagarde A E, Roder J C 1982 Human hybridomas constructed with antigen-specific Epstein-Barr virus-transformed cell lines. Proceedings of the National Academy of Sciences of the United States of America 79: 6651–6655

40. Steinitz M, Tamir S 1982 Human monoclonal autoimmune antibody produced in vitro: rheumatoid factor generated by Epstein-Barr virus-transformed cell line. European Journal of Immunology 12: 126–133

41. Steinitz M, Koskimies S, Klein G, Makela O 1979 Establishment of specific antibody producing human cell lines by antigen presentation and Epstein-Barr (EBV) transformation. Journal of Clinical and Laboratory Immunology 2: 1–7

42. Pickering J W, Gelder F B 1982 (letter) Journal of Immunology 129: 2314

43. Edwards P A W, Smith C M, Neville A M, O'Hare M J 1982 A human–human hybridoma system based on a fast-growing mutant of the ARH-77 plasma cell leukemia-derived line. European Journal of Immunology 12: 641–648

44. Milstein C, Cuello A C 1983 Hybrid hybridomas and their use in immunohistochemistry. Nature 305: 537–540

45. Crissman H A, Steinkamp J A 1973 Rapid, simultaneous measurement of DNA, protein, and cell volume in single cells from large mammalian cell populations. Journal of Cell Biology 59: 766–771

46. O'Hare M J, Smith C M, Edwards P A W 1983 A new human hybridoma system (LICR-LON-HMy2) and its use in the production of human monoclonal antibodies. In: Peeters H (ed) Protides of biological fluids, Colloquium 30. Pergamon Press, Oxford, pp 265–268

47. Sikora K, Alderson T St J, Ellis J 1983 A sensitive chain specific radioimmunoassay for human immunoglobulins using monoclonal antibodies. Journal of Immunological Methods 57: 151–154

48. Kohler G, Howe S C, Milstein C 1976 Fusion between immunoglobulin-secreting and nonsecreting myeloma cell lines. European Journal of Immunology 6: 292–295

49. Grillot-Courvalin C, Brouet J-C, Berger R, Bernheim A 1981 Establishment of a human T-cell hybrid line with suppressive activity. Nature 292: 844–845

50. Kozbor D, Roder J C 1983 The production of monoclonal antibodies from human lymphocytes. Immunology Today 4: 71–79

51. Nilsson K, Bennich H, Johansson S G O, Ponten J 1970 Established immunoglobulin producing myeloma (IgE) and lymphoblastoid (IgG) cell lines from an IgE myeloma patient. Clinical and Experimental Immunology 7: 477–489

52. Croce C M, Shander M, Martinis J, Cicurel L, D'Ancona G G, Dolby T W, Koprowski H 1979 Chromosomal location of the genes for human immunoglobulin heavy chains. Proceedings of the National Academy of Sciences of the United States of America 76: 3416–3419

53. Burk K H, Drewinko B, Trujillo J M, Ahearn M J 1978 Establishment of a human plasma cell line in vitro. Cancer Research 38: 2508–2513

54. Levy J A, Buell D N, Creech C, Hirshaut Y, Silverberg H 1971 Further characterization of the W1-L1 and W1-L2 lymphoblastoid lines. Journal of the National Cancer Institute 46: 647–654

55. Lever J E, Nuki G, Seegmiller J E 1974 Expression of purine overproduction in a series of 8-azaguanine-resistant diploid human lymphoblast lines. Proceedings of the National Academy of Sciences of the United States of America 71: 2679–2683

56. Moore G E, Kitamura H 1968 Cell line derived from patient with myeloma. New York State Journal of Medicine 68: 2054–2060

57. Olsson L, Kaplan H S 1980 Human–human hybridomas producing monoclonal antibodies of predefined antigenic specificity. Proceedings of the National Academy of Sciences of the United States of America 77: 5429–5431

58. Teng N N H, Lam K S, Riera F C, Kaplan H S 1983 Construction and testing of mouse–human heteromyelomas for human monoclonal antibody production. Proceedings of the National Academy of Sciences of the United States of America 80: 7308–7312

59. Abrams P G, Knost J A, Clarke G, Wilburn S, Oldham R K, Foon K A 1983 Determination of the optimal human cell lines for development of human hybridomas. Journal of Immunology 131: 1201–1204

60. Croce C M, Linnenbach A, Hall W, Steplewski Z, Koprowski H 1980 Production of human hybridomas secreting antibodies to measles virus. Nature 288: 488–489

61. Handley H H, Royston I 1982 A human lymphoblastoid B cell line useful for generating immunoglobulin-secreting human hybridomas. In: Mitchell M S, Oettgen H F (eds) Hybridomas in cancer diagnosis and treatment. Raven Press, New York, pp 125–132

62. Glassy M C, Handley H H, Hagiwara H, Royston I 1983 UC 729-6, a human lymphoblastoid B-cell line useful for generating antibody-secreting human–human hybridomas. Proceedings of the National Academy of Sciences of the United States of America 80: 6327–6331

63. Heitzmann J G, Cohn M 1983 The W1-L2-729-HF$_2$ human hybridoma system: stable hybrids at high frequency. Molecular Biology and Medicine 1: 235–243

64. Chiorazzi N, Wasserman R L, Kunkel H G 1982 Use of Epstein-Barr virus-transformed B cell lines for the generation of immunoglobulin-producing human B cell hybridomas. Journal of Experimental Medicine 156: 930–935

65. Olsson L, Kronstrom H, Cambon-De Mouzon A, Honsik C, Brodin T, Jakobsen B 1983 Antibody producing human–human hybridomas. I. Technical aspects. Journal of Immunological Methods 61: 17–32

66. Kaplan H S, Olsson L, Raubitschek A 1982 Monoclonal human antibodies: a recent development with wide-ranging clinical potential. In: McMichael A J, Fabre J H (eds) Monoclonal antibodies in clinical medicine. Academic Press, London, pp 17–35

67. Shoenfeld Y, Rauch J, Massicotte H, Datta S K, Andre-Schwartz J, Stollar B D, Schwartz R S 1983 Polyspecificity of monoclonal lupus autoantibodies produced by human–human hybridomas. New England Journal of Medicine 308: 414–420

68. Weiss R A 1982 Retroviruses produced by hybridomas. New England Journal of Medicine 307: 1587

69. Littlefield J W 1964 Selection of hybrids from matings of fibroblasts in vitro and their presumed recombinants. Science 145: 709–710

70. Pai G S, Sprenkle J A, Do T T, Mareni C E, Migeon B R 1980 Localization of loci for hypoxanthine phosphoribosyl-transferase and glucose-6-phosphate dehydrogenase and biochemical evidence of nonrandom X chromosome expression from studies of a human X-autosome translocation. Proceedings of the National Academy of Sciences of the United States of America 77: 2810–2813

71. Murray A W 1971 The biological significance of purine salvage. Annual Reviews of Biochemistry 40: 811–826

72. Siniscalco M, Klinger H P, Eagle H, Koprowski H, Fujimoto W Y, Seegmiller J E 1969 Evidence for intergenic complementation in hybrid cells derived from two human diploid strains each carrying an x-linked mutation. Proceedings of the National Academy of Sciences of the United States of America 62: 793–799

73. Szybalski W, Szybalska E H, Ragni G 1962 Genetic studies with human cell lines. National Cancer Institute Monographs 7: 75–89

74. Bertino J R 1975 Folate antagonists. In: Sartorelli A C, Johns D G (eds) Anti-neoplastic and immunosuppressive agents, part II, Springer Verlag, Berlin, Heidelberg, New York, pp 468–483
75. Seegmiller J E 1976 Inherited deficiency of hypoxanthine-guanine phosphoribosyltransferase in X-linked uric aciduria (the Lesch-Nyhan syndrome and its variants). In: Harris H, Hirshhorn K (eds) Advances in human genetics, vol 6. Plenum Press, New York, London, pp 75–163
76. Clements G B 1975 Selection of biochemically variant, in some cases mutant, mammalian cells in culture. In: Klein G, Weinhouse S (eds) Advances in cancer research, vol 21. Academic Press, New York, pp 273–390
77. Taggart R T, Samloff I M 1982 Stable antibody-producing murine hybridomas. Science 219: 1228–1230
78. Strauss G H, Albertini R J 1979 Enumeration of 6-thioguanine-resistant peripheral blood lymphocytes in man as a potential test for somatic cell mutations arising in vivo. Mutation Research 61: 353–379
79. Cox R, Masson W K 1978 Do radiation-induced thioguanine-resistant mutants of cultured mammalian cells arise by HGPRT gene mutation or X-chromosome rearrangement? Nature 276: 629–630
80. Evans H J, Vijayalaxmi 1981 Induction of 8-azaguanine resistance and sister chromatid exchange in human lymphocytes exposed to mitomycin C and X rays in vitro. Nature 292: 601–605
81. Steglich C, DeMars R 1982 Mutations causing deficiency of APRT in fibroblasts cultured from humans heterozygous for mutant APRT alleles. Somatic Cell Genetics 8: 115–141
82. Nelson J A, Carpenter J W, Rose L M, Adamson D J 1975 Mechanisms of action of 6-thioguanine, 6-mercaptopurine and 8-azaguanine. Cancer Research 35: 2872–2878
83. Van Zeeland A A, Simons J W I M 1975 The effect of calf serum on the toxicity of 8-azaguanine. Mutation Research 27: 135–138
84. Van Diggelen O P, Donahue T F, Shin S-I 1979 Basis for differential cellular sensitivity to 8-azaguanine and 6-thioguanine. Journal of Cellular Physiology 98: 59–72
85. Meyers M B, van Diggelen O P, van Diggelen M, Shin S-I 1980 Isolation of somatic cell mutants with specified alterations in hypoxanthine phosphoribosyltransferase. Somatic Cell Genetics 6: 299–306
86. Littlefield J W 1964 Three degrees of guanylic acid—inosinic acid pyrophosphorylase deficiency in mouse fibroblasts. Nature 203: 1142–1144
87. Albertini R J, DeMars R 1970 Diploid azaguanine-resistant mutants of cultured human fibroblasts. Science 169: 482–485
88. O'Brien S J, Shannon J E, Gail M H 1980 A molecular approach to the identification and individualization of human and animal cells in culture: isozyme and allozyme genetic signatures. In Vitro 16: 119–135
89. Dietz A A, Lubrano T 1967 Separation and quantitation of lactic dehydrogenase isoenzymes by disc electrophoresis. Analytical Biochemistry 20: 246–257
90. Van Diggelen O P, Phillips D M, Shin S-I 1977 Endogenous HPRT activity in a cryptic strain of mycoplasma and its effect on cellular resistance to selective media in infected cell lines. Experimental Cell Research 106: 191–203
91. McGarrity G J, Vanaman V, Sarama J 1978 Methods of prevention, control and elimination of mycoplasma infection. In: McGarrity G J, Murphy D G, Nichols W W (eds) Mycoplasma infection of cell cultures. Plenum Press, New York and London, pp 213–240
92. Beardsley T 1983 Contamination at Flow labs. Nature (News) 304: 674
93. Perlman D, Rahman S B, Semar J B 1967 Antibiotic control of mycoplasma in tissue culture. Applied Microbiology 15: 82–85
94. Boyle J M, Hopkins J, Fox M, Allen T D, Leach R H 1981 Interference in hybrid clone selection caused by mycoplasma hyorhinis infection. Experimental Cell Research 132: 67–72
95. Aula P, Nichols W W 1967 The cytogenetic effects of mycoplasma in human leukocyte cultures. Journal of Cellular Physiology 70: 281–290
96. Russell W C, Newman C, Williamson D H 1975 A simple cytochemical technique for demonstration of DNA in cells infected with mycoplasmas and viruses. Nature 253: 461–462
97. Hilwig I, Gropp A 1972 Staining of constitutive heterochromatin in mammalian chromosomes with a new fluorochrome. Experimental Cell Research 75: 122–126
98. Chen T R 1977 In situ detection of mycoplasma contamination in cell cultures by fluorescent Hoechst 33258 stain. Experimental Cell Research 104: 255–262
99. Del Guidice R A, Hopps H E 1978 Microbiological methods and fluorescent microscopy for the direct demonstration of mycoplasma infection of cell cultures. In: McGarrity G J, Murphy D G, Nichols W W (eds) Mycoplasma infection of cell cultures, Plenum Press, New York and London, pp 57–69

100. Hayflick L 1960 Decontaminating tissue cultures infected with pleuropneumonia-like organisms. Nature 185: 783-784
101. Schimmelpfeng L, Langenberg U, Peters J H 1980 Macrophages overcome mycoplasma infections of cells in vitro. Nature 285: 661-663
102. Marcus M, Lavi U, Nattenberg A, Rottem S, Markowitz O 1980 Selective killing of mycoplasmas from contaminated mammalian cells in cell cultures. Nature 285: 659-661
103. Van Diggelen O P, Shin S-I, Phillips D M 1977 Reduction in cellular tumorigenicity after mycoplasma infection and elimination of mycoplasma from infected cultures by passage in nude mice. Cancer Research 37: 2680-2687
104. Iscove N N, Melchers F 1978 Complete replacement of serum by albumin, transferrin, and soybean lipid in cultures of lipopolysaccharide-reactive B lymphocytes. Journal of Experimental Medicine 147: 923-933
105. Hansen D, Stadler J 1977 Increased polyethylene-glycol-mediated fusion competence in mitotic cells of a mouse lymphoid cell line. Somatic Cell Genetics 3: 471-482
106. Pontecorvo G 1975 Production of mammalian somatic cell hybrids by means of polyethylene glycol treatment. Somatic Cell Genetics 1: 397-400
107. Galfre G, Howe S C, Milstein C, Butcher G W, Howard J C 1977 Antibodies to major histocompatibility antigens produced by hybrid cell lines. Nature 266: 550-552
108. Gefter M L, Margulies D H, Scharff M D 1977 A simple method for polyethylene glycol-promoted hybridization of mouse myeloma cells. Somatic Cell Genetics 3: 231-236
109. Sharon J, Morrison S L, Kabat E A 1980 Formation of hybridoma clones in soft agarose: effect of pH and of medium. Somatic Cell Genetics 6: 435-441
110. Kadish J L, Wenc K M 1983 Contamination of polyethylene glycol with aldehydes: implications for hybridoma fusion. Hybridoma 2: 87-89
111. Honda K, Maeda Y, Sasakawa S, Ohno H, Tsuchida E 1981 The components contained in polyethylene glycol of commercial grade (PEG-6,000) as cell fusogen. Biochemical and Biophysical Research Communications 101: 165-171
112. Norwood T H, Zeigler C J, Martin G M 1976 Dimethyl sulfoxide enhances polyethylene glycol mediated somatic cell fusion. Somatic Cell Genetics 2: 263-270
113. Brodin T, Olsson L, Sjogren H-O 1983 Cloning of human hybridoma, myeloma and lymphoma cell lines using enriched human monocytes as feeder layer. Journal of Immunological Methods 60: 1-7
114. Kaufman E R, Davidson R L 1978 Biological and biochemical effects of bromodeoxyuridine and deoxycytidine on syrian hamster melanoma cells. Somatic Cell Genetics 4: 587-601
115. Fox R M, Tripp E H, Tattersall M H N 1980 Mechanism of deoxycytidine rescue of thymidine toxicity in human T-leukemic lymphocytes. Cancer Research 40: 1718-1721
116. Foung S K H, Sasaki D T, Grumet F C, Engleman E G 1982 Production of functional human T-T hybridomas in selection medium lacking aminopterin and thymidine. Proceedings of the National Academy of Sciences of the United States of America 79: 7484-7488
117. Foley G E, Lazarus H 1967 The response in vitro, of continuous cultures of human lymphoblasts (CCRF-CEM cells) to chemotherapeutic agents. Biochemical Pharmacology 16: 659-664
118. Bennett Jr L L 1975 Glutamine antagonists. In: Sartorelli A C, Johns D G (eds) Anti neoplastic and immunosuppressive agents, part II. Springer Verlag, Berlin, Heidelberg, New York, pp 484-511
119. Livingston R B, Venditti J M, Cooney D A, Carter S K 1970 Glutamine antagonists in chemotherapy. Advances in Pharmacology and Chemotherapeutics 8: 57-69
120. Buttin G, LeGuern G, Phalente L, Lin E C C, Medrano L, Cazenave P A 1978 Production of hybrid lines secreting monoclonal anti-idiotypic antibodies by cell fusion on membrane filters. In: Melchers F, Potter M, Warner N (eds) Lymphocyte hybridomas. Springer-Verlag, Berlin, Heidelberg, New York, pp 27-36
121. Wright W E 1978 The isolation of heterokaryons and hybrids by a selective system using irreversible biochemical inhibitors. Experimental Cell Research 112: 395-407
122. Clark S A, Stimson W H, Williamson A R, Dick H 1981 Hybridoma production by a human myeloma using biochemical selection. Journal of Supramolecular, Structural and Cellular Biochemistry, supplement 5, 100a
123. Kobayashi Y, Asada M, Higuchi M, Osawa T 1982 Human T cell hybridomas producing lymphokines. Journal of Experimental Medicine 128: 2714-2718
124. Kozbor D, Roder J C 1984 In vitro stimulated lymphocytes as a source of human hybridomas. European Journal of Immunology 14: 23-26
125. Astaldi G C B, Janssen M C, Lansdorp P, Willems C, Zeijlemaker W P, Oosterhof F 1980 Human endothelial culture supernatant (HECS): a growth factor for hybridomas. Journal of Immunology 125: 1411-1414

126. Subak-Sharpe J H, Bürk R R, Pitts J D 1969 Metabolic cooperation between biochemically marked mammalian cells in tissue culture. Journal of Cell Science 4: 353–367

127. deBruyn C H M M, Oei T L, Uitendaal M P, Hosli P 1977 Evidence of the existence of different types of metabolic cooperation. In: Müller M M, Kaiser E, Seegmiller J E (eds) Purine metabolism in man II. Plenum Press, New York, pp 172–185

128. Kozbor D, Dexter D, Roder J C 1983 A comparative analysis of the phenotypic characteristics of available fusion partners for the construction of human hybridomas. Hybridoma 2: 7–16

129. Sijens R J, Thomas A A M, Jackers A, Boeye A 1983 Clonal isolation of hybridomas by manual single-cell isolation. Hybridoma 2: 231–234

130. Zagury D, Morgan D A, Fouchard M 1981 Production of human T-lymphocyte clones. I. Monoclonal culture and functional cytotoxic maturation. Journal of Immunological Methods 43: 67–78

131. Dresser D W 1978 Assays for immunoglobulin-secreting cells. In: Weir D M (ed) Handbook of Experimental Immunology, 3rd edn. Blackwell Scientific Publication, Oxford, vol 2, pp 28.1–28.25

132. Kozbor D, Roder J C, Chang T H, Steplewski Z, Koprowski H 1982 Human anti-tetanus toxoid monoclonal antibody secreted by EBV-transformed human B cells fused with murine myeloma. Hybridoma 1: 323–328

133. Galfre G, Milstein C, Wright B 1979 Rat × rat hybrid myelomas and a monoclonal anti-Fd portion of mouse IgG. Nature 277: 131–133

134. Bankert R B, DesSoye D, Powers L 1980 Antigen-promoted cell fusion: antigen-coated myeloma cells fuse with antigen-reactive spleen cells. Transplantation Proceedings 12: 443–446

135. Moretta A, Pantaleo G, Moretta L, Cerottini J-C, Mingari M C 1983 Direct demonstration of the clonogenic potential of every human peripheral blood T cell. Journal of Experimental Medicine 157: 743–754

5

Immunofluorescence studies in leukaemia diagnosis

G. Janossy F. J. Bollum D. Campana

INTRODUCTION

The technical aspects of the newly emerging branch of cellular immunohaematology have been summarized in a previous volume of 'Methods in Haematology'[1]. Since the publication of the 'Leukaemic Cell', edited by D Catovsky in 1980–81, major advances have been made. During the late 70's and early 80's flow cytometry and fluorescence activated cell analysers were introduced for leukaemia studies[2,3] (see Ch.6) and conventional antisera were also established for the differential diagnosis of lymphoid leukaemia groups[4-7]. Around 1981 the first set of monoclonal antibodies (Mc Abs) was produced and was included in a technical summary of current developments[1]. At that time the Leukaemia Marker conferences[8] and WHO sponsored committees[9] deemed the following reagents to be as important in this area: (a) anti-ALL antiserum reacting with the common acute lymphoblastic leukaemia (cALL) antigen (MW 100 kd[10, 11]); (b) antisera to common core determinants of HLA-DR (Ia-like, p28,33) molecules[5,12-14]; (c) anti-T-cell reagents (anti-HuTLA)[15]; and (d) anti-immunoglobulin antisera[16,17]. At that time (e) anti-myeloid antisera could be successfully produced only in a handful of laboratories[18-20]. The newly arrived Mc Abs were being tested in combinations with the appropriately absorbed conventional reagents. While most of these antibodies were directed against membrane associated cell surface molecules, (f) one particular antiserum, made against a highly purified nuclear enzyme, terminal deoxynucleotidyl transferase (rabbit anti-TdT) complemented these reagents [21,22], and helped elucidate the 'normal equivalent' cells in the common form of ALL[23] as well as in the thymic variant of ALL (T-ALL[24,25]). The normal cells involved in many B-cell malignancies[26] still remained mysterious[27]. The main concepts of cellular immuno-haematology were however already accepted and used in clinical investigations[28].

Recent developments have not changed these ideas about leukaemia classification and origin, but rather dramatically expanded the volume of results and provided further confirmation as well as easier and more precise 'tools' for this area of research.

During the last 4 years further technical achievements have included (a) the wider introduction of new fluorescent dyes, such as Texas red and, more recently, phycoerythrin (PE)[29,30] (Ch.6); (b) the introduction of the immuno-gold method at both light and electron microscopic level[31]; (c) the development of very sensitive cytochemical methods, such as the immuno-alkaline phosphatase staining[32] (Ch.7), and the extension of all these techniques for analysing bone marrow trephine biopsies[33,34.]

Clearly, with such an arsenal of exciting methods available, the introduction of Mc Abs as essential diagnostic tools has progressed rapidly. It is also evident, however, that during these 'introductory' years in most laboratories the standardization of very large numbers of fully or partially characterized new reagents, and not merely the immuno-diagnosis of leukaemia, was the primary aim. In this situation the use of expanding 'panels' of Mc Abs has been inevitable. This sequence of events may create the impression that the immunodiagnosis of leukaemia will remain a field requiring the use of many antibodies in each case of disease. Nevertheless, new data, partly summarized in this communication, shows that there are a handful of 'winners' among the antibody panels. These special reagents acquire clinical roles on the basis of four criteria: (a) examples of these antibodies are reproducibly made in a number of laboratories, and available from the major immunodiagnostic companies; (b) these antibodies show a characteristic reactivity pattern, distinguishing major leukaemia groups; (c) the antibodies react, in most cases, with large proportions of leukaemic blasts, and (d) some of these antibodies might have a therapeutic role, either because of their intrinsic complement fixing capacity or because they are available in conjugated forms as immunotoxins. As expected, very few of these reagents are leukaemia—*specific* (but see ref.[35]), and the constraints on the interpretation of results, which have been developed for heterologous antisera[1,28], are still valid for the mouse and rat Mc reagents. It is likely that in the near future fewer but better 'established' reagents will be used which are known to react with 'familiar' antigens already investigated on thousands of cases of leukaemias. In difficult cases leukaemic populations will be studied with particularly informative combinations of reagents, in order to analyse the variation of antigen expression within the leukaemic clone, and for investigating samples with lower numbers of malignant cells. In this area, immunofluorescence analysis offers a quick reliable technology which is ideally suited for further investigative work with cell sorters.

IMMUNOFLUORESCENCE

The immunohistochemical and immunofluorescent methods represent excellent complementary techniques that should both be available in specialized immunohaematological laboratories, and used according to the clinical questions asked. The special features of immunofluorescence are as follows.

Immunofluorescence is an *extremely* rapid technique, particularly when directly labelled antibodies are used. When the cells are incubated with antibodies at room temperature (in the presence of 0.2% azide) the incubation time is only 5 minutes for each layer, providing that the samples are gently agitated once or twice in order to facilitate the mixing of reagents and cells.

The conjugated fluorochromes fluorescein isothiocyanate (FITC, green), tetra-ethyl-rhodamine isothiocyanate (TRITC, red) and texas red *do not fade* appreciably when simple chemicals are added to the mounting medium to retard the quenching caused by the ultraviolet (UV) light. Many of these chemicals have been described by Johnson et al[36], and p-Phenylene diamine (Cat.No 29500, BDH, Pools, UK) used at 0.1 per cent concentration in a 9:1 mixture of glycerol and phosphate buffered saline (PBS) is a practical formula. Alternatively, mountant media are available from

Citifluor Ltd. The City University, London, UK. A mountant that contains polyvinyl alcohol (PVA) for permanently setting has also been developed[37]. The recipe for the mountant which *sets and retards fading,* developed by Johnson, is as follows: 20 g PVA is dissolved in 80 ml PBS (overnight) and 40 ml glycerol is added. To a 100 ml of this mixture 2.5 g diazabicyclooctane (DABCO) is added and the pH is adjusted to 8.6[38]. Finally, phycoerythrin (PE; which fades quickly with filters for TRITC) can be better observed with filters for FITC when it fades slowly. In order to see the orange colour of PE with FITC filters it is necessary to remove the selective green barrier filter from the epifluorescence reflector housing.

A very important aim in all haematological studies is to obtain information about the phenotype of cells *in addition to cellular morphology.* This can be achieved, most satisfactorily, using the alkaline phosphatase anti-alkaline phosphatase (APAAP) technique (Ch.7). When immunofluorescence is used morphological details can be observed with phase contrast[1,39]. Furthermore, immunofluorescence labelling is compatible with haematoxylin staining without 'blocking' the fluorescence. After having been labelled with FITC and/or TRITC conjugated antibodies the cells are re-fixed in buffered formalin for 30 min and stained for 60 sec in Gill Haematoxylin[40]. The only important point here is that a batch of Haematoxylin free of autofluorescing impurities must be selected from the commercially available batches. Haematoxylin staining is feasible on cell smears as well as tissue sections[33].

The only genuine disadvantage of immunofluorescence methods (as compared to the immuno-histochemical approach) is the necessity to alternate between UV and conventional light.

This problem is considerably eased when the microscope is equipped with an electronically operated shutter system. Such a system is made by Vashaw Scientific Company, Atlanta, Georgia, USA. Rather than manually opening and closing separate shutters for UV and normal light, the electronically operated shutters are synchronously activated by pushing a button. Any one of the possible shutter-release and —closure combinations can be readily programmed on such a device. It is worth noting that on modern fluorescence microscopes or epifluorescence attachments switching between filter sets (fitted into a compact unit, capable of taking four or two sets of filters, respectively), is very simple and can be regarded as a prerequisite of modern immunofluorescence work (see below).

DOUBLE COMBINATIONS OF REAGENTS

When excellent histochemical methods such as the APAAP technique are available, the most important remaining advantage of immunofluorescence (using *single antibodies*) is the speed of investigation. On the other hand, *double-colour* immunofluorescence still has much to offer, because investigation of cells expressing two independent markers can readily be performed with this technique but not with double immunohistochemical techniques. This is because FITC and TRITC are viewed through separate filters, while the various shades of mixed histochemical colours are difficult to judge. (Of course, when the two markers are carried by *different* cells, e.g. during the study of κ and λ light chain expression by plasma cells or B-cells, double immuno-histochemistry with APAAP and immunoperoxidase gives clear results; Ch.7). Thus, it is important to discuss the technical aspects of double immunofluorescence analysis.

Double colour immunofluorescence can be achieved in four different ways: (a) with directly labelled antibodies used as single layers; (b) by using Mc Abs of different (sub)classes together with fluorochrome labelled second layer Abs specific for these; (c) by employing a Mc Ab (and the corresponding fluorochrome labelled second layer such as goat anti-mouse Ig) together with a heterologous antiserum (e.g. goat anti-human IgM for detecting B lymphocytes), and, finally, (d) by applying hapten-labelled Mc Abs together with fluorochrome labelled heterologous antihapten antisera. These combinations are equally useful, and reagents of excellent quality are commercially available. The details of these technical variants are as follows.

Directly labelled antibodies. These are used when the antigens are expressed on the cell surface at a relatively high density. These include Mc Abs to human Ig, HLA-DR and to antigens associated with natural killer (NK) cells and certain T-cell subsets such as T8+ (CD8) cells. Many reagents, directly labelled with FITC, TRITC and more recently with PE[29,30] within the Becton-Dickinson range are suitable for such analysis (Ch. 9). The investigator should be aware of the fact that some leukaemias may show a very weak expression of their characteristic membrane antigen. For example, some cases of chronic lymphocytic leukaemia exhibit only minute amounts of sIg. In other leukaemias, such as the common form of acute lymphoblastic leukaemia (ALL), the intensity of antigen expression (e.g. cALL antigen, MW: 100 kd, CD10) may be extremely variable within the malignant clone. Thus some positive cells might be missed when single layer direct tests are used. These Abs are best suited for analysis on sensitive fluorescence activated cell analysers (FACAs). The FITC- and PE-labelled Abs can be studied by using a single laser. Double colour display with directly labelled Mc Abs provides economical and discriminating technology (Ch. 6). In our laboratory the Mc Abs to the common core determinants of HLA-DR (p28, 33) antigens are very frequently applied as FITC, TRITC or PE conjugates.

Use of different isotypes. Mc Abs selected in pairs on the basis of their *different isotypes (IgM-IgG or IgG_1-IgG_2)* represent a practical application that gives both precision and high intensity. The crucial element here is the availability of (sub)class specific flurorochrome labelled second layers, preferably made in goats (and not in rabbits, because the latter Abs bind well to human Fc-receptors). These reagents need to be absorbed and eluted from sequential immunoadsorbent columns[1,41]. High quality reagents are available from companies such as Southern Biotechnology Associates Inc, (Birmingham, AL), Miles-Yeda, Israel and Meloy, Inc. The flexibility of this technology is demonstrated by the list of some Mc Abs which react with the same antigen but exhibit different (sub)classes and, for this reason, can be selected in various combinations (Table 5.1). This representative selection is compiled mainly from the Mc Ab panel submitted to the Second Workshop on Leukocyte Differentiation Antigens, held in Boston, Sept. 1984. Similar reagents are available from commercial sources. Some of the Abs from the authors' laboratory are also shown since they have been successfully used in (sub)class combinations in both cell suspensions and tissue sections (Fig. 5.1).

Heterologous antibody combinations. Combinations of Abs made *in different*

Table 5.1 The cluster designation and isotype of monoclonal antibodies to human leucocytes*†

	IgM		IgG$_2$		IgG$_1$	
T cell antibodies‡						
CD2 (T11)	9–2	(1)†	OKT11A	(3)	OKT11	(3)
pan-T	7T4	(2)	9.6	(4)	RFT11	(5)
					MT910	(6)
CD3 (T3)	VIT3		OKT3	(3)	UCHT1	(9)
periph.T (mitogenic)	T3/2	(2)	WT31	(8)	Leu-4	(10)
CD4 (T4)	BW264	(11)	OKT4	(3)	Leu-3a	(10)
helper	66.1	(4)	12T4	(2)	MT321	(6)
CD5 (T1)	n.a.		Leu-1	(10)	RFT1	(5)
pan-T + B-CLL			OKT1	(3)	MT215	(6)
CD6 (T12)	T12	(2)				
periph.T (not mitogenic)	RFT12	(5)	12.1	(4)	MT211	(6)
	MBG6	(12)				
CD7	n.a.		3A1	(13)	MT215	(6)
pan-T, strong on blasts			WT1	(8)		
			RFT2	(5)		
CD8 (T8)	RFT8μ	(5)	OKT8	(3)	RFT8γ	(5)
suppressor/cytotoxic			Leu2	(10)	MT415	(6)
Precursor cell associated†						
CD10	VILA1	(7)	J-5	(2)	RFAL1	(5)
common ALL antigen	RFAL3	(5)	RFAL2	(5)		
HLA-DR	RFDR1	(5)	RFDR2	(5)		
non-polymorphic						
B cell antibodies‡						
CD19		(14)	n.a.		B4	(2)
pre-B + B					HD37	(15)
CD20	RFB7	(5)	B1	(2)	—	
pan-B (mitogenic)			2H7	(16)		
CD21	B2	(2)	HB5	(17)	RFB6	(5)
C3d receptor						
CD22	n.a.		SHCL-1	(10)	RFB4	(5)
pan-periph B					To15	(18)
CD23 (B blast antigen)	PL-13	(1)	n.a.		Blast-2	(18)
Unclustered	Y29/55	(19)				

*The majority of monoclonal antibody clusters as defined at the two *Workshops on Leucocyte Differentiation Antigens* in Paris (1982) and Boston (1984) (reacting with the same cell populations and antigens of the same molecular weight and chemical characteristics) contain individual reagents of different isotypes. These antibodies can be used in combinations with (sub)class specific goat anti-mouse IgM, -IgG$_2$ and -IgG$_1$ second layers conjugated with -FITC and -TRITC fluorochromes. Although the Mc ABs shown include many commercially available reagents (such as Ortho, Becton-Dickinson and Coulter) the selection is essentially random and not exhaustive.

†The numbers in brackets refer to the Laboratories where the reagents are made or distributed from. *(1):* Naito & Dupont, New York; *(2):* Reinherz, Nadler, Ritz & Schlossmann (see Coulter range); (3): ORTHO, Raritan; *(4):* Hansen & Martin, Seattle; *(5):* Janossy, London; *(6):* Rieber, Münich; *(7):* Knapp, Vienna; *(8):* Tax, Nigmegen; *(9):* Beverley, London; *(10):* Becton-Dickinson; *(11):* Kurrle, Marburg; *(12):* McMichael, Oxford; *(13):* Haynes, Durham; *(14):* Poncelet, Montpelier; *(15):* Dorken, Heidelberg; *(16):* Clark, Seattle; *(17):* Tedder, Birmingham, AL.: *(18):* Mason, Oxford, *(19):* Forster, Basle.

‡One important conclusion from this Table is that Mc Abs of all three major isotypes are available for most of the T-cell clusters (CD2-CD8), against the common ALL antigen (CD10), and from the B-cell range (CD19-CD23) it is possible to make very strong B-cell cocktails which provide particularly strong staining intensity. The following antibodies may be mixed for this purpose: *IgM* class: RFB7 + B2;*IgG$_2$* subclass: B1 + HB5 + SCHL-1; *IgG$_1$* subclass: B4 + RFB6 + RFB4. Thus selected reagents of different isotypes can be used in combination with each other (e.g. T versus B) as well as any recently prepared Mc Abs detecting accessory cells of the immune system (e.g. follicular dendritic reticulum cells; (see, for example the Boston panel of myeloid reagents and Ch. 10).

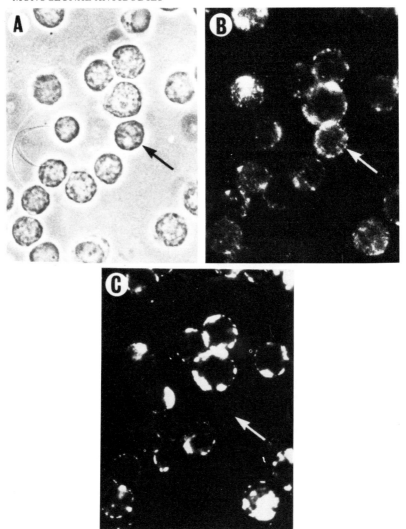

Fig. 5.1 Double staining technique for Abs of different class. The two Abs are B4 (CD19; p 35) from Coulter of IgG class in (B) and RFAL-3 (CD10; p100) of IgM to detect cALL antigen in (C). The second layers, specific for IgG and IgM, are conjugated to FITC and TRITC, respectively, and photographed with selective filters. The arrow points to a cell with is B4$^+$,cALL ag$^-$. (A): phase contrast. The goat anti-M-IgG and —IgM antibodies are from Southern Biotechnology Associates, Birmingham, AL.

species were used in earlier studies when exhaustively absorbed heterologous antisera were combined with the newly provided Mc Abs[14,23,24]. This is still an important combination when the Mc Abs are applied for investigation of the human B-cell subsets and plasma cells which exhibit Ig of different isotypes[42,43]. In essence, the murine Mc Ab bound to the surface or the cytoplasm of cells is visualized with fluorochrome labelled goat anti-mouse Ig, while a goat anti-human Ig isotype antiserum labelled with another fluorochrome identifies the relevant B-cell types upon which the study is focussed. With the help of such reagent combinations, the exact phenotypic profiles of pre-B and B-cell populations of the human bone marrow has recently been established (Fig. 5.2).

Chemically modified antibodies. Probably the most powerful system of double fluorochrome analysis is the use of *biotin-conjugated or hapten-labelled Mc Abs* in conjunction with appropriate fluorochrome labelled second layers. The two most prominent chemical alterations are the conjugation with biotin[44] and arsanilic acid, a hapten[45]. Biotin conjugated Mc Abs are visualized by fluorochrome labelled avidin molecules[46], while Mc Ab-arsanilic conjugates can be labelled by goat anti-arsanilic acid serum. This particular system has special power as the use of double colour fluorescence with *triple layer amplification* is also feasible (Fig. 5.3). The first fluorochrome 'arm' is: Mc Ab conjugated to arsanilic acid (first layer), rabbit anti-arsanilic acid (second layer, available from Becton-Dickinson; Cat. No. 9000) and goat or swine anti-rabbit Ig-FITC or TRITC (third layer, also available from Becton-Dickinson and other firms such as Dakopatt, Copenhagen). None of these layers cross-react with the components of the other arm: biotinated Mc Ab plus fluorochrome labelled avidin (available from Vector Ltd. and Seralab, UK). Streptavidin, a multivalent avidin compound with increased sensitivity[47] is also available in —FITC, —TRITC and —Texas red conjugated forms (Amersham Intern. Ltd UK).

Biotin conjugation

Principle
Biotin succinimide ester (BSE), dissolved in dimethylsulfoxide (DMSO), is conjugated to Mc Abs at pH 8.6[44].

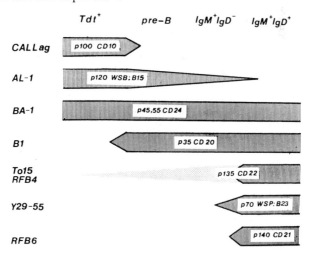

Fig. 5.2 Reactivity of B-cell Mc Abs with 'early' B lineage cells in the normal bone marrow. This figure demonstrates the use of combinations of directly labelled goat anti-human Ig-FITC reagents together with Mc Abs and goat anti-mouse-Ig-TRITC. The cells of IgM⁺ or IgD⁺ isotype in the bone marrow show different phenotypic patterns. The CD numbers refer to the provisional B-cell clusters established at the Boston workshop for Human Leucocyte Differentiation Antigens. WSB: unclustered reagent at the Boston Workshop 1984; WSP: unclustered reagent at the Paris Workshop, 1982. (From ref 42, Journal of Immunology, with permission of publishers.)

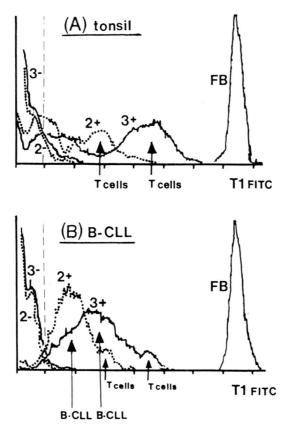

Fig. 5.3 Analysis of the increased sensitivity of fluorescein labelling using triple layers (3+) instead of double layer labelling (2+) on the fluorescence activated cell analyser. Tonsil cells in (A) and chronic lymphoid leukaemia cells in (B) are labelled with the T1 (CD5) T cell associated Mc Ab and goat anti-M-Ig-FITC (2+) as well as with T1 (CD5) —arsanilated Ab plus rabbit anti-arsanilic acid (Becton-Dickinson) and swine anti-rabbit-Ig-FITC (3+). When 3+ is used both the strong labelling on T-cells (in A) and the weak labelling on CLL cells (in B) is amplified fourfold over 2+. FB: fluorescein bead standards. (From ref 81 Journal of Immunology, with permission of publishers.)

Materials

Mc Ab solution (1 mg/ml) in 0.1M NaHCO$_3$ (pH 8.6) containing no azide or other preservative

BSE, dissolved immediately prior to use in DMSO: 1 mg/ml. The BSE is stored at 4°C in a dessicator.

phosphate buffered saline (PBS; pH7) with azide (0.2%)

Method
1. Take 3 samples (1 ml each) of the same Mc Ab solution. Mix these with 30, 60 and 120 μl BSE in DMSO, respectively.
2. Leave at room temperature for 4 hours.
3. Dialyze against PBS with azide overnight at 4°C.

4. Investigate which one of the three samples is the optimal conjugate (with bright staining using avidin FITC second layer) without non-specific fluorescence or loss of Ab activity.

Note. A similar method can be used to conjugate goat anti-mouse Ig second layers with biotin[46].

MONOCLONAL ANTIBODIES TO TERMINAL TRANSFERASE

During 1975 terminal deoxynucleotidyl transferase (TdT), a nuclear enzyme, was purified in sufficient quantities for immunizing rabbits and preparing a highly specific reagent (purified anti-TdT antibodies eluted from TdT-immunoadsorbent column). This reagent has proved to be suitable for immunofluorescence and — histochemical applications[21,22], and is marketed by Supertech, Inc. Bethesda, MD.

Heterologous anti-TdT antisera were made by other commercial companies such as Bethesda Research Labs, Bethesda, MD, and PL Biochemicals, Inc. Most of these antisera are specific for TdT and label only cortical thymocytes and a low proportion (0.1-10%) of cells (non-T, non-B lymphoid-like cells) in the fetal, infant and regenerating bone marrow[1,28] but less than 0.1% lymphoid-like cells in the circulating blood[48] and in the tonsil. These observations are in accord with the results of the biochemical assays for this thymic and bone marrow enzyme[22], and are also echoed in the high TdT levels of thymic ALL and common ALL, respectively[14,22,49]. Some 'anti-TdT' antisera, however, show strong nuclear staining of tonsil lymphocytes as well (for example, ref.[50]) indicating non-specificity. It can be misleading to use these reagent batches for leukaemia diagnosis, as with these reagents some normal lymphoid cells and inflammatory infiltrates would be classified as 'leukaemic'. In our laboratories we regularly test anti-TdT reagents on thymus, bone marrow, blood and tonsil. Commercial batches with extra-thymic and —medullary activities are then discarded. In addition, even the batches of rabbit anti-TdT antisera which are apparently specific for nuclear TdT on the relevant normal and leukaemic cells when used in conventional immuno-fluorescence assays, may show extra activities when applied in more sensitive and slightly different test systems.

Because of the difficulty in obtaining consistent polyclonal anti-TdT it is advantageous to replace rabbit anti-TdT reagents with mouse Mc Abs to TdT. Mouse monoclonals against human TdT have now been prepared[51] and have already been applied to human material (Lanham, et al personal communication). We tested four Mc Abs available from Supertechs, Bethesda, MD, in immunofluorescence and immunohistochemical assays. Mc Abs HTdT-1, —2, —3, and —4 gave clear, moderately strong staining on cortical thymocytes and 3% of bone marrow cells in the samples analysed without showing any detectable activity on normal blood and tonsil lymphocytes (Campana & Janossy, manuscript in preparation). When tested in common ALL, all these Mc Abs gave the expected positive results (Fig. 5.4). HTdT-1 gave the strongest staining (Fig. 5.4a) but, as might be expected, a combination of monoclonals was required (Fig. 5.4d) to produce a staining intensity comparable to the polyclonal rabbit anti-TdT (Fig. 5.4e). It will probably be best to use a mixture of the Mc anti-TdTs for routine staining procedures.

Using immunofluorescence the predominant staining with all monoclonals tested was nuclear, and only traces of cytoplasmic TdT staining could be observed in the leukaemic samples analysed. When the APAAP technique[32] was used in our

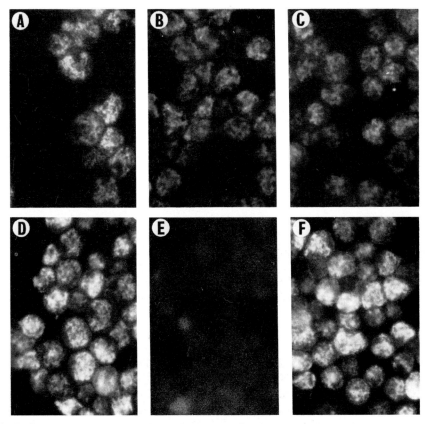

Fig. 5.4 Standardization of immunofluorescent staining with mouse Mc Ab to terminal deoxynucleotidyl transferase (TdT) and goat-anti-mouseIg-FITC (51). The Mc Abs HTdT-1 (A), HTdT-3 (B) and HTdT-4 (C), on their own, give moderately strong staining on cells from a patient with common ALL. When the three Abs (1 + 3 + 4) are mixed the staining intensity on ALL is very strong (D), while on the control case of AML no staining is observed (E). The figure at the lower right corner (F) is the positive control: staining with the rabbit anti-TdT and swine anti-rabbit Ig-FITC. For further details of the Hu anti-TdT Mc Abs see ref 51.

laboratory HTdT-4 (but not HTdT-1, HTdT-2 or HTdT-3) gave distinct cytoplasmic labelling in 6 out of 11 leukaemic samples tested. This is probably due to detection of separate epitopes by the Mc Abs, resulting in the detection of TdT breakdown products or newly-sythesized TdT molecules that might be present in the cytoplasm. The increased sensitivity of immuno-enzymatic methods must be appreciated for appropriate interpretation of these results, and a formal comparative investigation between the new APAAP anti-TdT method and the enzyme levels detectable by biochemical assays is warranted. The IF assays for TdT have been verified by this type of comparative study.[52]

TRIPLE COMBINATIONS OF REAGENTS

Triple marker combinations are difficult to read during diagnostic procedures, but reveal important details in leukaemia and stem cell research when it is desired to detect rare haemopoietic and lymphoid precursor cells in developing fetal and normal tissues. These simple but delicate methods are important for investigating the differentiation linked appearance of antigens detected by newly developed Mc Abs. Although in these studies the markers are used as identity tags, it is preferable to concentrate on antibodies which detect *molecules with known function,* including TdT, immunoglobulin (Ig) and molecules that are part of the T-cell receptor detected by T3-like (CD3) antibodies. It is also clear that some of these studies need to be followed up by double colour cell sorting (Ch. 6) for further functional assessment.

The rationale of these investigations is as follows. Two markers are usually needed to define the position of a single cell within its developmental lineage: (a) One of these is for identifying immature cells. TdT and early antigens such as RFB1[53], 3C5[54] and, under defined conditions, HLA-DR[3,13,28] serve this purpose; (b) The second is the relevant *maturity marker* which includes Ig (first cytoplasmic and later membrane Ig) or the mitogenic B1-like antigen (p35; CD20 in Table 5.1) for the B cell lineage[55], and the mitogenic T3-like antigen (p19,29; CD3 in Table 5.1) for the T-cell lineage. It is interesting to note that T3 is first expressed in the cytoplasm of thymocytes before being detectable in the membrane of T lineage cells (Campana and Janossy; unpublished results). The markers (a) and (b) are mostly expressed on different, i.e. immature and mature cells, respectively, with a minor overlap. TdT+ cytoplasmic μ+ (very rare) cells[23] and TdT+, T3+ thymocytes[56] represent these transitional forms. The question remains then: (c) how the expression of any *third* marker can be mapped into this lineage maturation scheme?

Using this scheme a whole series of Abs can be analysed within both the B and the T lineage[23,53,56,57]. In the myeloid lineage the technique is also, in theory, useful but here there is one major problem. The marker for immaturity in this case should be an antibody reacting with the human pluripotential precursor cells. An optimist might say that such markers already exist and may include RFB1[53], 3C5[54] and My10, described by Civin et al[58] as well as possibly My-9, described by Griffin et al (Ch. 10). But there is as yet no established assay in vitro for human pluripotent immature cells. It is therefore not possible to verify the whole range of the functional activities expressed by the cells reactive with these selected Mc Abs (Ch. 10).

The technical points of these triple assays are as follows. Anti-TdT and anti-Ig and B1(CD20) or T3(CD3) antibodies label structures that are at different sites (in the nucleus versus cytoplasm or membrane) and are also expressed mostly on different cells. One can safely use the same fluorochrome (e.g. FITC) to visualize both antibodies. This is demonstrated in Figure 5.5, taken from the work of Bodger et al[53]. Consequently, the third antibody is used with the other fluorochrome (e.g. TRITC).

A more sophisticated technique is to employ FITC, TRITC and a *third* type of identity tag. Unfortunately, the third, stilbene based blue fluorochrome does not emit strong enough light. The immunogold technique[31] is a better option. This triple technique has recently been described by van Dongen et al[59]. Goat(G) anti-mouse(M) Ig is conjugated with colloidal gold particles of 30 nm (G30). This reagent is available from Janssen Pharmaceutica, Beerse, Belgium. The incubation steps are as follows. The cells are first incubated with Mc Ab, washed and mixed with G-anti-M-Ig-G30. After further washes the free anti-M-Ig binding sites on the G30 are blocked by normal mouse serum. The second Ab, this time *directly* labelled with

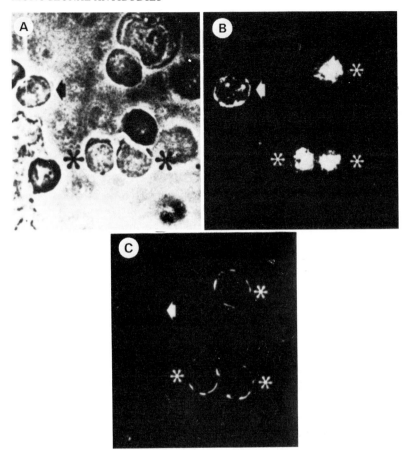

Fig. 5.5 Demonstration of the basic technique for triple-labelling using a marker for 'immaturity': nuclear staining for anti-TdT, together with the marker of 'maturity': membrane staining for anti-IgM on the same FITC channel (b), and labelling with a Mc Ab RFB1 on the TRITC channel (c). (a): phase contrast. Asterisks show the TdT^+, IgM^- immature cells reacting with RFB1 Ab, and arrow points to the TdT^-, IgM^+ mature B-cells unreactive with RFB1. (From ref 61 Blood, with permission of publishers.)

TRITC (anti-Ig or anti-HLA-DR or anti-T), is added. Finally, smears are made in a cytocentrifuge and stained for nuclear (e.g. TdT) or cytoplasmic antigens with FITC-labelled reagents. In these studies the double-colour epifluorescence attachment is complemented with a third compact unit which works according to the same Ploem's principle but emits polarized light instead of fluorescence. In this particular unit designed for polarized light: the first filter is a polarizer for the excitation light, followed by a beam splitter and analyzer filter. The latter extinguishes reflected light which still has the same polarization as the excitation beam[31].

With the triple marker combinations the 'normal equivalent' cells of common ALL[23,28] and thymic (or T-) ALL[24] have been found. The methods have also been used to dissect the development of B-lineage cells in the human fetus[57,61,62] (see Fig. 5.5) and in the normal bone marrow (reviewed in Fig. 5.2). More recently van

Dongen et al[60] have presented their observations that rare TdT+ cells are seen in the bone marrow of patients undergoing maintenance therapy for other diseases than T-ALL. Some of the rare TdT+ cells express HLA-DR antigens together with the 3A1-like (CD7; WT1 or RFT2) antigen. The latter is an interesting antibody which almost invariably reacts with >99% of blast cells in T-ALL (see below). Further cell separation and functional studies will be necessary to prove the hypothesis that these rare cells include human prothymocytes, a rather elusive population of cells.

IMMUNODIAGNOSIS OF LEUKAEMIA

With the variety of available techniques it is not easy to find an universally optimal method for immunodiagnosis. Also, the number of samples received and the degree of instrumentation (including computerization) of the laboratory are modifying factors. The basic possibilities are: microscopic analysis with immunofluorescence or immuno-histochemistry (Ch. 7) and flow cytometery on fluorescence activated analysers (Ch. 6). In our laboratory all three methods are used but in a complementary fashion. Here an economical version of the immunofluorescence analysis is described with the following consideration in mind. Many samples arrive for immunological studies because they represent a clinical problem for an experienced haematologist. These samples may contain only a small proportion of malignant cells. A single run of routine immunological investigation may not give the full answer immediately. On the contrary, it is best to plan a rapid first phase of investigation, with the knowledge that an additional specially designed second study with reagents selected from a much larger pool of antibodies may be required. The method described here is regarded as a convenient *first round.* Depending on the results obtained the investigation may need more detailed morphological study (with the help of immuno-histochemistry) or 'spread' into the area of quantitative flow cytometry and cell sorting (with the help of a cell sorter, assisted by a powerful computer).

A RAPID MICROPLATE METHOD

Principle
Five elements contribute to the economy of this test: (a) microplates with U-wells are used to provide a vehicle simulaneously staining and washing 96 samples[63]; (b) Antibody panels are constructed as multiples of six tests, and Titertek multipipettes are employed to handle six reagents and six samples simultaneously. These samples are transferred onto slides, for viewing, in a pre-arranged pattern of 2 × 6; (c) Large thin coverslips or, alternatively, 12-well multitest slides, after having been coated with *poly-L-lysine*[64], receive the 12 droplets of cells. The cells attach to the coated surface whilst preserving their membrane integrity; (d) We have two choices: one is to view the labelled and attached cells, very rapidly, on an *inverted microscope;* the other is to fix the 12 spots of cells onto the coverslip or onto a 12-well multitest slide in formalin vapour and allow to dry. After preparing a conventionally mounted sample, the cells can be viewed on a standard microscope. In both instances identical

epifluorescence attachments and lenses (bright 63 × Phaco objectives with numerical apertures 1.3) are used and there is no compromise on optical quality; (e) Depending on the results, it is possible (i) to *re-stain* the residual cells left in the microplate wells with directly labelled second Ab (e.g. anti-HLA-DR) in order to see individual results more precisely with double staining; (ii) to prepare cytospins from selected microwells and stain these with anti-TdT, etc; (iii) to analyse cells from selected microwells on the cell sorter.

Equipment

1. Microplate carriers (MSE; Cat. No. 41159-1900) and centrifuge (Mistral 3000, MSE; Cat. No. 41151-3058)

2. Microscopes, inverted and/or normal version with epiillumination, filter sets for FITC and TRITC, phase contrast condenser and objective 63 Phaco N.A. 1.3

Materials

Microplates with U-bottom wells (Sterilin; Cat. No. M24A)

Plate shaker (Dynatech; Cat. No. AM69)

Adhesive microplate cover (Flow Labs. Cat. No. 77-400-05)

Plastic stoppers for individual wells (e.g. from Pierce & Warriner Ltd)

Titertek 8-fold multi-pipettes: 5-50 μl (Cat. No. 77-858-00); 50-200 μl (Cat. No. 77-869-00; both from Flow Labs.), together with trays for solutions; also tips in unlimited quantity, changed after each operation. Note that only 6 out of the 8 chanels of the Titertek pipettes are used.

Microplates with V-bottomed wells (in order to contain the reagents in a pre-established order).

Repette repeating dispensers, 2 ml total volume with teflon piston (Jencons Scientific; Cat. No. H9/255/22) for rapid repeated delivery of 50 μl cell suspensions

Racks for holding 12-24 large coverslips (22 × 64 mm, only slightly smaller than normal slides)

Alternatively 12-well multitest Slides (Flow Labs. Cat. No. 60-412-05)

Moisture chambers with small edges to hold coverslips

Coverslip holders fitted onto the stage of inverted microscope

PBS with 0.2% bovine serum albumin and 0.2% sodium azide

Solution of poly-L-lysine, 1mg/ml in distilled water (MW: 15-30 000, Sigma; Cat. No. P7890)

Formalin vapour (40% formaldehyde in a tight moist chamber)

Permanent mountant: 20 g poly-vinylalcohol in a 80 ml PBS + 40 ml glycerol containing 3 g diaza-bicyclooctane (DABCO), pH 8.6[42];

or semipermanent mountant: PBS and glycerol in 1:1 ratio.

Method

1. Preparation of poly-L-lysine coated coverslips: load a few dozens of coverslips into racks and dip the individual racks into poly-L-lysine solution. Leave the coverslips in a horizontal position for 15-30 minutes in a moist chamber and wash the slips briefly in PBS. Keep the dried coated slides wrapped in clingfilm at 4°C until use.

2. Leukaemia analysis: remove red blood cells and granulocytes on a Ficoll-Isopaque gradient. Adjust the concentration of cell suspension to $2-4 \times 10^6$ cells/ml. Distribute 50 μl of this cell suspension from each patient into 12 microwells of a U-bottom plate using a repeating dispenser.

3. Add 50 μl of Mc Abs appropriately diluted in PBSA containing 0.2% azide. Deliver the reagents with the Titertek multi-pipette. These reagents are taken from the V bottomed microplates. Multiple rows of reagents are prepared at the beginning of each week in sufficient amount and in the correct concentration in order to cover the laboratory's requirement for that week (see below). After adding the reagents cover the plates carefully with an adhesive sheet in order to seal all wells. Shake the plate gently while incubating it for 10 min at 20°C.

4. Top up the microwells with 100 μl PBSA (using Titertek pipette) and spin the plate for 30 sec at 1500 r.p.m. Remove supernatant with quick gentle inversion of the plate. Resuspend gently on a plate shaker and add 150 μl cold PBSA. Wash cells 4 ×.

5. Add 50 μl goat anti-mouse-Ig-FITC (with 0.2% azide) at appropriate dilution (after having established this at the beginning of the week). Incubate for 10 min at 20°C.

6. Spin and wash plate as in 4. After the final wash, add 5-6 μl PBSA plus azide to the small pellet with Titertek, and transfer approximately 2 μl of the concentrated cells (i.e. about one third of cell suspension) onto the poly-L-lysine coated coverslip. Transfer two rows of 6 samples: 12 samples for each patient. In the meanwhile cover the microplate again with adhesive sheet and place it onto ice.

7. Place the coverslips with the 12 little droplets into their carrier on the stage of the inverted microscope. These can be viewed almost immediately with UV light and phase contrast, as the cells sediment and attach to the coated coverslips.

8. If the evaluation of 12 samples cannot be completed within 20-25 min (before the droplets dry out), the cells in the droplets can be fixed to the coverslip in formalin vapour. After 5 min the coverslip is removed and let dry at 20°C (10-15 min). Then it is turned over with the cells facing downwards and mounted on a slide either as a permanent preparation using PVA or as a semi-permanent sample using 1:1 mix of PBS and glycerol as a mountant. These slides are viewed on a conventional UV epifluorescence microscope. An alternative is to put the 2 × 6 samples on 12-well multitest slides, fix in formalin, dry and study on a conventional UV microscope.

9. Two-thirds of each sample is still in the microplate. After recording the first results, cytospin preparations are made from selected wells for nuclear TdT staining with TRITC conjugated reagents (see above).

10. If the results are difficult to interpret (e.g. due to low proportions of leukaemic blasts) the samples in the wells are incubated with 5% mouse serum (in order to saturate cell-bound goat anti-mouse Ig activity) and then double stained for strong membrane antigens such as HLA-DR, IgM, etc. In this case a new coverslip with a set of a further 12, this time double-labelled, droplets is made and viewed with two colour filter sets.

The most relevant antibodies

The technique described above is rapid and versatile enough, so that after having learned the results from the first with 12 reagents, further investigations can be performed on the same day. The first set of reagents is essentially a 'safe' panel of antibodies including the best standardized diagnostic reagents (Table 5.2). These are arbitrarily classified as (a) *stem cell-associated;* (b) *myeloid;* (c) *common ALL-* and *B-lineage-* associated and; finally (d) T-lineage-related. These terms are merely convenient phrases to describe the most obvious reactivity patterns shown in more detail in Table 5.2.

(a) The characteristics of individual reagents are as follows: the *stem-cell related* ABs such as 3C5 [54] and anti-HLA-DR are found on immature cells without discriminating between acute myeloid (AML) and the common form of acute lymphoid leukaemias (cALL). Large numbers of positive cells in a sample immediately indicates a preponderance of 'immature' leukaemic cells. In addition, as documented before[1,5,13,14], anti-HLA-DR is reactive with B-cell disorders. Rare leukaemias of activated peripheral TdT-negative T cells can also be HLA-DR+[14]. The characteristics of *pluripotent* stem cells, in man, are unknown (see above) and in this respect the reactivities of 3C5 and anti-HLA-DR (just as any other reagents) are still enigmatic[65]. Another reagent, RFB1 was also used previously for identifying 'immature' cells[53]. This anti-[thymocyte plus myeloid] antibody is however not used routinely because B-chronic lymphocytic leukaemias (B-CLL, but curiously not pre-B ALL) were also found to be RFB1 positive[66].

(b) The two *myeloid* antibodies which may be included in the first screening range are My9 and Mo2 (both available from Coulter). These Abs have been described by Griffin et al[67]; (see Ch. 10). The former is the single reagent with the highest percentage reactivity on AML[67], although only 70-90% of all cases of AML are positive[68]. Mo-2 indicates monocytic differentiation within the myeloid leukaemia[67]. Amongst the antibodies tested at the Second Workshop on Human Differentiation Antigens in Boston no additional reagent cluster has emerged which would react predominantly with myeloblasts (but see below for clusters reacting with mature myeloid and megakaryocytic cells).

(c) There are four groups of antibodies within the *common ALL-B cell* associated category. The widest 'cover' from early precursors through cALL+,TdT+ cells to B-lymphocytes is provided by the CD19 cluster of antibodies, with the B4 and Leu-12 Abs as prominent representatives[30,69]. These Abs, available from Coulter and Becton-Dickinson, are reactive with an antigen of 95 kd which is expressed even on 'null' ALL cases which do not express the cALL[81] (p100, CD10) antigen. B4 is negative with AML blasts. A further important group of antibodies is the CD10 cluster. These reagents include Abs to the common ALL Ag (cALL; 100 kd). The first in this group was J-5 (IgG2 class) made by Ritz et al[70]. This Ab, now available from Coulter, was soon followed by VIL-A1 Ab of IgM class[71] and a series of very robust rat anti-cALL Abs including AL-2 and AL-3[72]. Many other similar reagents are available (see e.g. Table 1 for a set of Abs with different (sub) classes). The next group includes reagents with strong anti-B cell reactivity (without reacting with cALL+ cells). This is the CD20 cluster of Abs, with an antigen of 35 kd. The B1 antibody available from Coulter is an excellent representative of this group[73]. In our laboratory we use, for the same purpose, a 'cocktail' of two anti-B Abs: one pan-B RFB7 (35 kd; CD20) together with RFB4 Ab (CD22 cluster). Our rationale for using the cocktail is that it permits the identification of B-cells in *both* suspension and tissue sections of bone marrow biopsies (see below) as well as in lymph node biopsies[33]. As shown in Table 5.2 the most conventional B-cell marker completes this range: this is Mc Ab to IgM (e.g. those available from Unipath).

(d) Finally, a few *T-cell associated* markers are included. In the field of acute leukaemia diagnosis one of the most prominent group of reagents is the CD7 Ab group detecting an antigen of 40 kd. This group includes 3A1, described by Haines[74] and WT1 characterized by Tax et al[75] and RFT2[76]. The Becton-Dickinson equivalent is Leu-9[30] and is included in ORTHO range as OKT16. These Abs react strongly with T-blasts and are positive in virtually all cases of T-ALL, including those which are negative with sheep erythrocyte rosetting and the corresponding T11-like CD2 antibodies[77]. On the other hand, virtually all cases of common ALL are CD7-ve. It is interesting to note that CD7 Abs show reactivity with some cases of AML[74,77]. The next two reagents used in our laboratory are the T-cell specific CD2 (T11-like) and CD3 (T3-like) Abs. These are powerful pan-T reagent. In our hands, the question whether T-leukaemias show the phenotype of thymic (CD2+, CD3- or ±) or peripheral T-cells (CD2+,CD3+) is decided by these cells' TdT positivity (thymic) or negativity (peripheral T) rather than by the membrane reactivity pattern with T-cell associated Abs. As pointed out above, samples pre-stained with FITC using the *first round reagents* can be selected for double staining with anti-TdT plus TRITC labelled second layer Abs. When the suspicion of a T cell disorder is raised, the CD7 and CD2+CD3 stained samples are certainly amongst those doubly labelled for TdT. The last reagent, CD5 (OKT1, Leu-1, T101-like), is an interesting one. This particular Ab recognizes an antigen of 65k. This is expressed on thymocytes (and T-ALL) weakly, T-cells strongly and on typical B-CLL cells weakly[78,79]. Thus, among B-cell malignancies, this Ab is, paradoxically, a convenient marker for B-CLL, and suitable for establishing the diagnosis at a very early stage of the disease (i.e. in the differential diagnosis of lymphocytosis *versus* B-CLL). The CD5+ B cells are also seen in centrocytic lymphomas[80], which may spill over to the blood. The normal equivalents of these peculiar CD5+(T1+) B-cells are found in the fetal lymph nodes within the primary nodules of the fetal lymph nodes[62] and the fetal spleen[81].

As the reactivity pattern with the first 12 antibodies emerge, further tests might be required. These are largely dependent upon the location of the laboratory (i.e. leukaemia centre, general hospital or pediatric oncology group, etc.). An immediate task is double staining for TdT. Table 5.2 shows some of the expected patterns of reactivity in leukaemias. In cases of non-lymphoid HLA-DR positive stem-cell associated disorders additional myeloid reagents might be studied, as discussed in chapter 10. If the HLA-DR reagent is negative, erythroid and megakaryocytic leukaemias are among the definite possibilities, and, indeed, some megakaryocytic leukaemias may masquerade in the form of ALL[82]. In the Boston Workshop clusters of antibodies emerged that react with mature granulocytic cells (CD11) and with megakaryocytes and platelets (CD12). Useful panels of anti-myeloid Abs have also been worked out by Knapp et al[83] and Griffin et al[68] (see also Ch. 10). The latter is available through Coulter.

If the diagnosis of cALL is made, three further Abs are of interest. The Mc Abs BA2 (CD9) and BA1 (CD24) indicate further heterogeneity within the cALL group[84], and staining for cytoplasmic Ig heavy chain should precisely map the block of differentiation.

The diagnosis of B-cell malignancy would not be complete without assessing the

Table 5.2 Diagnostic reagents in leukaemia ('first round')[a]

Ab (feature)	MW	cALL	AML	T-ALL	peripheral T leukaemia	B-NHL	B-CLL	ref.
stem cell associated								
1. 3C5		+	+	–	–	–	–	54, 58
2. Class II anti-HLA-DR	28,33k	+	+(–)[b]	–	–	+	+	1, 5, 7,13, 14
myeloid								
3. My9		–	+	–	–	–	–	67
4. Mo2		–	some +	–	–	–	–	67
common ALL and B								
5. CD19 ('B4-like')	95k	+	–	–(±)[c]	–	+	+	69, 81
6. CD10 (cALLag)	100k	+	–		–	–	–	2, 10, 11, 70–72, 107
7. CD20 ('B1-like')	35k	–	–	–	–	+	+	73
or B cocktail (RFB7 + CD22)								42
8. anti-IgM		–	–	–	–	+	+	1, 16, 17
T cell associated								
9. CD7 (3A1, WT1, RFT2)	40k	–	–(±)[d]	+	+ or –[e]	–	–	30, 74–77
10. CD2 (T11-like)	50k	–	–	+	+	–	–	30, 118
11. CD3 (T3-like)	19–29k	–	–	–[f]	+	–	–	105,118
12. CD5 (T1-like)	65k	–	–	+	+[g]	–	+[h]	78, 80, 81, 105, 118
TdT		+	–	+	–	–	–	1, 21, 57

[a] Used in a microplate assay system. On the basis of the results additional Abs are used for further analysis (see text).

[b] AML-s are heterogeneous in terms of HLA-DR expression[5, 13, 14].

[c] A few T-ALL blasts weakly express cALL antigen[28, 107].

[d] Some AML-s carry p40 antigen[74, 77].

[e] Sezary cells are p40 negative[88].

[f] A few T-ALL cases are weakly CD3 (T3) positive and also express T3 cytoplasmically.

[g] T-CLL is frequently CD5 (T1) negative[86].

[h] See text.

intensity of IgM staining (low in CLL and high in prolymphocytic. leukaemia). The monoclonality test for κ or λ light chain expression is an immediate task, and the expression of Ig isotypes (μ, δ, γ, α, ϵ) may also be important. Finally, it should be appreciated that plasma cell disorders may be detected by anti-plasma cell Abs such as PCA1[85] from Coulter and express only cytoplasmic Ig. Hence the need for restaining samples in cytospin preparations with the anti-Ig isotype panel.

In the case of T-cell malignancies and immuno-regulatory disorders[86] the Abs included in the clusters established in Paris and Boston (CD2-CD8 in Table 5.1) are the obvious choice. This panel should also include Abs to T-activation antigens, such as IL-2 receptor detected by the Tac antibody[87]. The cluster designation of this reagent is CD25 (available commercially from Becton-Dickinson). It is interesting to note that CD7, strongly positive with T-ALL is frequently unreactive with T-cells in Sezary syndrome[88]. Chronic disorders, e.g. those with the CD8(T8)+, CD5(T1)-phenotype frequently progress slowly and may represent, at least in a sizeable proportion of cases non-malignant immunoregulatory disorders rather than frank malignancies[86]. One must be extremely careful not to confuse *true monoclonality* (as established on the ground of κ and λ testing in cases of B/plasma cell malignancies) with the observation of *shifted T4/T8 ratios,* which may represent an immunoregulatory disorder as well as an expansion of a single clone of T-cells that may be malignant[86].

DETECTION OF RESIDUAL LEUKAEMIC CELLS

For the detection of minimal disease large numbers of cells have to be screened, and it has been claimed that fluorescence activated cell analysis (FACA) is particularly suitable[89] for this analysis. Modern flow cytometry is very rapid and important parameters related to the cells' size and granularity such as forward angle and 90° scatter profiles and fluorescence intensity of single cells are recorded. The background noise is, however, fairly high (0.5-1%). Without additional corroborating evidence from another independent antibody in a double colour system, or without a positive sort of the suspicious rare cells — followed by the scrutiny of these cells' morphological features, the identification of low count residual leukaemia can be risky. By contrast, microscope analysis during immunofluorescence work is performed in conjunction with the assessment of phase contrast morphology. With the APAAP method the reactivity of Mc Abs together with light microscopical analysis is possible. When the tumour cell contamination is low, morphological and immunological analysis of the samples are performed on whole cytospin preparations, which contain at least 10 000 cells. (Normally one cytospin has 25-30 000 cells). If the marker is strong, 100 fields containing 100-200 cells each, can be studied reasonably quickly. Thus these observations can be performed on fairly large numbers of cells. It is essential to formally compare the sensitivity of flow cytometry and microscopy by controlled dilution experiments.

The discussion here is only concerned with the technical aspects of detecting small numbers of antibody reacting cells. Whether this technology can be used, and under what conditions, for identifying leukaemia-associated changes will be discussed below. Here we simply select a favourable situation for analysis. Bradstock et al[24,25] have demonstrated that the blast cells in T-ALL reflect the features of thymocytes, which normally do not circulate and are absent in peripheral lymphoid tissues and

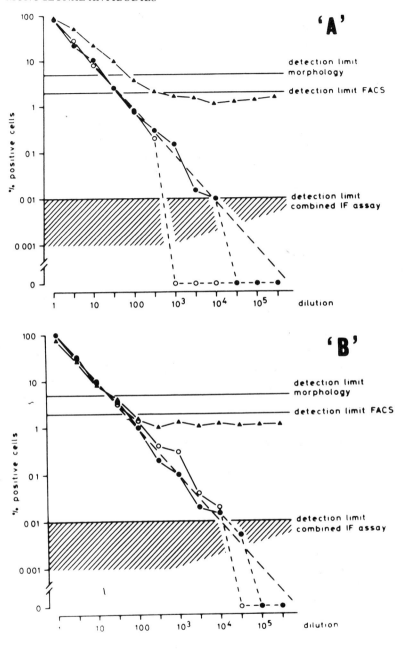

Fig. 5.6 Sensitivity of fluorescence activated cell analysis and the immunofluorescence test performed on the microscope. Thymocytes ('A') and non-Hodgkin lymphomas cells of convoluted T type ('B') were labelled for T6 cortical thymocyte antigen and analysed on FACA (▲) and on the microscope (●, ○). The samples (▲) and (○) are suspension preparations. The samples (●) were spun in a cytocentrifuge and double labelled for T6 and TdT. The samples represent artificial mixtures of thymocytes ('A') and T-NHL cells ('B') diluted with normal peripheral blood cells in the ratios shown. (From ref 90 with permission of publishers.)

bone marrow. Cells with thymic features that appear in patients who have been treated for T-ALL are likely to be residual or relapsing malignant cells. This is therefore a model system for investigating the sensitivity of fluorescence activated cell analysis *versus* the fluorescence microscope.

Two types of experiments were conducted by van Dongen and his colleagues using cortical thymocytes, and malignant cells of T-ALL type[90]. The latter were from a case of convoluted T-cell non-Hodgkin lymphoma (T-NHL) with general dissemination and positivity for T6 (CD1) cortical thymocyte antigen. These cells were mixed with mononuclear blood cells of a normal healthy donor, that in normal individuals contain no T6 (CD1) cells. The thymocytes and NHL cells were identified by counting the numbers of cells exhibiting T6. The results show that with the cell sorter the detection limits of both the cortical thymocytes and the NHL cells of thymic type were in the range of 1-2%. The reason for this is that the instrument used regularly recorded a non-specific noise around this level. Microscopic study of cell suspensions was capable of reliably detecting 0.1% tumour load in this particular type of disorder, and <1% cortical thymocytes.

The result of the microscopical analysis is reasonable but can be improved still further if a second marker for 'lymphoid immaturity' such as nuclear TdT, is used in combination with T6-like Ab. This is now an unfair comparison with cell sorter analysis, because since the early studies by McCaffrey[91] anti-TdT staining has not been reliably performed on suspensions of cells, and this valuable extra parameter cannot be analysed by flow cytometry with current techniques. The detection limits of NHL cells and cortical thymocytes with the combined assay on the microscope are below the 0.01% level (Fig. 5.6). In other words, a single malignant cell per cytospin preparation can be picked out if the scientist is industrious enough to take the time for scanning. Essentially similar observations were reached by analysis for rare tumour cells in bone marrow and exudate fluids when the APAAP technique is applied for analysing carcinoma associated antigens such as cytokeratin or reactivity with anti-milk fat globule Mc Abs (Ch. 7).

The sensitivity of this analysis puts the question of 'normality' into sharp focus. In the first studies a heterologous anti-human T-cell antiserum (anti-HuTLA) was used to establish that cells of cortical thymocyte phenotype (TdT+, HuTLA+) were absent outside the human thymus[24]. Similar findings were made with the monoclonal T6(CD1) plus anti-TdT combination. No doubles were recorded in the bone marrow, blood, tonsil and cerebrospinal fluid[24,25,92]. The fact that only T-cells of medullary type, but not those of cortical type, migrate out from the thymus has also been confirmed in animal experiments[93]. Nevertheless, there have been reports of the presence of T6+ cells in the blood, particularly after bone marrow transplantation[94], and also in the bone marrow. When this question was re-investigated using T6/TdT double staining, these rare T6+ bone marrow cells have been found to be TdT-negative[95], and are therefore not typical thymocytes. The T6+ cells in cord blood and in the blood after bone marrow transplants are also mostly TdT-negative[96].

During these studies it has become obvious that the T6(CD1) antigen is not a very reliable marker for T-ALL blasts[24]. Recently a clinically more useful antibody was found to replace the rabbit-HuTLA. These are the reagents in the CD7 (p40) group, including antibodies such as 3A1[74], WT1[75] and RFT2[76], Leu-9[30] and 4A[36]. These Abs are almost invariably positive with T-ALL cases (>95% of patients in this group) and

>98% of blasts are reactive. Tax et al[75] have shown that strongly WT1+(CD7+),TdT+ large blasts are present in the infant thymus and may represent the normal cell equivalent of T-ALL. No CD7+, TdT+ doubles were found in the bone marrow or in the circulation, in samples taken from normal bone marrow donors or from patients with regenerating bone marrow off chemotherapy[75]. More recently, van Dongen et al[60] reinvestigated this question and confirmed the findings by Tax et al[75], and made two additional observations: in the bone marrow of eight patients on maintenance therapy *for non-T malignancy* (but, curiously, not in the samples off maintenance therapy) extremely few (0.01-0.13% of all nucleated cells) CD7+,TdT+ cells were seen. The frequency of these doubles in healthy adult volunteers was as low as 0.001-0.006%. The second finding is that these CD7+,TdT+ cells are peculiar, because they carry HLA-DR antigens[59], while typical CD7+,TdT+ cells in the thymus (as well as T-ALL blasts) are HLA-DR-negative. The simplest explanation is therefore that these exquisitely rare cells are prothymocytes or their close relatives[60].

The conclusions are two-fold: (a)the methods shown are very sensitive for finding rare cells, and with the improving quality of Abs and second layers this technology is becoming more accessible; (b)The CD7+,TdT+ combination is not leukaemia specific at a single cell level, but these cells are normally so rare that in the bone marrow they always constitute <10% of all TdT+ cells present, the remainder being the TdT+,cALL+ putative pre-B-cell precursor population[1,23]. Thus, if the percentage of CD7+TdT+ doubles within the TdT+ pool is >20%, the suspicion of residual T-ALL disease arises. These detection limits are more sensitive than conventional morphology and flow cytometry.

The final comment is in regard to early TdT+ precursors in fetal liver and the bone marrow. These represent large proportions of the lymphoid and lymphocyte-like cells present[61,81] and are believed to be pre-B-cell precursors showing an identical phenotype to common ALL: TdT+, HLA-DR+, CD10(cALL)+, CD9(BA-2)+, CD24(BA-1)+, RFB-1+, CD19(B4)+[53,57,81,84]. In previous studies it was emphasized that these cells are almost totally restricted to the bone marrow[23,28]. For that reason, as has been pointed out, the TdT test is not suitable for predicting relapse in the marrow, but on the other hand, it might be used to identify leukaemia at an extramedullary site, such as the cerebrospinal fluid, blood and testis[92,98]. Recent studies by Froehlich et al[48] and van Dongen et al[90] have established that very rare normal TdT+ cells are present in the circulation, but the percentage is always lower than 0.2% of mononuclear cells. TdT+ cells above this limit in the blood suggest leukaemic involvement. The conclusion is less clear in the study of the cerebrospinal fluid from 35 patients studied in full remission. Three samples had low (<0.2% TdT+ contamination, and none of these patients relapsed during the 6 month follow-up period[90]. These cells could have been normal cells, and the results, although preliminary, seem to suggest that a single TdT+ cell in the body fluids is not necessarily an indication for drastic medical intervention.

ELIMINATION OF 'UNWANTED' CELLS

One of the first therapeutic applications where Mc Abs may play a prominent part is the elimination of unwanted cells (e.g. residual leukaemic cells or T-lymphocytes) from the bone marrow during bone marrow transplantation. This procedure is referred to in the press as *'purging'*, *'cleansing'* or *'laundering'*. In order to use efficiently the various Abs for purging, three conditions have to be met: (a) the method of purging must be *simple*. A number of groups perform autologous bone marrow transplants without purging[99], and only simple techniques will persuade most groups to perform controlled investigations in sufficiently large numbers of patients to establish whether the purging is necessary and beneficial; (b) There is a need to analyse which antibodies perform well and under which particular condition(s). Here methods are needed that are sufficiently *sensitive* and capable of identifying as low as 0.01-0.1% residual cells. Finally, (c) it is a great advantage if the assay system is *rapid* and the results are obtained on the same day, e.g. prior to the re-infusion of the donor bone marrow into the recipient patients during the purging of T-lymphocytes. The effects of cytolytic complement are indeed very quick, and phenotypic analysis of the residual populations can be performed together with rapid analysis of cell viability using dye-exclusion tests. Similarly, as pointed out above, combination analysis for membrane Ag and nuclear TdT is particularly suitable for this purpose as a sensitive assay (Fig. 5.6) for analysing the efficacy of single Abs or mixtures for destroying the leukaemic populations of individual patients. This technology is important during preliminary studies for autologous transplantation, because the rapidly obtained but detailed results give a firm indication whether single Abs are capable of providing the expected results or, alternatively, whether combinations of reagents are required for quantitative and total lysis of all leukaemic cells.

ELIMINATION OF LEUKAEMIC CELLS

Two comments are relevant here. Firstly, it is well documented that Mc Abs of IgG_2 class most frequently fix rabbit complement, while those of IgM class are not only able to lyse cells in the presence of rabbit complement, but, in a proportion of cases also work with human complement[100] and can therefore be applied with the patients' own serum. On the other hand, Abs of IgG_1 class are preferred for the purpose of conjugation with toxins or their derivations, such as Ricin-A chain[101]. Secondly, the fraction of the whole leukaemic population from which the disease may regenerate (clonogenic cells) can be very small, while the bulk of the leukaemia present, particularly in the circulating blood, can be a mere collection of irrelevant end-cells on their way to perish. Clearly, the antibodies which bind to and destroy clonogenic cells are of primary importance. The major problem here is that there is no proof to show that a clonogenic assay under artificial in vitro conditions represents the same populations as the precursor cells from which leukaemic clones may grow in the special micro-environments of the bone marrow or at sites of extramedullary relapse. The establishment of relevant assays in vitro may not be impossible. It is already known that the composite environment where normal precursor cells proliferate in the bone marrow shows great similarity to the multi-layered elements of the Dexter-type culture system in vitro [102]. In our view, however, these assays for clonogenic cells will remain difficult for clinical studies, in spite of their immense theoretical interest. There is, however, another way of selecting the most important Abs for purging the leukaemic populations.

It is an attractive hypothesis that the leukaemic clonogenic cells most probably represent the earliest forms identifiable within the lineage[103,104]. Two examples demonstrating this possibility are T-ALL and common ALL. The first studies on the thymic form of ALL demonstrated that HTA-1 (T6-like) antigen (detected by the Abs of the CD1 group) is not fully expressed on large populations of T-ALL blasts[24,105], and is indeed absent on the corresponding normal thymic blast cell populations[24,56,76]. Thus the CD1 Abs, although specific for T-ALL, would not be suitable for purging, because one could even enrich for the T6-negative T-ALL blasts. T11-like (CD2) Abs show a much better cover of T-ALL than T6 (CD1), but a small population of T-ALL blasts (TdT+) and of normal thymic blasts are still T11-negative[27]. On the other hand, reagents in the CD7 group (3A1, WT1, 4A, Leu-9, RFT-2) are positive in the vast majority of T-ALL cases[75,77], as well as with normal thymic blasts[76]. Other observations also indicate that the CD7 marker is on early thymic precursor cells, some of which might be clonogenic. In young embryos around the 9th gestational week, a few days before the thymus becomes lymphoid, CD7-positive cells with no other T-cell associated markers gather around the thymic rudiment[106]. The CD7 reagents are therefore likely to cover the relevant population of thymic precursors, most probably including clonogenic T-ALL blasts as well.

An identical argument can be presented for selecting Abs which react with early B cell types in the common form of ALL. Many cases are effectively covered by Mc Abs to the common ALL (cALL) antigen[107], but its expression can be heterogeneous, with a variable number of cALL-,TdT+,HLA-DR+ blast cells present[108,109]. Particularly in adults, cALL-negative, TdT+ so-called null cases with no detectable cALL+ blast cells are relatively frequently seen[110]. Thus, in addition to CD10 Abs, reactive with the cALL Ag, further reagents are also required. The Abs CD9 (BA-2) and CD24 (BA-1) are amongst these[84], but the most promising ones are the CD19 Abs (e.g. B4) which reliably pick up cALL-negative TdT+ cells in the leukaemic population (Fig. 5.1)[81].

It is interesting to note that putative early cells with clonogenic potential in tests in vitro are also being identified in other diseases such as B-CLL and multiple myelomatosis. The B-cell type relevant in B-CLL has, again, been found during the early stage of development.[62,81]

IMMUNOFLUORESCENT ASSAY FOR TESTING THE EFFICACY OF PURGING IN ALL

Principle

The rapid diagnosis of cALL and T-ALL, using a microplate method, has been described above (Table 5.2). When the range of Mc Abs reacting with the TdT+ leukaemic population is established, a further study for analysing the efficacy of leukaemia cell removal is set up. The cell suspension containing known numbers of TdT+ leukaemic cells is mixed with known numbers of 'inert' cells (HL60, human or chicken erythrocytes: rbc) which are TdT-ve and do not express ALL-associated antigens. The cell mixture is incubated with complement fixing Abs and rabbit or human serum, as a source of cytolytic complement. The 'inert' cells are necessary for two reasons. Without them in high count leukaemia insufficient numbers of cells would be recovered for making a slide, and by counting the ratios of TdT+ and 'inert' cells the exact proportions of residual leukaemia can be estimated. Further details are as follows. The best negative control is the [leukaemic + inert cell] mixture incubated with an irrelevant Mc Ab with complement. The results are evaluated in cytospin preparations after staining for nuclear TdT (FITC; Fig. 5.7, see also above) and for membrane-bound Mc Ab (G-anti-M-Ig-TRITC). The *first result* (the percentage of residual leukaemia resistant to lysis) is obtained as follows: in the sample incubated with the *relevant* antibody and complement the number of TdT+ cells (N1) is counted within an area of 5000 'inert' cells. Then a similar count is made in the sample incubated with the irrelevant Mc Ab and complement (N2). N1/N2 × 100 = % of residual TdT+ cells. The *second result* is the phenotypic analysis of this residual TdT+ population: these cells may have failed to bind the Ab; or might have bound the Ab which, however, was incapable of mediating a cytolytic action through complement activation.

Equipment
   1. Waterbath, 37°C
   2. Bench centrifuge
   3. Fluorescence microscope

Materials
   Sterile suspension of HL60 cell line, human or chicken red cells in 5% BSA.
   Hanks balanced salt solution (with Ca++; HBSS)
   PBS with 0.2% azide (PBS-A)
   Rabbit serum as complement source, previously selected for efficient lysis with Mc Abs (from Pelfreeze, UK representative: Northeast Biomedical Co., Uxbridge), stored at —70°C in small aliquots after only one thawing.
   If required, fresh human serum as complement source.
   Anti-cALL and anti-T-ALL Mc Abs of IgM or IgG_2 class.
   Rabbit anti-TdT antiserum (Supertech. Bethesda, MD, USA) and goat or swine anti-R-Ig-TRITC.
   Goat anti-mouse Ig-FITC.
   Deoxyribonuclease (DNA-ase; Sigma), 100 units/ml stock solution, frozen in small aliquots and diluted 1:10 in HBSS prior to use.
   LP3 tubes (Luckham).

Method
   1. Prepare mononuclear cell suspension on Ficoll-Isopaque from the bone marrow (or if it is not available: from peripheral blood). Wash these cells in HBSS and resuspend at $2×10^7$/ml.
   2. Similarly, wash HL60 or rbc in HBSS and resuspend at $2×10^7$/ml.
   3. Mix 1 and 2, 50μl each in LP3 tube; the number of tubes depends upon the amount of sample available and the number of conditions (individual Abs and their cocktails, worked out according to the results of a prior microplate assay). Negative controls: irrelevant Mc Ab.
   4. Add Mc Abs in excess, 4-10 times the saturation dose in 100 μl HBSS; incubate for 20 min at 20°C.

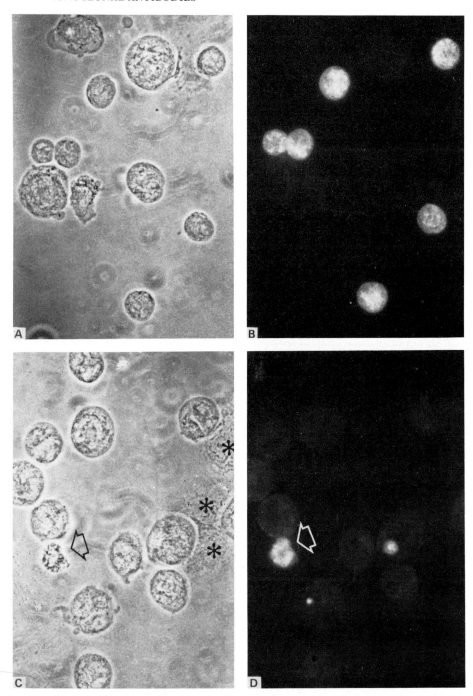

Fig. 5.7 Detection of minimal residual leukaemia in the bone marrow samples after purging with antibody and complement. Leukaemic samples are taken at presentation. Smears are made from pre-incubation samples. The intermediate-sized cells (A) are leukaemia blasts identified by labelling for terminal deoxynucleotidyl transferase (TdT, a nuclear enzyme) in (B). After incubation with anti-common-ALL antibody and complement, the vast majority of TdT$^+$ cells have disintegrated (asterisk) and only one residual damaged TdT$^+$ cell (D) is seen (see the ragged appearance of cells in phase contrast; arrow in (C)).

5. To individual tubes add equal amount (200 μl; 50%) of rabbit complement. Alternatively, add two different doses of human complement: 100 μl (33%) and 50 μl (20% final C' concentration). Cap tubes and incubate at 37°C for 45 min.

6. Add DNA-ase, 10 units in 1 ml to each tube and incubate for a further 10 min at 37°C, followed by two washes in PBS-A containing 0.2% azide.

7. After one wash in HBSS, resuspend in 200 μl and add complement again as in 5.

8. Resuspend the cells in 50 μl PBS-A, add G-anti-M-Ig-FITC, incubate for 10 min (with gentle shaking on ice) and wash twice in PBS-A.

9. Resuspend in 200-250 μl and make at least 5 cytospin preparations. Fix these for 30 min in cold methanol, and stain two of these for nuclear TdT with R-anti-TdT and Sw(or G) anti-R-Ig-TRITC.

10. Stain one further cytospin with May-Grünwald-Giemsa.

11. On the cytospin, count: (a) the number of WBC per 5000 rbc or HL60; (b) the number of TdT+ cells per 5000 rbc or HL60; (c) the number of Mc Ab positive cells within the TdT+ population. Also investigate whether there are: (d) considerable numbers of lymphoblasts, Mc Ab negative and also TdT-negative, or (e) lymphoblasts, Mc Ab positive, TdT-negative.

Note. In our laboratory 50 cases of leukaemia were tested recently with this method. Five representative cases are shown in Table 5.3. Seventeen of the patients had T-ALL based on the phenotypes of the blast cells (Table 5.2): Class II antigen negative (HLA-DR-), p40(CD7) positive as shown by the reactivity of RFT2 antibody, and positivity with TdT in the majority of blasts (>80%). In 15 patients these blast populations were destroyed by the RFT2 Ab plus rabbit complement, as illustrated in the case of patient 1 in Table 5.3. In the two remaining cases 8 and 41% of blast cells survived the complement 'kill'. Twenty seven patients had a non-T ALL. These patients were more heterogeneous than the T-ALL group and showed a distribution pattern of Ab reactivity similar to those published by Greaves et al[107,111], Kersey et al[84] and Nadler et al[81]. Four patients had null ALL unreactive with anti-cALL (CD10) Abs RFAL-1, —2, —3 and BA3. Another 8 patients reacted only partially with these Abs (Patient 5 in Table 5.3) and additional reagents such as BA-1 and BA-2 were necessary to provide >99% reactivity[84,112]. In 15 cases, however, the 'cover' of blasts was >99% with the RFAL-2 Ab alone and in 10 of these patients this Ab + rabbit complement removed all identifiable TdT+ cells (e.g. Patient 3 in Table 5.3). It is interesting to note that some patients had >99% RFAL-2 reactivity and still a few TdT+,RFAL-2+ cells did in fact escape lysis. In patient 2 of Table 5.3 (but not in Patients 1 and 3) these cells were nevertheless efficiently eliminated with another Ab, CAMPATH-1[100]. The conclusion of this part of the analysis is that the cases of null and common ALL require individual study with the available reagents. The new B4-type Abs (CD19) may also be important (Fig. 5.1) and should be added to the anti-cALL (CD19), BA-1 or VIB-C5 (CD24), BA-2 (CD9) and CAMPATH-1 antibodies[113]. Finally, six cases of B-ALL-s and bone marrow samples involved in generalized non-Hodgkin lymphomas were analysed. In these cases the Y29/55 antibody[114] has effectively eliminated all identifiable malignant B-cells. Unlike in ALL, in B-cell malignancy the residual cells were investigated by their κ or λ chain expression. In five out of the six cases no B-lymphocyte with the relevant light chain could be identified as a potential malignant cell.

The surprising overall conclusion from this study is therefore that from the total 50

Table 5.3 Elimination of leukaemic bone marrow cells with Ab + C'

	Patient 1 (AT)	Patient 2 (CF)	Patient 3 (SC)	Patient 4 (JB)	Patient 5 (AMcG)
WBC (10^9/l)	(60)	(50)	(75)	(30)	(5)
Total no. of blasts in BM[a] %	85	97	97	86	48
Ab reactivity:					
HLA-DR, Class II RFDR-1	2	96	95	n.t.	59[i]
cALL Ag (CD10)RFAL-2	80 (weak)	94 (strong)	82	92	14[i]
p40 (CD7)RFT-2	95 (strong)	2	3	<1	34[i]
leucocyte AG, CAMPATH-1	94	97	n.t.	88	n.t.
TdT	94	80	87	94	42[i]
Complement lysis (% of tripan blue positive dead cells):					
RFAL2 + rabbit C'	n.t.	79	84	89	20
RFT2 + rabbit C'	97	n.t.	8	10	20
CAMPATH-1 + rabbit C'	90	98	n.t.	83	n.t.
Combined complement lysis and TdT test (% of TdT$^+$ cells):					
RFAL2 + rabbit C'	(N2) 3500[b]	38[f]	(N1) <1[c]	(N1) 20[g]	(N1) 3200
RFT2 + rabbit C'	(N1) <1[c]	(N2) 4000[b]	(N2) 4400[b]	(N2) 5000[b]	(N2) 4500[b]
CAMPATH-1 + rabbit C'	150[d]	(N1) <1[c]	n.t.	120[h]	n.t.
N1/N2 (%)	<0.1[e]	<0.1[e]	<0.1[e]	0.4	71%
Conclusion	T-ALL for purging with RFT2	cALL for purging with CAMPATH-1	cALL for purging with RFAL-2	cALL with few residual TdT$^+$ cells	'null' ALL anti-cALL is ineffective

[a] BM: bone marrow

[b] The number of TdT$^+$ cells counted in the population of 5000 'inert' cells (see text for explanation).

[c] No TdT$^+$ cells can be detected on the whole slide (>5000 cells). All the residual white blood cells are granulocytes, plasma cells and occasional small lymphocytes with no nucleoli. These are present in variable proportions.

[d] 150/3500 = 4% of the original TdT$^+$ input is resistant to Ab + C'.

[e] Relevant Ab in the presence of C'/irrelevant Ab with C' = % of surviving TdT$^+$ cells (probably residual leukaemia, not lysed by Ab). For further explanation: see text.

[f] 38/4000 = 1% of the original TdT$^+$ input is resistant to Ab + C'.

[g] 20/5000 = 0.4% of the original TdT$^+$ input is resistant to Ab + C'.

[h] 120/5000 2.4% of the original TdT$^+$ input is resistant to Ab + C'.

[i] The TdT$^+$ population is HLA-DR$^+$, partially cALL$^+$. T-ALL is excluded by the absence of RFT2$^+$/TdT$^+$ blasts.

n.t. not tested

cases 30 samples contained malignant populations which were totally destroyed with the available antibodies. This is an unexpected result because the range of complement fixing Abs is still limited. It is likely that with the addition of just a few reagents, including cytolytic CD19, these results will still further improve. The technique for cell elimination (i.e. complement lysis) is simple and the detection system is sensitive enough to pick up very small numbers of residual cells (see above).

ELIMINATION OF T-CELLS FROM BONE MARROW

Antibodies to T-cells are also used for purging bone marrow in order to prevent graft versus host disease in recipients of allogeneic bone marrow[115]. The analysis of residual T-cells can be performed by investigating the mitogenic response to T-cell mitogens such as PHA[116,117]. These investigations are optimally complemented by the immunofluorescence analysis of viable T-cells because the latter is a rapid test.

Principle

The method is conveniently performed by combining membrane staining (with FITC labelled reagents) with ethidium bromide (EB) staining. This dye gives bright red fluorescence in the nucleus of dead cells. Thus the investigation can be focused to see whether the residual anti-T Ab reacting cells (FITC, green membrane staining) are still viable or, in fact, dead (EB, nuclear positivity).

Materials

Cells, 2×10^7/ml
PBS with 10% FCS
Ethidium bromide (EB; 1:500 dilution of 0.01 mg/ml stock solution)

Procedure

1. After complement mediated lysis using T cell reactive Abs of IgG$_2$ or IgM class (CD2-CD8) stain cells (1×10^6 in 50 μl PBS + 10% FCS) with goat-anti-mouse Ig-FITC.

2. Add 20 μl EB and analyse the cells on the microscope immediately (within 5-10 minutes). Count cells with phase contrast and fluorescence. Study the membrane labelled cells (FITC) and record those with no EB nuclear stain (residual viable T-cells).

Note. EB can be toxic, and for this reason it is best to investigate the tubes individually. The membrane (FITC) and EB (red fluorescence) is also optimal for two-colour flow cytometry analysis where double labelled (dead) and FITC-labelled (only FITC, still viable) T-lymphocytes can be counted rapidly. The latter population can be sorted to investigate the presence of functionally active T-cells in cultures following the lytic procedure.

CONCLUSION

The great advance of applying Mc Abs in leukaemia diagnosis and therapy has been paralleled by the diagnostic application of molecular genetics for the detection of gene rearrangements. In monoclonal lymphoid populations the genes of membrane receptors such as surface Ig and T-cell receptor are analysed. When a collection of DNA fragments from a heterogeneous population of cells is analysed on a southern blot no single rearranged band can be detected because each rearrangement is below the threshold of detection. Nevertheless, the method is very sensitive and as low as 5-10% of cells with uniform ('monoclonal') rearrangements can be detected as a positive band. This sensitivity poses problems. In leukaemias of pluripotent stem cell origin, for example, cells of myeloid appearance may exist in the company of 5-10% otherwise unremarkable B-lymphoid cells. These may also belong to the malignancy and carry Ig rearrangements[118]. This sort of finding may lead to the erroneous impression that myeloid cells exhibit B-cell features. These questions will be resolved when immunological phenotyping of subpopulations and programmed cell sorting based on these criteria are followed by gene rearrangement studies of the sorted populations. Similar analysis with normal cells will also be performed. These two major technologies, combined, will lead to the mapping of genes and their products during a process abundantly documented: the orderly acquisition of membrane (and other, e.g. TdT) differentiation antigens. It may then be that malignancy-related changes, in genes and their products, will be clearly defined.

ACKNOWLEDGEMENTS

This work has been supported by the Leukaemia Research Fund (Grant No.81/21) and the Medical Research Council of Great Britain (Grant No.SPG8417830). Mrs Elizabeth Price-Jones, Dr Margarita Bofill and Mrs Kamal Ivory have helped in the diagnostic work, and Ms Judy Wynne and Mrs Eira Rawlings assisted in producing the Mc Abs. We are grateful to Dr Ian Hann, Royal Hospital for Sick Children, Glasgow, and to our colleagues in the North East Thames Region for supplying leukaemia samples, and to the members of the Haematology Department, Royal Free Hospital, for helpful discussions. We also acknowledge the help from our colleagues who supplied us the following monoclonal antibodies: Dr H. K. Forster (Basel): Y29/55; Dr A. M. Lebacq (Bruxelles): AL-2 and AL-3; Dr H. Waldmann (Cambridge): Campath-1; Dr T. LeBien (Minneapolis): BA-1 and BA-2; Dr R. W. Tindle (Crawley): 3C5 antibody. Drs J. J. M. VanDongen (Rotterdam), H. G. Drexler and J. Minowada (Chicago) have kindly allowed us to see their papers prior to publication.

REFERENCES

1. Janossy G 1980 Membrane markers. In: Catovsky D (ed) Methods in haematology. Churchill Livingstone, Edinburgh, vol. 2, 129–183
2. Greaves M F 1975 Clinical applications of cell surface markers. Progress in Haematology 9: 255–303
3. Janossy G, Roberts M M, Capellaro D, Greaves M F, Francis G E 1978 Use of the fluorescence activated cell sorter in human leukaemia. In: Knapp W, Holubar K, Wick G (eds) Immunofluorescence and related staining techniques. Elsevier/North-Holland Biomedical Press, 111–122
4. Greaves M F, Brown G, Rapson N T, Lister T A 1975 Antiserum to acute lymphoblastic leukaemia cells. Clinical immunology and immunopathology 4: 67–84
5. Schlossman S F, Chess L, Humphreys R E, Strominger J L 1976 Distribution of Ia-like molecules on the surface of normal and leukaemic human cells. Proceedings of the National Academy of Sciences USA 73: 1288–1299

6. Rodt H, Netzel B, Thiel E, Jager G, Huhn D, Haas R, Gotze D, Thierfelder S 1977 Classification of leukemic cells with T- and O-ALL-specific antisera. In: Thierfelder S, Rodt H, Thiel E (eds) Immunological diagnosis of leukemias and lymphomas. Springer-Verlag, Berlin/Heidelberg/New York, 87–107
7. Janossy G, Greaves M F, Sutherland R, Durrant J, Lewis C 1977 Comparative analysis of membrane phenotypes in acute lymphoid leukaemia and in lymphoid blast crisis of chronic myeloid leukaemia. Leukaemia Research 1: 289–300
8. Knapp W 1981 Leukemia markers. Academic Press, London/New York
9. Belpomme D, Borella L, Braylan M, Greaves M, Herberman R, Hitzig W, Kersey J, Petrov R, Ritts R, Seligmann M 1978 Immunological diagnosis of leukaemia and lymphoma. British Journal of Haematology 38: 85–97
10. Brown G, Capellaro D, Greaves M F 1975 Leukaemia-associated antigens in man. Journal of the National Cancer Institute 55: 1281–1289
11. Sutherland R, Smart J, Niaudet P, Greaves M F 1978 Acute lymphoblastic leukaemia associated antigen. II. Isolation and partial characterization. Leukaemia Research 2: 115–123
12. Billing R, Minowada J, Cline M, Clark B, Lee K 1978 Acute lymphocytic leukaemia-associated membrane antigen. Journal of the National Cancer Institute 61: 423–429
13. Winchester R J, Ross G D, Jarowski C I, Wang C Y, Halper J, Broxmeyer H E 1977 Expression of Ia-like antigen molecules on human granulocytes during early phases of differentiation. Proceedings of the National Academy of Science USA 74: 4012–4016
14. Janossy G, Hoffbrand A V, Greaves M F, Ganeshaguru K, Pain C, Bradstock K, Prentice H G, Kay H E M 1980 Terminal transferase enzyme assay and immunological membrane markers in the diagnosis of leukaemia — a multi-parameter analysis of 300 cases. British Journal of Haematology 44: 221–234
15. Greaves M F, Janossy G 1976 Antisera to human T lymphocytes. In: Bloom B R, David J R (eds) In vitro methods in cell mediated and tumor immunity. Academic Press, London/New York p 89–104
16. Seligmann M, Brouet J C, Preud'homme J L 1977 The immunological diagnosis of human leukaemias and lymphomas; an overview. In: Thierfelder S, Rodt H, Thiel E (eds) Immunological diagnosis of leukemias and lymphomas. Springer-Verlag, Berlin, 1–16
17. Catovsky D, Frisch B, Van Noorden S 1975 B, T and null cell leukaemias. Electron microscopy and surface morphology. Blood Cells 1975 1: 115–117
18. Roberts M, Greaves M F 1978 Maturation linked expression of a myeloid cell surface antigen. British Journal of Haematology 38: 439–452
19. Jager G, Hoffman-Fezer G, Rodt H, Huhn D, Thiel E 1977 Myeloid antigens and antigen densities in mice and men. Haematology and Blood Transfusion 20: 109–116
20. Baker M, Falk R S, Falk J, Greaves M F 1976 Detection of a monocyte specific antigen in human acute leukaemia cells. British Journal of Haematology 32: 13–21
21. Bollum F J 1975 Antibody to terminal deoxynucleotidyl transferase. Proceedings of the National Academy of Science USA 72: 4119–4122
22. Bollum F J 1979 Terminal deoxynucleotidyl transferase as a hematopoietic cell marker. Blood 54: 1203–1215
23. Janossy G, Bollum F J, Bradstock K F, McMichael A, Rapson N, Greaves M F 1979 Terminal transferase positive human bone marrow cells exhibit the antigenic phenotype of common acute lymphoblastic leykemia. Journal of Immunology 123: 1525–1529
24. Bradstock K F, Janossy G, Pizzolo G, Hoffbrand A V, McMichael A, Pilch J R, Milstein C, Beverley P, Bollum F J 1980 Subpopulations of normal and leukemic human thymocytes: an analysis using monoclonal antibodies. Journal of the National Cancer Institute 65: 33–42
25. Bradstock K F, Janossy G, Tidman N, Papageorgiou E S, Prentice H G, Willoughby M, Hoffbrand A V 1981 Immunological monitoring of residual disease in treated thymic acute lymphoblastic leukaemia. Leukaemia Research 5: 301–309
26. Salmon S E, Seligmann M 1974 B cell neoplasia in man. Lancet 2: 1230–1233
27. Catovsky D, Pittman S, O'Brien M, Cherchi M, Costello C, Foa R, Pearce E, Hoffbrand A V, Janossy G 1979 Multiparameter studies in lymphoid leukaemias. American Journal of Clinical Pathology 72: 736–745
28. Greaves M F, Janossy G 1978 Patterns of gene expression and the cellular origins of human leukaemias. Biochemica et Biophysica Acta 516: 193–230
29. Oi U T, Glazer A N, Stryer L 1982 Fluorescent phycobiliprotein conjugates for analyses of cells and molecules. Journal of Cell Biology 93: 981
30. Becton Dickinson 1982–1984 Monoclonal Antibody Source Book
31. De May J 1983 The immunogold staining method used with monoclonal antibodies. In: Polak J M, Van Noorden S (eds) Immunocytochemistry, practical application in pathology and biology. Wright P S G, Bristol 82–102

32. Moir D J, Ghosh A K, Abdulaziz Z, Knight P M, Mason D Y 1983 Immunoenzymatic staining of haematological samples with monoclonal antibodies. British Journal of Haematology 55: 395–410

33. Chilosi M, Pizzolo G, Fiore-Donati L, Bofill M, Janossy G 1983 Routine immunofluorescent and histochemical analysis of bone marrow involvement of lymphoma/leukaemia the use of cryostat sections. British Journal of Cancer 48: 763–775

34. Falini B, Martelli M F, Tarallo F, Moir D J, Cordell J L, Gatter K C, Loreti G, Stein H, Mason D Y 1984 Immunohistological analysis of human bone marrow trephine biopsies using monoclonal antibodies. British Journal of Haematology 56: 365–386

35. Naito K, Knowles R W, Real F X, Morishima Y, Kawashima K, Dupont B 1983 Analysis of two new leukemia-associated antigens detected on human T-cell acute lymphoblastic leukemia using monoclonal antibodies. Blood 62: 852–855

36. Johnson G D, Nogueira A G M 1981 A Simple method of reducing the fading of immunofluorescence during microscopy. Journal of Immunological Methods 43: 349–353

37. Freer S M 1984 Permanent mount for immunofluorescence. Journal of Immunological Methods 66: 187–190

38. Johnson G D, Holborow E J 1984 Immunofluorescence. In: Weir D M, Herzenberg L A (eds) Handbook of experimental immunology, 4th edn. (in press). Blackwell Scientific Publications, London

39. Bessis M 1973 Living blood cells and their ultrastructure. Springer-Verlag, Heidelberg, Berlin, p 686–690

40. Chilosi M, Pizzolo G, Vincenzi C 1983 Haematoxylin counterstaining of immunofluorescence preparations. Journal of Clinical Pathology 36: 114–126

41. Gathings W E, Lawton A R, Cooper M D 1977 Immunofluorescence studies of the development of pre-B cells, B lymphocytes and immunoglobulin isotype deversity in humans. European Journal of Immunology 7: 804–810

42. Campana D, Janossy G, Bofill M, Trejdosiewicz L K, Ma D, Hoffbrand A V, Mason D Y, Lebacq A-M, Forster H 1985 Human B cell development. I. Phenotypic differences of B lymphocytes in the bone marrow and peripheral lymphoid tissue. Journal of Immunology 134: 1524–1530

43. Tedder T F, Fearon D T, Gartland G L, Cooper M D 1983 Expression of C3b receptors on human B cells and myelomonocytic cells but not natural killer cells. Journal of Immunology 130: 1668–1673

44. Guesdon J L, Ternyuck T, Avrameas S 1979 The use of avidin-biotin interaction in immunoenzymatic techniques. Journal of Histochemistry and Cytochemistry 27: 1131–1139

45. Simmonds R G, Smith W, Marsden H 1982 3-phenylazo-4-hydroxyphenyl-isothiocyanate: versatile reagent for the efficient haptenation of Ig and other carrier molecules. Journal of Immunological Methods 54: 23–30

46. Warnke R, Levy R 1979 Detection of T and B cell antigens with hybridoma monoclonal antibodies: a biotin-avidin-horseradish peroxidase method. Journal of Histochemistry and Cytochemistry 28: 771–776

47. Hoffman K, Wood S W, Brinton C C, Montibeller J A, Finn F M 1977 Iminobiotin affinity columns and their application to retrieval of streptavidin. Proceedings of the National Academy of Science USA 77: 4666–4668

48. Frölich T W, Buchanan G R, Cornet J A M, Sartain P A, Graham-Smith R 1981 Terminal transferase containing cells in peripheral blood: implications for the surveillance of patients with lymphoblastic leukaemia or lymphoma in remission. Blood 58: 214–220

49. Hoffbrand A V, Ganeshaguru K, Janossy G, Greaves M F, Catovsky D, Woodruff R E 1977 Terminal deoxynucleotidyl transferase levels and membrane markers in the diagnosis of acute leukaemia. Lancet 520–523

50. Barr R D, Koekebakker M, Mahony 1984 Demonstration of TdT in single cells by indirect immunofluorescence. II. An examination of specificity. Leukaemia Research 8: 429–434

51. Bollum F J, Augl C, Chang L M S 1984 Monoclonal antibodies to human terminal transferase. The Journal of Biological Chemistry 259: 5848–5850

52. Bradstock K F, Janossy G, Hoffbrand A V, Ganeshaguru K, Llewellin P, Prentice H G, Bollum F J 1981 Immunofluorescence and biochemical studies of terminal deoxynucleotidyl transferase in treated acute leukaemia. British Journal of Haematology 47: 121–131

53. Bodger M, Francis G E, Delia D, Thomas J A, Granger S M Janossy G 1981 A monoclonal antibody specific for immature human haemopoietic cells and T lineage cells. Journal of Immunology 127: 2269–2274

54. Tindle R W, Nichols R A B, Chan L, Campana D, Catovsky D, Birnie G T 1984 A novel monoclonal antibody B1-3C5 recognises myeloblasts and non-T, non-B lymphoblasts in acute leukaemia and chronic granulocytic leukaemia blast crisis and reacts with immature cells in normal bone marrow. Leukaemia Research 9: 1–9

55.   Clark E A, Shu G, Ledbetter J A 1984 Role of the Bp35 cell surface polypeptide in human B cell activation. Proceedings of the National Academy of Science USA (in press)
56.   Tidman N, Janossy G, Bodger M, Granger S, Kung P C, Goldstein G 1981 Delineation of human thymocyte differentiation pathways utilizing double staining techniques with monoclonal antibodies. Clinical and Experimental Immunology 45: 457–467
57.   Hokland P, Rosenthal P, Griffin J, Nadler L, Daley J, Hokland M, Schlossman S F, Ritz J 1983 Purification and characterization of fetal hematopoietic cell that express the common acute lymphoblastic leukaemia antigen (CALLA). Journal of Experimental Medicine 157: 114–129
58.   Civin C I, Strauss L C, Brovall C, Feckler M J, Schwartz J F, Shaper J H 1984 Antigenic analysis of hematopoiesis. III. A hematopoietic progenitor cell surface antigen defined by a monoclonal antibody raised against KG-la cells. Journal of Immunology 133: 1–10
59.   Van Dongen J J M, Hooijkaas H, Comans-Bitter W M, Benne K, Van Os T M, De Josselin de Jong J. 1985 Triple immunological staining using colloidal gold, fluorescein and rhodamine as labels. Journal of Immunological Methods. In press
60   Van Dongen J J M, Hooijkaas H, Comans-Bitter W M, Hählen K, Van Zanen G E 1985 The small subpopulation of T cell marker +/TdT+ cells in the human bone marrow may represent prothymocytes. Advances in Experimental Biology and Medicine. In press
61.   Bodger M P, Janossy G, Bollum F J, Burford G D 1983 The ontogeny of terminal deoxynucleotidyl transferase positive cells in the human fetus. Blood 61: 1125–1131
62.   Bofill M, Janossy G, Janossa M, Burford G D, Seymour G J, Wernet P, Kelemen E 1985 Human B cell development. II. Subpopulations in the human fetus. Journal of Immunology 134: 1531–1538
63.   Uchanska-Ziegler B, Wernet P, Ziegler A 1980 Standardization of the microplate method for screening monoclonal antibodies. Journal of Immunological Methods 39: 85–89
64.   Bross K J, Pangalis G A, Staatz C G, Blume K G 1978 Demonstration of cell surface antigens and their antibodies by the peroxidase-antiperoxidase method. Transplantation 25: 331–334
65.   Moore H A S, Broxmeyer H E, Sheridan A P C, Meyers P A, Jacobsen N, Winchester R J 1980 Continuous human bone marrow culture: Ia antigen characterization of probable pluripotential stem cell. Blood 55: 682–690
66.   Melo J V, Catovsky D, Bodger M 1984 Reactivity of the monoclonal antibody RFB1 in chronic B-cell leukaemias. Scandinavian Journal of Haematology 32: 417–422
67.   Griffin J D, Linch D, Sabbath K, Larcom P, Schlossman S F 1984 A monoclonal antibody reactive with normal and leukemic human myeloid progenitor cells. Leukaemia Research 8: 521–534
68.   Matutes E, Rodriguez B, Polli N, Tavares de Castro J, Passera A, Andrews C, Griffin J D, Tindle R W, Catovsky D 1984 Characterization of myeloid leukaemias with monoclonal antibodies 3C5 and MY9. Journal of Haematological Oncology (in press)
69.   Nadler L M, Anderson K C, Marti G, Bates M, Park E, Daley J F, Schlossman S F 1983 Human B lymphocyte-associated antigen expressed on normal mitogen-activated and malignant B lymphocytes. Journal of Immunology. 131: 244–258
70.   Ritz J, Pesando J M, Notis-McConarty J, Lazarus H, Schlossman S F 1980 A monoclonal antibody to human acute lymphoblastic leukaemia antigen. Nature 283: 583–585
71.   Liszka K, Majdic O, Bettelheim P, Knapp W 1981 A monoclonal antibody (VIL-A1) reactive with common acute lymphatic leukaemia cells. In: Knapp W (ed) Leukaemia Markers. Academic Press, London/New York, 61–64
72.   Lebacq A M, Ravoet A M, Bazin H, Sutherland D R, Tidman N, Greaves M F 1983 Rat AL2, AL3, AL4 and AL5 monoclonal antibodies bind to the common acute lymphoblastic leukaemia antigen. International Journal of Cancer 32: 273–279
73.   Stashenko P, Nadler L M, Hardy R, Schlossman S F 1980 Characterization of a human B lymphocyte-specific antigen. Journal of Immunology 125: 1678–1685
74.   Haynes B F, Eisenbarth G S, Fauci A S 1979 Human lymphocyte antigens: production of a monoclonal antibody that defines functional thymus-derived lymphocyte subsets. Proceedings of the National Academy of Science USA 76: 5829–5837
75.   Tax W J M, Tidman N, Janossy G, Trejdosiewicz L K, Willems R M, Leeuwenberg J F M, De Witte T, Capel P J A, Koene R A P 1984 Monoclonal antibody (WT1) directed against a T cell surface glycoprotein: characteristics and immunosuppressive activity. Clinical and Experimental Immunology 55: 427–436
76.   Janossy G, Trejdosiewicz L K, Price-Jones E et al 1985 Standardization of antibodies for bone marrow transplantation. Leukaemia Research (in press)
77.   Vodinelich L, Tax W, Bai Y, Pegram S, Capel P, Greaves M 1982 A monoclonal antibody WT1 for detecting leukaemias of T cell precursors. Blood 60: 742–750
78.   Martin P J, Hansen J A, Siadak A W, Nowinski R C 1981 Monoclonal antibodies recognizing

human T lymphocytes and malignant human B lymphocytes: a comparative study. Journal of Immunology 127: 1920–1926

79. Royston I, Majda J A, Baird M S, Meserve B L, Griffiths J C 1980 Human T cell antigens defined by monoclonal antibodies: the 65,000 -Dalton antigen of T cells (T65) is also found on chronic lymphocytic leukaemia cells bearing surface immunoglobulin. Journal of Immunology 125: 725–731

80. Stein H, Gerdes J, Mason D Y 1982 The normal and malignant germinal centre. Clinics in Haematology 11: 531–559

81. Nadler L M, Korsmeyer S J, Anderson K C, Boyd A W, Slaughenhoupt B, Park B, Jensen J, Coral F, Meyer R J, Sallan S E, Ritz J, Schlossman S F 1984 B cell origin of non-T cell acute lymphoblastic leukemia. A model for discrete stages of neoplastic and normal pre-B cell differentiation. Journal of Clinical Investigation 74: 332–340

82. Vainchenker W, Deschamps J F, Bastin J M, Guichard J, Titeux M, Breton-Gorius J, McMichael A J 1982 Two monoclonal antiplatelet antibodies as markers of human megakaryocyte maturation: immunofluorescent staining and platelet peroxidase detection in megakaryocyte colonies. Blood 59: 514–519

83. Knapp W, Bettelheim P, Majdic O, Liszka K, Schmidmeier W, Lutz D 1984 Diagnostic value of monoclonal antibodies to leukocyte differentiation antigens in lymphoid and non-lymphoid leukemias. In: Bernard A, Boumsell L (eds) Leucocyte/Typing. Springer-Verlag, Berlin

84. Kersey J H, Goldman A, Abramson C, Nesbit M, Perry G, Gajl-Peczalska K, LeBein T 1982 Clinical usefulness of monoclonal antibody phenotyping in childhood acute lymphoblastic leukaemia. Lancet 2: 1419–1421

85. Anderson K C, Park E K, Bates M P, Leonard R C F, Hardy R, Schlossman S F, Nadler L M 1983 Antigens on human plasma cells identified by monoclonal antibodies. Journal of Immunology 130: 1132–1138

86. Catovsky D, Linch D, Beverley P B L 1984 T cell disorders in haematological diseases. Clinics in Haematology 11: 661–695

87. Uchiyama T, Broder S, Waldmann T A 1981 A monoclonal antibody (anti-Tac) reactive with activated and functionally mature human T cells. I. Production of anti-Tac monoclonal antibody and distribution of Tac positive cells. Journal of Immunology 126: 1393–1397

88. Catovsky D, San Miguel G F, Soler G, Matutes E, Melo G V, Bouricas J, Haynes B S 1984 T cell leukaemias, immunological and clinical aspects. Journal of Experimental and Clinical Cancer Research 2: 229–233

89. Ault K A 1979 Detection of small numbers of mononuclear B lymphocytes in the blood of patients with lymphoma. New England Journal of Medicine 30: 1401–1405

90. Van Dongen J J M, Hooijkaas H, Hahlen K, Benne K, Bitter W M, Van Der Linde-Preesman A A, Tettero I L M, Van De Rijn M, Hilgers J 1984 Detection of minimal residual disease in TdT positive T cell malignancies by double immunofluorescence staining. In: Lowenberg B, Hagenbeck J (eds). Minimal residual disease in acute leukaemia. Martinus-Nijhoff B V, The Hague, Netherlands, p 167–81

91. McCaffrey R P, Harrison A, Parkman B S, Baltimore D 1975 Terminal deoxynucleotidyl transferase activity in human leukaemic cells and normal thymocytes. New England Journal of Medicine. 292: 775–780

92. Bradstock K F, Papageorgiou E S, Janossy G 1981 Diagnosis of meningeal involvement in patients with acute lymphoblastic leukaemia using immunofluorescence for terminal transferase. Cancer 47: 2478–2481

93. Scollay R G, Butcher E C, Weissman I L 1982 Thymus cell migration: cells migrating from thymus to peripheral lymphoid organs have a 'mature' phenotype. Journal of Immunology 128: 1566–1570

94. De Bruin H G, Astaldi A, Leupers T, van de Griend R J, van Dooren L, Schellekens P T A, Tanke H J, Roos M, Vossen J M 1981 T lymphocyte characteristics in bone marrow transplanted patients. Analysis with monoclonal antibodies. Journal of Immunology 127: 244–254

95. Kluin-Nelemans J C, Bolhuis R L H, Lowenberg B, Sizoo W, Campana D 1984 Identification of normal and regenerating bone marrow cells with a panel of monoclonal antibodies. Submitted for publication

96. Campana D, Michaelewicz R, Favrot M, Janossy G 1984 Features of immature lymphoid cells in the cord blood. Personal communication

97. Batory G, Bofill M, Petranyi G G, Janossy G, Hollan S R 1984 Comparative analysis of monoclonal antibodies of workshop T series on suspensions and tissue sections. In: Bernard A et al (eds) Leucocyte typing. Springer-Verlag, Berlin, p 409–475

98. Thomas J A, Janossy G, Eden O B, Bollum F J 1982 Demonstration of nuclear terminal

transferase deoxynucleotidyl transferase (TdT) in leukemic infiltrates of testicular tissue. British Journal of Cancer 45: 709–717

99. Gorin N C, David R, Stachowiak J, Salmon Ch, Petit J C, Parlier Y, Najman A, Duhamel G 1981 High dose chemotherapy and autologous bone marrow transplantation in acute leukaemias, malignant lymphomas and solid tumours. A study of 23 patients. European Journal of Cancer 17: 557–568

100. Hale G, Bright S, Chumbley G, Hoang T, Metcalf D, Munro A, Waldmann H 1984 Removal of Tcells from bone marrow for transplantation: a monoclonal antilymphocyte antibody that fixes human complement. Blood 62: 873–882

101. Filipovitch A H, Vallera D A, Youle R J, Quinones R R, Neville D M, Kersey J H 1984 Ex-vivo treatment of donor bone marrow with anti-T cell immunotoxins for prevention of graft-versus-host disease. Lancet i: 469–472

102. Allen T D 1981 Haemopoietic microenvironments in vitro: ultrastructural aspects. Ciba Foundation Symposium 84, Pitman, London, p 38–67

103. Greaves M F 1979 Tumour markers, phenotypes and maturation arrest in malignancy: a cell selection hypothesis. In: Boelzma E, Rumke P (eds) Tumour markers. Impact and prospects. Elsevier/North Holland Biomedical Press, 201–212

104. Griffin J D, Larcom P, Schlossman S F 1983 Use of surface markers to identify a subset of acute myelomonocytic leukaemia cells with progenitor cell properties. Blood 62: 1300–1303

105. Reinherz E L, Kung P C, Goldstein G, Levey R H, Schlossman S F 1980 Discrete stages of human intrathymic differentiation: analysis of normal thymocytes and leukemic lymphoblasts of T-cell lineage. Proceedings of the National Academy of Science USA 77: 1588–1592

106. Lobach D F, Hensley L L, Ho W, Haynes B F. Ontogeny of human T cell antigens 1985. In: Reinherz E, Hansen J A (eds). Leucocyte typing II (in press)

107. Greaves M F, Hariri G, Newman R A, Sutherland D R, Ritter M A, Ritz J 1983 Selective expression of the common acute lymphoblastic leukemia (gp100) antigen on immature lymphoid cells and their malignant counterparts. Blood 61: 628–639

108. Greaves M F, Paxton A, Janossy G, Pain C, Johnson S, Lister I A 1980 Acute lymphoblastic leukaemia associated antigen. III. Alteration in expression during treatment and in relapse. Leukaemia Research 4: 1–14

109. Greaves M F, Janossy G, Peto J, Kay H E M 1981 Immunologically defined subclasses of acute lymphoblastic leukaemia in children: their relationship to presentation features and prognosis. British Journal of Haematology 48: 179–192

110. Barnett M J, Greaves M F, Amess J A L, Gregory W M, Rohatiner A Z S, Dhalival H S, Slevin M L, Biruls R, Malpas J S, Lister T A 1985 Treatment of acute lymphoblastic leukaemia in adults. British Journal of Haematology (in press)

111. Greaves M F, Delia D, Newman R, Vodinelich L 1982 Analysis of leukaemic cells with monoclonal antibodies. In: McMichael A, Fabre J (eds) Monoclonal antibodies in clinical medicine. Academic Press, London, 129–165

112. Janossy G, Campana D, Price Jones E Efficacy of complement lysis on ALL blasts. Manuscript in preparation

113. Janossy G 1984 'Purging' of bone marrow and immunosuppression. In: Lennox H (ed) Clincial Applications of Monoclonal Antibodies. British Medical Bulletin. Churchill Livingstone, Edinburgh, p 247–253

114. Forster H K, Gudat F G, Girard M F, Albrecht R, Schmidt J, Ludwig C, Obrecht J P 1982 Monoclonal antibody against a membrane antigens characterizing leukemic human B lymphcytes. Cancer Research 42: 1927–1939

115. Prentice H G, Blacklock H A, Janossy G, Gilmore M J M L, Price-Jones L, Tidman N, Trejdosiewicz L K, Skeggs D B L, Panjwani D, Ball S, Graphakos S, Patterson J, Hoffbrand A V 1984 Depletion of T lymphocytes in donor marrow prevents significant graft versus host disease in matched allogeneic leukaemia marrow transplant recipients. Lancet 1: 472–476

116. Granger S M, Janossy G, Francis G, Blacklock H A, Poulter L W, Hoffbrand A V 1982 Elimination of T lymphocytes from human bone marrow with monoclonal anti-T antibodies and cytolytic complement. British Journal of Haematology 50: 367–374

117. Hansen J A, Martin P J, Kamoun M, Torok-Storb B, Newman W, Nowinski R C, Thomas E D 1981 Monoclonal antibodies recognizing human T cells: potential role for preventing GvH reactions following allogeneic marrow transplantation. Transplantation Proceedings 13: 1133–1137

118. Rovigatti U, Mirro J, Kitchingman G, Dahl G, Ochs J, Murphy S, Stass S 1984 Heavy chain immunoglobulin rearrangement in acute non-lymphoid leukaemia. Blood 63: 1023–1027

119. Ortho Diagnostic. Catalogue of Monoclonal Antibodies. 1983

6

Cell surface antigen and morphological characterization of leucocyte populations by flow cytometry

M. R. Loken

INTRODUCTION

The discrimination between cell types in a standard microscope requires the observer to assess several features of each cell. Cell size and shape, nuclear size and shape, the presence or absence of granules, as well as intensity and colour of stain are all integrated in the viewer's mind in order to identify a particular cell. This multidimensional approach is also being used in flow cytometry to identify and to characterize multiple populations of leucocytes. In this technique cells flow rapidly through a sensing region illuminated by a laser or a mercury arc lamp. Several detectors, each assessing a different optical or electronic characteristic of the cells, are focused on this small area. By correlating these multiple features of a cell as it flows through the detection system, the precise identification of that cell can be made.

As the optical detection systems of the flow cytometers become increasingly sophisticated, more parameters can be assessed simultaneously as a cell passes through the sensing area. Originally flow systems had a single fluorescence channel and discriminated between cells based on differences in the amount of fluorescence observed in that single channel.[1] A forward light scattering detector then was added and could be used to discriminate between live and dead lymphocytes.[2] The light scatter signal could also be used to identify size differences between the particles as they flowed through the instrument.[3] Studies of light scattering indicated that detectors set at different angles with respect to the laser beam identified different physical characteristics of the particles being examined.[4] By adding a second light scatter detector at 90° from the laser beam, lymphocytes, monocytes and neutrophils could be distinguished on unstained cells.[5] Additional fluorescence channels were then added in order to correlate the cell surface expression of more than one antigen in the population.[6] By adding a second laser and thus a second sensing region to the systems it is possible to quantify three and four colours of immunofluorescence.[7,8] The combination of physical parameters (light scattering) with immunological probes (immunofluorescence using monoclonal antibodies) provides a powerful tool for the study of heterogenous populations of cells.

The analysis of leucocyte populations in a flow cytometer has several advantages over conventional microscopy. The cells are analyzed much more rapidly than by microscope. Cells can be processed at speeds of 1000 cells or more per second so that in a short period of time a large number of cells can be assessed. This increased number of cells permits more accurate statistical analysis of the proportion of different cell types comprising the population. In addition the data are quantitative both in determining the number of cells binding a particular label as well as in assessing the amount of label per cell. The ability to quantify the amount of antigen per cell is an additional parameter for distinguishing different cell populations. Cells are no longer simply classified as positive or negative, but can be grouped according to amount of probe attached to the cell.

In this article a standard four parameter flow cytometer will be described. The discrimination of lymphocytes, monocytes and neutrophils using light scattering will be discussed. The procedure for performing two colour immunofluorescence on the lymphocyte population will be presented with an emphasis on the compensation required for the correction of spectral overlap between the two fluorophores. Additional information about flow cytometry can be found in other review articles[9,10,11,12,13] and the journal, 'Cytometry.'

DESCRIPTION OF A FLUORESCENCE ACTIVATED CELL SORTER

Several commercial instruments are used in flow cytometric experiments (Becton Dickinson FACS Systems, Sunnyvale, CA; Coulter Electronics, Hialeah, FL; Ortho Diagnostics Systems, Westwood, MA). Although a mercury arc lamp is used in some instruments, the discussion here will be limited to the laser-based flow cytometers.

When peripheral blood leucocytes are to be analysed on a flow cytometer they are first prepared and stained by standard immunofluorescence techniques.[10] Then, instead of preparing a microscope slide, the cells are introduced into the flow cytometer. The single cell suspension is forced under pressure to a nozzle. The cells are centered in the stream coming out of the nozzle by a concentric flow of cell free sheath fluid within the nozzle. Some instruments examine the cells within the nozzle (cuvette) while others interrogate the cells after they exit (stream-in-air). The laser light intersects the path of the cells at right angles to their flow and is focused to a spot of between 25 and 50 microns. When the cells are passing this spot in the stream-in-air instrument, they are travelling at a speed of approximately 10 metres per second. All of the measurements on the cell must be made simultaneously during the approximately five microseconds that the cell is within the laser beam. Therefore all the detectors are focused onto that point and the electronics are synchronized in order to process all four signals simultaneously.

As the cells pass through the laser, they scatter some of the laser light. This scattered light differs from fluorescence in that scattered light is of the same wavelength as the laser. The amount of light scattered by the cell is dependent on the angle that the detector is placed with respect to the laser beam.[4] In the stream-in-air flow cytometer illustrated in Figure 6.1 two different scatter detectors are used. The forward light scattering detector (FLS) is positioned looking into the laser beam. Direct laser light is blocked from entering this detector by a beam stop. This forward light scatter detector observes light scattered just off axis from the laser beam.

The second light scatter detector is part of a complete detector system positioned at right angles to both the laser and the stream. As shown in Figure 6.1, a microscope objective is focused on the intersection of the stream and the laser. The light is directed through a series of mirrors and dichroic mirrors onto three (or more) detectors. The first detector observes light of the same wavelength as the laser,

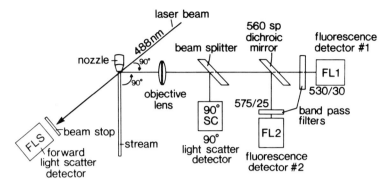

Fig. 6.1 Schematic diagram depicting the optical arrangement of a laser based four parameter flow cytometer. In this stream-in-air flow cytometer the laser beam intersects the stream carrying the cells just outside the nozzle. The forward light scatter detector (FLS) detects light of the same wavelength as the laser, just off axis from the beam. Three other detectors are positioned 90° from both the laser beam and the stream. An objective lens collects the light and directs it onto a light scatter detector and two fluorescence detectors. The 90° light scatter detector (90° SC) detects 488 nm light scattered from the laser beam. The 560 SP dichroic mirror transmits light below 560 nm while reflecting light with longer wavelengths. Green light is detected in fluorescence detector #1 (FL1) through a band pass filter 530/30. Orange light is detected in fluorescence detector #2 (FL2) through a bandpass filter 575/25.

scattered light. This light scatter detector is termed a '90° detector' (90° SC) since it is positioned at right angles to the incident laser beam.

Two other detectors are arranged to observe fluorescence with longer wavelengths than the exciting light. Chromophores attached to the cells are induced into an excited state by the laser light with subsequent emission of longer wavelength light. In the configuration depicted in Figure 6.1, different portions of the light spectrum fall on each of the two fluorescence detectors (FL1 and FL2). The optical filters shown in this figure are optimally designed to detect fluorescein (FITC) and phycoerythrin (PE). The 560 SP dichroic mirror transmits wavelengths below 560 nm while reflecting wavelengths greater than 560 nm. The 530/30 bandpass filter transmits green light through a window 30 nm wide centered on 530 nm (530 ± 15 nm). Similarly, the 575/25 bandpass filter transmits orange light through a 25 nm wide window (575 ± 12.5 nm). Other optical filters can be selected for use with other fluorophores.

Signals are generated in all four detectors simultaneously as an individual cell passes through the laser beam. These four signals are then processed by the electronics of the flow cytometer. The signals are amplified using linear or logarithmic amplifiers, are digitized, and are stored for later quantitative analysis. Under different experimental conditions it may be necessary to look at only one of the signals or it may be necessary to look at two or possibly all four signals to quantify the population under investigation.

If only one of the four cellular parameters is to be studied, the data are usually collected as a histogram. An example of a histogram is shown in Figure 6.2. Peripheral blood mononuclear cells were stained with the monoclonal antibody anti-Leu 3a conjugated with PE (Becton Dickinson Monoclonal Center, Mountain View, CA). The relative fluorescence from each individual cell is stored in a pulse

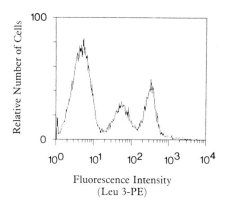

Fig. 6.2 Fluorescence histogram of peripheral blood mononuclear cells stained with anti-Leu 3a conjugated with phycoerythrin (PE). Three populations of cells (bright, mid-intensity, and unstained) are identified in this single parameter histogram.

height analyzer. The resulting histogram is in actuality a probability distribution in which the numbers of cells with any given fluorescence intensity is plotted as a function of increasing fluorescence. In this figure it is clear that three populations are identifiable; one with bright fluorescence with a peak of approximately 250 units, a mid-intensity peak centered at 50 units, and a third population with the same fluorescence as unstained cells of approximately 5 units. (These fluorescence units are relative although through proper calibration the fluorescence units can be directly related to the number of fluorochromes on each cell.)

It may be important in a particular experiment to correlate two parameters on a cell population. Such a correlation can be displayed as a 'dot plot' or 'scattergram.' A dot plot illustrating the correlation between forward light scattering and anti-Leu 3a staining of peripheral blood mononuclear cells is shown in Figure 6.3. Each dot represents a single cell with the position of the dot representing the size of the signal identified by the two detectors as the cell passes through the system. The clustering of dots indicates a grouping of cells with similar characteristics. Three populations of cells are evident in this dot plot. The dimmest and brightest populations are small by forward light scattering while mid-intensity cells are significantly larger by forward light scattering. It has been shown that the dim, large cells reactive with anti-Leu 3a are monocytes while the other two populations are small lymphocytes[14].

The correlation between two parameters can also be depicted by a contour plot. In this representation the data are collected as a two dimensional histogram. The numbers of cells of each intensity are collected and stored in a two dimensional array. The mountains and valleys identified by a two dimensional histogram are then depicted in the contour plot. The data collected as a dot plot in Figure 6.3A are redrawn as a contour plot in Figure 6.3B. Individual lines connect equivalent cell numbers much as a contour map illustrates altitude. The same three clusters of cells are evident in Figure 6.3B as are identified in Figure 6.3A.

In some experiments it may be important to correlate all four parameters for each cell as it passes through the system. This is accomplished by using a process called

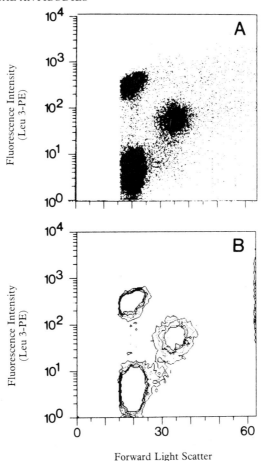

Fig. 6.3 Correlation between light scattering and fluorescence for peripheral blood mononuclear cells stained with anti-Leu 3a-PE. (A) In this plot each cell is represented by a dot. The position of the dot is directly related to the signal in the forward light scatter and fluorescence detectors for that individual cell. Populations of cells can be identified by clustering of dots. The small cells by light scattering can be split into two groups, bright and unlabelled cells. The larger cells by light scattering have mid-intensity fluorescence. (B) The same cell populations are displayed in a contour plot or two dimensional histogram. The height of the peaks are represented by the contour levels drawn at 5, 10, 15, 20, and 25 cells. Cell populations are identified by concentric contour lines.

'list mode.' In list mode the four parameters for each cell are stored together. For each cell passing through the system all parameters are digitized and stored in the computer in a lengthening list. When a sufficient number of cells has been analyzed, the data are stored on some permanent medium such as magnetic tape or floppy disk. At a later time the experiment can be replayed cell by cell and the correlations between any of the parameters can be identified. This analysis using list mode allows all the information for an experiment to be collected without preselection so that the correlation between two or more parameters can be made after the fact. In addition, list mode permits the analysis of very few cells in a sample. By collecting all parameters for all of the cells in a small sample it is necessary to only run the sample once through the flow cytometer.

DISCRIMINATION OF CELL TYPES BY LIGHT SCATTERING

The two light scattering detectors illustrated in Figure 6.1 (FLS and 90°SC) observe quite different characteristics of the cells. Forward light scattering, just off axis from the laser beam, discriminates cells primarily by size[3]. Because this signal is a complex interaction of defraction and refraction of the cell, one is not able to obtain a true cellular volume[4]. It has been shown, however, that the light scattering signal can be used in a relative manner to discriminate between larger and smaller cells[15]. This ability to discriminate cells by size is critically dependent upon the angle at which the detector collects the light with respect to the laser beam. The best size discrimination results when the light scatter detector collects light very close to the axis of the laser beam[11]. The predominant cellular characteristic that is observed in the 90° light scattering detector is reflection. The incident laser beam is reflected from the nucleus, the granules included in the cytoplasm, and from irregularities in the cell surface membrane. The properties identified by the two light scatter detectors are then quite different, one detector observing size while the other detector independently assessing reflectivity.

The combination of these two independent parameters permits the differential analysis of cell types in peripheral blood without staining the sample. It is possible to distinguish lymphocytes, monocytes and granulocytes from each other based solely on their light scattering properties[5]. Such an analysis of peripheral blood leucocytes in which the erythrocytes have been lysed using ammonium chloride[16] is shown in Figure 6.4A. Three populations can be identified corresponding to lymphocytes, monocytes and granulocytes. Sorting of these populations confirms this identification. A comparison of the light scattering pattern of whole blood (with erythrocytes lysed by ammonium chloride) with a mononuclear cell preparation using Ficoll-Paque (Pharmacia, Piscataway, NJ) is shown in Figure 6.4B. The population of granulocytes is missing from the mononuclear cell preparation. The clear distinction between these cell types using light scattering is consistent for normal individuals. However, when examining clinical patient blood, i.e. leukemic, one of the populations usually predominates over the others. With chronic lymphatic leukemia almost all of the cells lie within the lymphocyte population, whereas with acute myelogenous leukemia most of the cells lie within the monocyte peak. In patients undergoing immunotherapy or other drug treatments, the discrimination between lymphocytes and monocytes may be blurred. A large number of blast cells makes it difficult to discriminate between the lymphocytes and monocytes.

The importance of discriminating cells based on light scattering is illustrated by Figure 6.3. It is clear that the mid intensity anti-Leu 3 positive cells are large by light scattering and therefore can be identified as monocytes. This staining is quite distinct from that observed on lymphocytes which are the smaller cells by light scattering. Of the three populations identifiable in the histogram in Figure 6.2, only the dimmest and the brightest are lymphocytes.

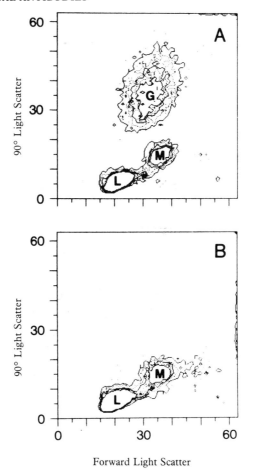

Fig. 6.4 Discrimination of leucocyte populations by forward and 90° light scattering. **A** Leucocytes were prepared by lysis of the erythrocytes using ammonium chloride. Three populations of cells can be identified among the remaining cells, lymphocytes (L), monocytes (M), and granulocytes (G). **B** When a mononuclear cell fraction is isolated using a density gradient only the lymphocytes (L) and the monocytes (M) are present.

MULTI-COLOUR IMMUNOFLUORESCENCE

Until recently the two chromophores most frequently used in immunofluorescence were fluorescein and rhodamine. A new pair of dyes, the phycobiliproteins, is now being used in immunofluorescence[17]. One of these proteins, B-phycoerythrin, can be used with fluorescein to yield two-colour fluorescence with only a single wavelength of excitation. The phycobiliproteins are naturally-occurring pigments used by algae and cyanobacteria as auxiliary chromophores in the photosynthetic apparatus. B-phycoerythrin which is a large molecule of 250 000 daltons has an extremely high extinction coefficient thereby efficiently trapping light[18,19]. In addition, the quantum yield (number of photons emitted/number of photons absorbed) approaches the theoretical maximum of one. This compound is soluble in water and the fluorescence is unaffected by a wide range of pH.

Since phycoerythrin and fluorescein efficiently absorb 488 nm light, both fluorescein and phycoerythrin can be excited at the same wavelength. Their emission spectra, however, are quite separate. A comparison of the spectral properties of fluorescein and B-phycoerythrin is shown in Figure 6.5. The peak of fluorescein excitation is 495 nm while that for phycoerythrin is 545 nm. Fluorescein has a broad emission spectrum, peaking at 520 nm, while phycoerythrin has a relatively narrow emission spectrum with a maximum at 575 nm. Because of this spectral overlap of fluorescein and phycoerythrin, optical filters cannot completely separate the emission of one chromophore from the other. As shown in Figure 6.5, the 530/30 filter used in the first fluorescence channel (FL1 Figure 6.1) transmits a large portion of the fluorescein emission while the 575/25 filter used in the second fluorescence channel (FL2 Figure 6.1) transmits the orange phycoerythrin signal. Since the fluorescein emission is rather broad, some of this fluorescence is able to pass the 575/25 filter. This means that a small part of the fluorescein emission will be detectable in the FL2 fluorescence channel (Figure 6.5). Since phycoerythrin has very little green light in its emission spectrum, only fluorescein will be detectable in the FL1 channel.

When cells are stained with only FITC, signals will be observed in both of the detectors (Fig. 6.6A). The very brightest green cells yield a significant signal in the

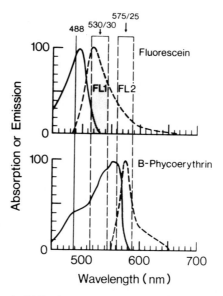

Fig. 6.5 Relative absorption (solid lines) and emission (dashed lines) spectra of fluorescein and B-phycoerythrin. Since both dyes absorb blue light, an argon ion laser operating at 488 nm can be used to excite both fluorescein and phycoerythrin. The optical filters used to discriminate the fluorescence emission (FL1 and FL2) are depicted in the spectra by the vertical dashed lines. The 530/30 bandpass filter used in FL1 transmits light from fluorescein almost exclusively whereas the 575/25 band pass filter used in FL2 transmits both fluorescein and phycoerythrin fluorescence. This spectral overlap in the FL2 channel necessitates the use of an electronic compensation network to identify fluorescein and phycoerythrin independently.

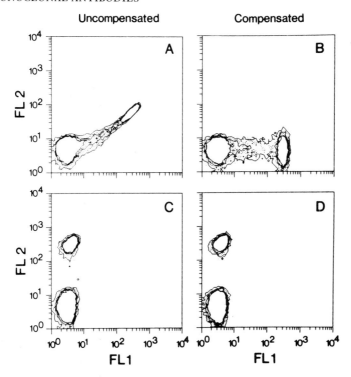

Fig. 6.6 Comparison of two colour fluorescence before and after compensation of cells singly stained with either fluorescein or phycoerythrin. (A) Mononuclear cells from human peripheral blood were labelled with anti-Leu 2a FITC. The lymphocytes, as identified by forward light scattering, were then analyzed in the two colour system using the filters shown in Figure 6.5. The positive cells identified in FL1 are also seen in FL2. The identification of the FITC labelled cells in FL2 can be eliminated using a compensation network (B). In (C) and (D), lymphocytes labelled with anti-Leu 3 PE were analyzed. Without compensation (C) the positive cells can be identified only in the FL2, not the FL1 channel. Therefore compensation is not needed between the FL2 and FL1 channels. The contour plot shown in (D) was collected with the same compensation as was used in (B) showing that compensation of one channel does not affect the other.

orange, FL2 channel. Cells which are labelled with only phycoerythrin will produce signals only in the FL2 channel (Fig. 6.6C). The comparison of FITC and PE single labelled cells is shown in Figure 6.6A and 6.6C. The FITC labelled cells do not lie along the axis but curve up and are seen in the PE channel. When phycoerythrin is used to label the cells the PE stained cells are not observed in the FL1 channel.

The detection of fluorescein fluorescence in the phycoerythrin channel is dependent on the emission spectra of the chromophores used to stain the cells and upon the optical filters used to detect those stains. There is a linear correlation between the amount of stain detected in one channel with that detected in the other. Because of this linear relationship it is possible to compensate for the spectral overlap using an electronic circuit[6]. The purpose of this circuitry is to subtract a portion of the signal observed in the fluorescein detector (FL1) from that observed in the phycoerythrin detector (FL2). This circuitry can be easily set so that cells stained only with FITC will not give a signal in the FL2 channel, Figure 6.6B. The FITC labelled cells lie along the X axis after compensation. Since phycoerythrin has very

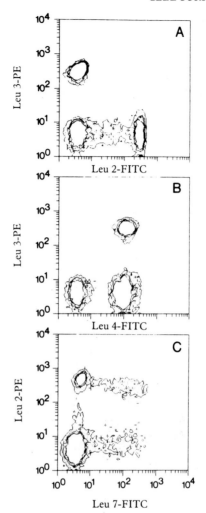

Fig. 6.7 Peripheral blood lymphocytes, as identified by forward angle light scattering, were assessed for two colours of immunofluorescence after compensation.
(A) Mononuclear cells were simultaneously stained with anti-Leu 3a PE and anti-Leu 2 FITC.
(B) Lymphocytes were double labelled for anti-Leu 4 FITC and anti-Leu 3 PE.
(C) The correlation between anti-Leu 2 PE and anti-Leu 7 FITC on peripheral lymphocytes.

low leakage into the fluorescein channel, no compensation is required in the other direction. (When PE conjugated antibodies are used to identify very dense antigens, e.g. anti-HLA, compensation of the PE signal must be made.) Compensation of the FITC channel does not affect the PE signal since the contour plots for the PE labelled cells are identical whether compensated or uncompensated. (Figure 6.6C,D)

Since the system can now be adjusted to detect the two chromophores independently, the flow cytometer can be used to correlate the expression of two different cell surface antigens. An example of this correlated staining can be shown by labelling peripheral blood mononuclear cells with both the anti-Leu 2 FITC and the anti-Leu 3 PE antibodies. Since the anti-Leu 2 antibody reacts with the T cytotoxic/suppressor cell[20] while the anti-Leu 3 antibody binds to the helper/inducer T-cell[21], the two populations identified by these two antibodies are separate and nonoverlapping (Fig. 6.7A). Among normal individuals three populations of cells are observed when mononuclear cells are double labelled with anti-Leu 2 and anti-Leu 3: 3^+2^-, 3^-2^+, and 2^-3^-. A very low number of overlapping immature T-cells, 3^+2^+, are observed in the normal patient. However, among patients undergoing immunosuppression the double labelled 2^-3^+ cell may form a significant proportion of the lymphocytes in that individual (R. Guttman, personal communication). By performing the two colour fluorescence it is possible to obtain a helper/suppressor ratio using only one sample. By correlating the two stains on one sample it is also possible to identify the overlapping population of 3^+2^+ cells which could not be obtained using single colour reagents.

An illustration of overlapping populations identifiable by two colour fluorescence is shown in Figure 6.7B where peripheral blood mononuclear cells were stained with anti-Leu 3 PE and anti-Leu 4 FITC. Since anti-Leu 4 identifies all T-cells[23], while anti-Leu 3 reacts with only the helper T-cells, all of the Leu 3^+ cells are Leu 4^+. There are cells that are Leu 4^+ that are not Leu 3^+, presumably the cytotoxic/suppressor T-cells. The Leu 3^-4^- population of lymphocytes is also identifiable in this contour plot. There are, however, no lymphocytes that are of the 3^+ 4^- phenotype. Using this combination of reagents one is able to determine the total number of T-cells as well as the proportion of helper T-cells in one sample. The proportion of cytotoxic suppressor cells can be estimated by subtracting the proportion of helper cells from the total T-cell population.

It is possible to see all combinations of populations identified by two colours. The results of an experiment in which peripheral blood mononuclear cells were labelled with anti-Leu 2 PE and anti-Leu 7 FITC are shown in Figure 6.7C. The anti-Leu 2 antibody identified the cytotoxic/suppressor T-cell while the anti-Leu 7 binds to the large granular lymphocyte (LGL)[24]. In the correlation between these two antibodies, cells which express Leu 2 only and cells which express Leu 7 only are readily apparent. There are cells which express both antigens while a significant proportion of cells express neither antigen. Cells within each of these populations can be isolated for further functional studies as described in Chapter 9.

SUMMARY

The use of the quantitative aspects of flow cytometry coupled with the specificity of monoclonal antibodies provides a powerful tool for the study of individual cells and heterogenous cell populations. Discrimination of cells based on physical parameters, i.e. light scattering, allows the characterization of cells based on morphological difference. Monoclonal antibodies on the other hand identify differences in biochemical structures on the cell surfaces thus providing an independent method of discriminating between cells. Two or more monoclonal antibodies can be identified using the multi-colour fluorescence capabilities of flow cytometry so that cells can be distinguished based upon multiple cell surface markers. By combining these multiple parameters one is able to identify not only differences between cell types based on morphological differences, but also to identify functional, maturational and activation differences between cell types. Full utilization of these probes requires multi-parameter analysis in order to precisely correlate the cellular characteristic with an individual cell. By combining four or more parameters simultaneously differences between cells can be identified where fewer parameters would not allow the discrimination.

REFERENCES

1. Bonner W A, Hulett H R, Sweet R G, Herzenberg L A 1972 Fluorescence activated cell sorting. Review of Scientific Instruments 43: 404–426
2. Julius M H, Sweet R G, Fathman C G, Herzenberg L A 1975 Fluorescence activated cell sorting and its application. In: Richman C R, et al (eds) Cells: probes and problems. Los Alamos, US Energy Research and Development Administration. (CONS 73-1007)
3. Mullaney P F, Dean R N 1970 Small angle light scattering of biological cells. Biophysical Journal 10: 764–775
4. Salzman G C, Mullaney P F, Price B J 1979 Light scattering approaches to cell characterization. In: Melamed M, Mullaney P F, Mendelsohn M (eds) Flow cytometry and sorting. John Wiley, New York
5. Salzman G C, Crowell J M, Martin J C, Trujillo T T, Romero A, Mullaney P F, LaBauve P M 1975 Cell classification by laser light scattering; identification and separation of unstained leucocytes. ACTA Cytologica 19: 374–386
6. Loken M R, Parks D R, Herzenberg L A 1977 Two colour immunofluorescence using a fluorescence activated cell sorter. Journal of Histochemistry and Cytochemistry. 25: 899–910
7. Loken M R, Lanier L L 1984 Three colour immunofluorescence analysis of leu antigens on human peripheral blood using two lasers on a fluorescence activated cell sorter. Cytometry 5: 151–158
8. Parks D R, Hardy R R, Herzenberg L A 1984 Three colour immunofluorescence analysis of mouse B lymphocytes sub populations. Cytometry 5: 159–167
9. Melamed M, Mullaney P F, Mendelsohn M (eds) 1979 Flow cytometry and sorting. John Wiley, New York
10. Loken M R, Stall A M 1982 Flow cytometry as an analytical and preparative tool in immunology. Journal of Immunological Methods 50: R85–92
11. Horan P K, Loken M R 1985 A practical guide to the use of flow systems. In: Ploem J S, Van Dilla M A, Dean P R (eds) Methods of flow cytometry, Academic Press, New York (In press)
12. Parks D R, Lanier L L, Herzenberg L A 1985 Flow cytometry and fluorescence activated cell sorting. In: Weir D A (ed) Handbook of experimental immunology, 4th edn. Blackwell Scientific, Edinburgh (In press)
13. Parks D R, Herzenberg L A 1984 Fluorescence activated cell sorting: theory, experimental optimization and application in lymphoid cell biology. In: Kolwich S P, Kaplan N O (eds) Methods in Enzymology. Academic Press, New York Vol 108: 197–241
14. Wood G S, Warner N L, Warnke R A 1983 Anti-Leu 3/T4 antibodies react with cells of monocytes/macrophage and langerhans lineage. Journal of Immunology 131: 212–217
15. Loken M R, Sweet R G, Herzenberg L A 1976 Cell discrimination by multi-angle light scattering. Journal of Histochemistry and Cytochemistry 24: 284–290
16. Mishell B B, Shiigi S M (eds) 1980 Selected methods in cellular immunology. WH Freeman and Co., San Francisco
17. Oi V T, Glazer A M, Stryer L 1982 Fluorescent phycobiliprotein conjugates for analyses of cells and molecules. Journal of Cell Biology 93: 981–990
18. Glazer A N, Hixson C S 1977 Subunits structure and chromophore composition of rhodophytan phycoerythrins: *porphyridium cruentum* B phycoerythrin and b phycoerythrin. Journal of Biological Chemistry 252: 32–40
19. Grabowski J, Gantt E 1978 Phycophysical properties of phycobiliproteins from phycobilisomes: fluorescence lifetimes quantum yields and polarization spectra. Photochemistry and Photobiology 28: 39–47
20. Engleman E G, Benike C J, Glickman E, Evans R L 1981 Antibodies to membrane structures that distinguish suppressor/cytotoxic and helper T cell lymphocyte subpopulations block the mixed leucocyte reaction in man. Journal of Experimental Medicine 154: 193–205
21. Evans R L, Wall D W, Platsoucas C D, Siegal F P, Fikrig S M, Testa C M, Good R A 1981 Thymus dependent membrane antigens in man: inhibition of cell mediated lympholysis by

monoclonal antibodies to the TH$_2$ antigen. Proceedings of the National Academy of Sciences 78: 544–550

22. Rienhertz E L, Schlossman S 1980 The differentiation in function of the human T lymphocytes. Cell 19: 821–824

23. Leadbetter J A, Evans R L, Lipinski M, Cunningham-Rundles C, Good R A, Herzenberg L A 1981 Evolutionary conservation of surface molecules that distinguish T lymphocytes helper/inducer and T cytotoxic suppressor subpopulations in mouse and man. Journal of Experimental Medicine 153: 310–322

24. Abo T, Balch C M 1981 A differentiation antigen of human NK and K cells identified by a monoclonal antibody (HNK-1). Journal of Immunology 127: 1024–1029

7

Immuno-enzymatic labelling of haematological samples with monoclonal antibodies

D. Y. Mason W. N. Erber B. Falini H. Stein K. C. Gatter

INTRODUCTION

The introduction in the early 1970's of immunocytochemical methods for studying human haematological neoplasms led to a rapid increase in knowledge concerning the origin and nature of these disorders. However these immunocytochemical procedures were performed in only a small number of specialist laboratories. This restriction was due in part to the limited availability of satisfactory immunocytochemical reagents (e.g. primary antisera and fluorochrome conjugates), and partly to the fact that these studies were based on indirect immunofluorescent labelling of living cells in suspension, a technique which requires the constant availability of experienced technical staff.

The first of these obstacles to the widespread use of immunocytochemical techniques in haematological diagnosis began to be removed towards the end of the 1970's, with the introduction of monoclonal antibodies against antigens on human blood and bone marrow cells, and with their commercial distribution. However the immunocytochemical techniques by which these antibodies were used remained unchanged and this constituted a continuing obstacle to their use in the routine haematological laboratory.

In the present Chapter we describe a variety of simple immunocytochemical techniques which enable antigens recognised by monoclonal antibodies to be demonstrated in blood, bone marrow and tissue samples. These procedures have the advantage that samples may be stored (following minimal processing) for unlimited periods before labelling: this is of particular importance for the routine laboratory in which staff may not be available at all times to perform immunocytochemical labelling. Furthermore all of the reagents used in the procedure described in this Chapter are commercially available. Thus many of the previous barriers to the use of immunocytochemical procedures for analysing human haematological disorders are removed, and it is hoped that these techniques will come to be used in the future on an increasingly wide scale in diagnostic laboratories.

IMMUNO-ENZYMATIC LABELLING TECHNIQUES

Advantages

The techniques described in this chapter are all immuno-enzymatic procedures, in which the sites to which a primary monoclonal antibody binds are revealed by labelling with either horseradish peroxidase or calf intestinal alkaline phosphatase.

Immuno-enzymatic techniques offer two major advantages over immuno-fluorescent procedures, particularly in the context of analysing haematological samples:

1. The reaction product of the enzyme can be examined with a conventional light microscope, and counterstaining of labelled preparations is possible. As a result the microscopist is no longer in the dark (literally) concerning the nature and location of positively stained cells, as he is when examining immunofluorescently labelled preparations.

2. Immuno-enzymatic reaction products are stable on storage so that slides may be examined (and if necessary re-examined) over a period of time. In contrast, immunofluorescent preparations tend to fade with time (although not as rapidly as is sometimes suggested). An important practical consequence is that the complex immunohistological staining patterns which are often seen in lymphoid tissue biopsies can be analysed in detail. The fact that conventional counterstaining is possible (see above), greatly facilitates this detailed analysis.

The question is sometimes raised as to whether immuno-enzymatic techniques are more sensitive than immunofluorescent procedures (or vice versa). There have been numerous claims in the past from both sides, but in practice there is (at least at present) little to choose between the two techniques. This is indicated by the fact that none of the human cellular antigens recognised with currently available monoclonal antibodies have proved detectable by one technique but not by the other. However it should be added that new immunoalkaline phosphatase techniques of enhanced sensitivity (as described below) may change this state of affairs in the future.[1]

Principles of immuno-enzymatic staining procedures
The methods used for the immuno-enzymatic staining of haematological samples are summarized in Figures 7.1 and 7.13, and described in detail in the *Technical Appendix* to this chapter.

Immunoperoxidase labelling
Two simple immunoperoxidase procedures are used in the authors' laboratory.[2] In the two-stage indirect immunoperoxidase procedure (Fig. 7.1a), the cell or tissue sample is incubated first with a monoclonal antibody, and then with peroxidase-conjugated anti-mouse Ig. This procedure gives good staining of a wide range of antigens in human tissues. However when greater sensitivity is required a three-stage indirect immunoperoxidase technique is used (Fig. 7.1b). This procedure is identical in its initial steps to the two-stage method, differing only in that a third stage, consisting of peroxidase-conjugated anti-rabbit Ig, is added. This method is substantially more sensitive than the two-stage indirect technique and it should be used whenever immunoperoxidase labelling of maximal sensitivity is required.

Attempts in the past (in the premonoclonal era) to increase the sensitivity of labelling reactions by creating multilayer immunocytochemical sandwiches often led to problems of excessive background staining, and at first sight the three-stage indirect sandwich immunoperoxidase technique (Fig. 7.1b) appears to run this risk. However background labelling was due in part to the excess of nonspecific antibody which is present in all polyclonal antisera. Monoclonal antibodies are inherently much purer reagents than polyclonal antisera, and contain little or no mouse

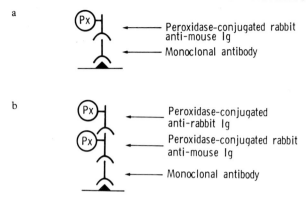

Fig. 7.1 Schematic representation of the two immunoperoxidase procedures used in the authors' laboratory for labelling monoclonal antibodies showing (a) two stage and (b) three stage immunoperoxidase procedures. For further details see the main text and the *Technical Appendix.*

immunoglobulin other than specific antibody. Hence the type of triple sandwich shown in Figure 7.1b may be created with minimal risk of background labelling.

A variety of alternative immunoperoxidase labelling procedures have been employed in other laboratories for staining tissue sections with monoclonal antibodies. One procedure is a four stage PAP technique, in which the monoclonal antibody is followed by rabbit anti-mouse Ig, an unlabelled 'bridging' anti-rabbit Ig antibody, and PAP immune complexes (formed between peroxidase and rabbit anti-peroxidase). A second technique which has been used in several laboratories is the ABC procedure, in which the second stage anti-mouse Ig antibody is labelled with biotin, and this reagent is recognized by a third stage complex consisting of avidin and biotin-labelled peroxidase. We have only limited experience of these two techniques. However our impression is that they are not more sensitive than the indirect methods outlined above, and their popularity may stem more from their novelty than from any demonstrable advantages in terms of sensitivity or specificity.

Immuno-alkaline phosphatase labelling
For many years immunoperoxidase labelling was by far the most widely used immuno-enzymatic procedure. However recently it has become apparent that alkaline phosphatase offers several advantages relative to peroxidase as an antibody label[3]:

1. The vivid red immuno-alkaline phosphatase reaction product (see Figs. 7.2–7.8) is more easily visualised than are the reaction products produced in immunoperoxidase preparations. This makes the technique particularly suitable for staining surface antigens in cell smears (Figs. 7.2, 7.7, 7.9–7.11)[4,5,6].

2. The maximal intensity of labelling which can be produced in the immuno-alkaline phosphatase procedure is greater than can be achieved by immuno-peroxidase staining.

3. Endogenous peroxidase present in granulocytes, erythroid cells or macrophages may on occasion give rise to unwanted background staining in immunoperoxidase procedures. It is difficult to abolish this activity by exposing samples to peroxidase inhibitors (such as methanol) without causing antigenic denaturation. In contrast endogenous alkaline phosphatase activity survives poorly in tissue sections or cell

Fig. 7.2 Immuno-alkaline phosphatase staining with monoclonal anti-T cell antibody of a buffy coat smear from normal blood. Note the strongly labelled T cells, contrasting with unstained red cells and leucocytes.

Fig. 7.3 Immuno-alkaline phosphatase labelling with monoclonal anti-cytokeratin of a cryostat section from a bone marrow trephine. Strongly labelled clusters of metastatic mammary carcinoma cells are seen, lying in a negative background (of fibrotic normal marrow).

Fig. 7.4 Bone marrow smears from a case of metastatic carcinoma: (a) A single clump of carcinoma cells (arrowed) is seen in the routinely stained smear; (b) and (c) Immuno-alkaline phosphatase labelling of air dried smears from the same case with anti-cytokeratin reveals the clumps of carcinoma cells, but shows no reactivity with normal marrow cells.

Fig. 7.5 Immuno-alkaline phosphatase labelling of cytocentrifuged cells from a case of chronic myeloid leukaemia in blast crisis, using monoclonal anti-HLA-DR. Many of the cells are stained, but their reactivity is limited to small clumps of labelling, probably intracytoplasmic in localization.

Fig. 7.6 Immuno-alkaline phosphatase labelling of a peripheral blood smear from a case of acute lymphoblastic leukaemia using anti-TdT. Several strongly stained blast cells are seen, together with one unlabelled normal myeloid cell (arrowed).

Fig. 7.7 Immuno-alkaline phosphatase labelling of blood smears from a case of chronic lymphocytic leukaemia with three monoclonal antibodies (anti-HLA-DR, anti-T3 antigen, and anti-T1 antigen). (a) HLA-DR antigen is present on all the leukaemic cells seen, but absent from a polymorph (arrowed). (b) Three normal T-cells are labelled for the T3 antigen, but the leukaemic cells are negative; (c) T1 antigen is strongly expressed on two normal lymphocytes (arrowed), but also weakly expressed on the CLL cells. This pattern is typical of chronic lymphocytic leukaemia.

Fig. 7.8 Air dried bone marrow smears from a case of rhabdomyosarcoma: (a) The Romanovsky stained smear shows infiltration with primitive vacuolated cells, which had been diagnosed as lymphoblasts; (b) Staining with monoclonal anti-desmin (the intermediate filament characteristic of muscle) shows that the neoplastic cells are strongly labelled. Note the two unstained normal cells (arrowed).

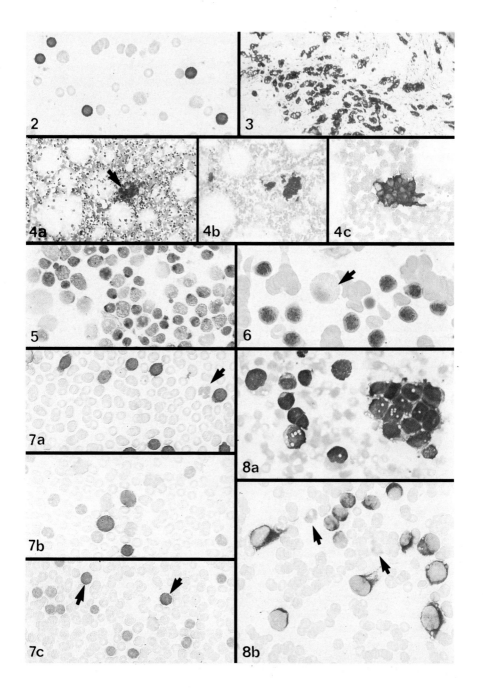

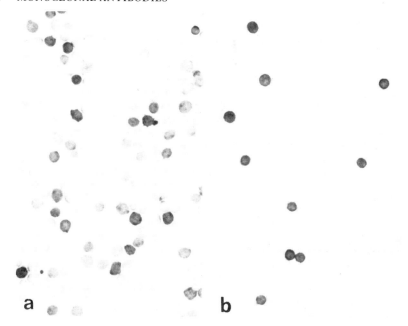

Fig. 7.9 Immuno-alkaline phosphatase staining of cytocentrifuged cells from the cerebrospinal fluid of a patient with acute lymphoblastic leukaemia: (a) Staining for common acute lymphoblastic leukaemia antigen (monoclonal antibody J5) shows a population of positive cells, varying in the intensity of staining; (b) Staining for T-cells (monoclonal antibody UCHT1) shows a smaller number of T-cells, which are presumably reactive.[6]

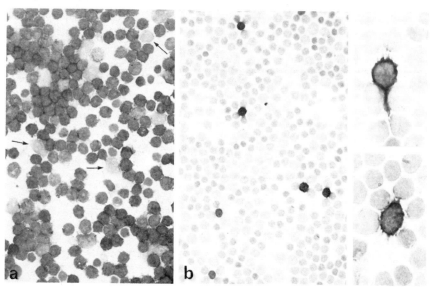

Fig. 7.10 Immuno-alkaline phosphatase staining of two haematological samples with monoclonal anti-IgM: (a) Peripheral blood from a case of prolymphocytic leukaemia shows intense labelling of the majority of cells, although occasional unstained cells (arrowed) can be seen; (b) Bone marrow aspirate from a case of acute lymphoblastic leukaemia shows occasional strongly IgM-positive normal lymphoid cells lying among a background of unstained leukaemic cells. Two of the IgM-positive cells in this sample are shown in high magnification revealing villous processes projecting from their surfaces.[6]

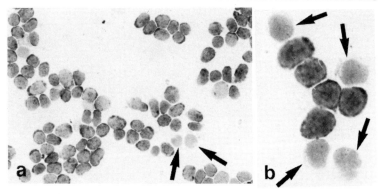

Fig. 7.11 Immuno-alkaline phosphatase staining of bone marrow cells from a case of acute lymphoblastic leukaemia, using monoclonal antibody specific for the common-acute lymphoblastic leukaemia antigen (antibody J5): (a) At low magnification, it is evident that the majority of cells are strongly labelled. Two non-reactive cells are indicated by arrows (b) a high power view shows five positively labelled leukaemia cells, together with four unlabelled cells (arrows)[6].

smears and any residual activity may be selectively inhibited by including levamisole in the enzyme substrate solution[7]. The absence of endogenous enzyme activity in the immuno-alkaline phosphatase procedure is of importance when staining lymphoid tissue rich in infiltrating eosinophils (as shown in Fig. 7.12), or blood or bone marrow smears (Figs. 7.2, 7.4, 7.6–7.8), or when attempting to detect antigen-positive cells in sections of human bone marrow trephines (Figs. 7.3, 7.13–7.16).

Immuno-alkaline phosphatase labelling is performed in the authors' laboratory by two different methods (Fig. 7.17), one of which is analogous to the three-stage indirect immunoperoxidase technique described above, while the other (the APAAP procedure[1]) is analogous to the PAP immunoperoxidase technique. These two procedures are of comparable sensitivity. However substantial enhancement of sensitivity can be attained in the APAAP technique by repeating the second and third incubation stages (Fig. 7.18) making it possible to detect antigens which are present at levels too low to be reliably demonstrated by other methods.

STAINING OF TISSUE SECTIONS

The use of immuno-enzymatic procedures for staining human tissue samples in cryostat section represents a relatively recent advance, since the majority of studies of cell surface markers in lymphoid tissue and bone marrow samples carried out before the late 1970's were performed on cell suspensions. This latter approach suffers from several disadvantages.

1. When a cell suspension is prepared from a tissue sample, information concerning the topographical relationships between different elements present in the sample is lost. It is thus not possible, when studying neoplastic lymphoid tissue, to assess the degree to which normal tissue architecture has been effaced, or whether there is preferential involvement of one or other region within the tissue (e.g. B-cell follicles, T-cell areas, etc). Furthermore, when staining human bone marrow, the presence of stromal cells or the relationship of antigen-positive cells to tissue

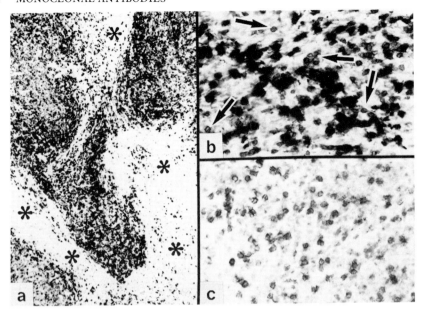

Fig. 7.12 Illustration of the way in which background staining due to endogenous tissue enzyme activity may obscure immunohistological labelling reactions in immunoperoxidase procedures, but may be eliminated by employing the immuno-alkaline phosphatase method. A cryostat section of nodular sclerosing Hodgkin's disease tissue is shown, stained with a monoclonal anti-T-cell antibody by an immunoperoxidase procedure (a and b) and by an immuno-alkaline phosphatase technique (c). In the low power view of the immunoperoxidase reaction (a) areas of lymphoid tissue, lying among fibrous tissue bands (asterisks) contain numerous strongly peroxidase-positive eosinophils. A high power view of one of these areas (b) shows these cells in greater detail and also reveals more weakly stained T lymphocytes (arrowed), characterized by a ring-like staining reaction. In a corresponding area of the sample stained by the immuno-alkaline phosphatase technique (c) the eosinophils are no longer visualized and the only labelled cells are T lymphocytes.[1]

landmarks (e.g. bone trabeculae or fat spaces) cannot be assessed (Fig. 7.13–7.16, 7.19).

2. Extraction of cells in suspension from solid tissue introduces the risk of selectively depleting one cell population relative to another, e.g. a population of fragile neoplastic cells in a lymph node biopsy may be under-represented in the final cell suspension. Furthermore some types of malignant cells (e.g. Reed-Sternberg cells) and also adherent 'framework' cells (e.g. follicular dendritic reticulum cells—Figures 7.15, 7.20) may be difficult to isolate in suspension in high yield.

3. Solid tissue samples are considerably more convenient to handle than are cell suspensions, since the former type of sample may be rapidly prepared for future study by freezing, whereas cell suspensions are conveniently analysed in the living state. In consequence, surface labelling of cells in suspension must be carried out within a short period of obtaining the sample, whereas frozen tissue samples are stable for very long periods and sections may be cut at the convenience of the laboratory.

It is important to note that the labelling methods described in this Chapter are applied principally to cryostat sections rather than to paraffin sections. Conventional fixation techniques denature most of the antigenic markers recognised by currently

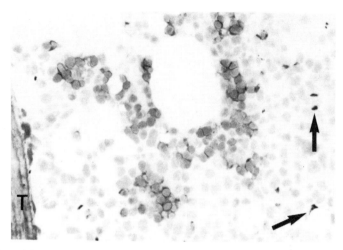

Fig. 7.13 The staining of bone marrow (cryostat section) from a case of myeloproliferative disease with monoclonal anti-glycophorin antibody, showing islands of positively labelled erythroid precursors. Red blood cells (arrowed) are also strongly stained. T indicates a bone trabecula.[8]

available monoclonal antibodies. Attempts have been made in a number of laboratories to unmask these denatured antigens (e.g. by proteolytic digestion of paraffin sections) but in the authors' experience the antigenicity of very few human white cell surface markers can be recovered in this way. It should be added however that there are a number of important exceptions to the rule that surface antigens do not survive routine tissue processing. Two such fixation-resistant antigens (leucocyte common antigen and milk fat globule membrane antigen) are of diagnostic value and are discussed below under *Practical applications of immuno-enzymatic labelling.*

It may also be noted that recently the use of freeze-dried paraffin embedded tissue for immuno-enyzmatic labelling has been explored in this laboratory[10,11]. This approach offers the advantages of using paraffin embedded tissue (i.e. good morphology and convenience of storage) combined with preservation of the great majority of antigens detectable with currently available monoclonal antibodies.

Handling of tissue samples
Something of a mystique surrounds the initial freezing step in immunocytochemical studies of cryostat sections. In practice it is found unnecessary to freeze tissue samples immediately after surgical excision, and in most instances there is little, if any, deterioration in antigenicity or morphological preservation following storage for a period of up to 24 hours at either room temperature or 4°C. However, if tissue is to be stored before freezing, it is important that it is kept moist, e.g. in tissue culture medium or physiological saline.

It appears to be unimportant how the tissue is frozen, provided that this step is achieved rapidly. It is not necessary to use an intermediate cooling medium such as isopentane, and our practice (see *Technical Appendix*) is to immerse a tube containing the tissue sample directly in liquid nitrogen.

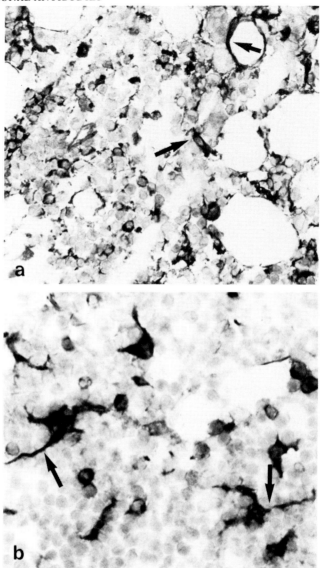

Fig. 7.14 Bone marrow (cryostat sections) stained by the immuno-alkaline phosphatase technique with monoclonal anti-HLA-DR: (a) Normal bone marrow shows the presence of strongly labelled cells (arrowed) characterized by long cytoplasmic processes lining the fat globules; (b) In a case of acute leukaemia similar cells (arrowed) are seen more clearly[8].

Storage of tissue samples

Tissue samples do not show morphological or antigenic deterioration if stored in the frozen state. We normally keep the tissue at −70°C, although satisfactory results are obtained if the tissue is kept at −20°C. Storage in liquid nitrogen gives results which are as good as (but no better than) storage at −70°C.

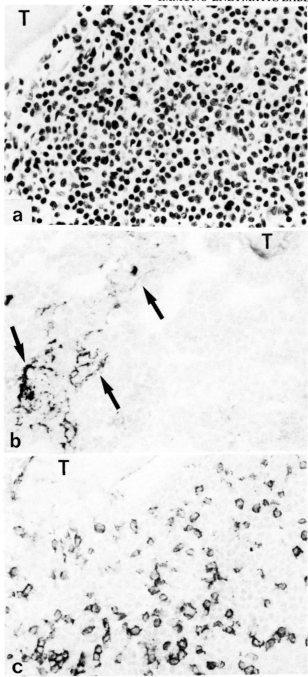

Fig. 7.15 Bone marrow involved by a germinal centre derived lymphoma (centroblastic/centrocytic type): (a) Note the presence of paratrabecular infiltration by small cells with indented nuclei (paraffin section); (b) Bone marrow cryostat section from the same case stained by the immuno-alkaline phosphatase technique with monoclonal anti-C3b complement receptor. Note the presence of dendritic reticulum cells (arrowed) within a neoplastic follicle; (c) Immuno-alkaline phosphatase staining for T cells reveals the presence of plentiful darkly stained cells within the neoplastic follicle. T indicates a bone trabecula.[8]

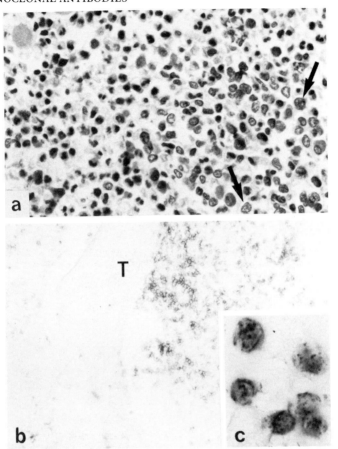

Fig. 7.16 Blast transformation in a case of chronic myeloid leukaemia: (a) The paraffin-embedded marrow trephine biopsy reveals an area containing numerous scattered blast cells (arrowed) intermingled with more mature myeloid elements; (b) Immuno-alkaline phosphatase staining of bone marrow (cryostat section) from the same case with anti-TdT antibody. Clusters of positively stained blast cells are seen; T indicates a bone trabecula; (c) At high magnification the granular nuclear pattern of cells staining is seen.[8]

Cryostat sectioning

This is performed using a conventional laboratory cryostat and no special precautions are necessary. Trephine sections of human bone marrow are more difficult to prepare than are sections from other tissues, (reflecting the small size of the sample and the presence of bone trabeculae) but with perseverance good sections can be obtained in the great majority of samples[8].

Storage of frozen sections

Cryostat sections can be stored for a period of several weeks at $-20°C$ without loss of antigenic reactivity or morphological detail. On longer storage some deterioration of the sections may occur.

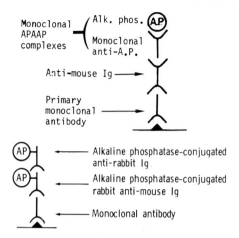

Fig. 7.17 Schematic representation of the two immuno-alkaline phosphatase procedures used in the authors' laboratory for labelling monoclonal antibodies. For further details see the main text and the *Technical Appendix*.

Primary monoclonal antibodies

Table 7.1 lists some of the antibodies which are used in the authors' laboratory for the analysis of human lymphoid tissue biopsies and trephine marrow sections. All of these reagents are available commercially, and can provide much information concerning the nature of neoplastic and reactive disorders affecting these tissues.

Whenever it is possible to obtain a monoclonal antibody as either tissue culture supernatant or ascites (or immunoglobulin purified from ascites) it is preferable to use the former type of preparation. Ascitic fluid inevitably contains contaminating polyclonal immunoglobulin, and non-specific staining will usually occur if the antibody is used at too high a concentration. In contrast most, and usually all, of the Ig present in a hybridoma tissue culture supernatant consists of specific antibody and there is consequently little risk of nonspecific staining. Unfortunately the majority of commercially available monoclonal antibodies against human tissue antigens are produced in the form of material purified from ascitic fluid. However one supplier (Dakopatts) now produces antibodies in the form of tissue culture supernatant designed specifically for immunocytochemical use.

Controls

It is important when labelling cryostat sections of human tissue that both negative and positive controls are included. A negative control should consist of a slide in which either the primary antibody has been omitted and replaced by buffer alone, or a slide in which an irrelevant antibody, unreactive with the tissue preparation, is substituted for the primary antibody. If any staining is seen in negative controls it indicates that the immuno-enzymatic revealing system is giving rise to nonspecific labelling. The only exception is that scattered endogenous peroxidase-positive granulocytes (Fig. 7.12a) will often be seen in negative control sections.

Positive controls should consist of tissue sections known to contain the antigen under investigation. Tonsil provides a convenient control tissue when analysing human lymphoid tissue antigens, whilst the reactivity of many epithelial markers may

Table 7.1 Monoclonal antibodies used for the immuno-enzymatic analysis of cell and tissue samples

Specificity	Source
Anti-B-cell	
Pan-reactive anti-B	1
Anti-IgM	1, 2
Anti-IgD	1, 2
Anti-T-cell	
Pan-reactive (Tl-like)	1, 3
Pan-reactive (T3-like)	2, 3
Pan-reactive (T11-like, anti-SRBC receptor)	1, 4
Pan-reactive, DAKO T2	1
Anti-helper/inducer T-cells	1, 3
Anti-cytotoxic/suppressor T-cells	1, 3
Anti-epithelial	
Anti-cytokeratin	1
Anti-milk fat globule membrane (anti-EMA)	1, 2
Miscellaneous	
Anti-HLA-DR	1, 3
Anti-leucocyte common	1
Anti-dendritic reticulum cell	1
Anti-CALLA	1, 5
Anti-C3b receptor	1
Anti-TdT (polyclonal)	6

1 = Dakopatts   4 = New England Nuclear
2 = Unipath   5 = Coulter
3 = Becton Dickinson   6 = Supertechs

Monoclonal antibodies are now available from an increasing number of commercial sources, and this list does not represent a definitive selection of these reagents, but rather those reagents which the authors have found of value in their own laboratory.

be checked on sections of breast tissue. Positive control sections should always show clearcut staining of antigens in the expected distribution patterns: in the absence of such positive reactions the labelling of pathological tissue cannot be interpreted.

STAINING OF CELL SMEARS

Most of the previously published work on the detection of cellular antigens in haematological samples has been based on immunofluorescent labelling of cell suspensions. However this technique has a number of disadvantages in the context of the routine haematological laboratory. Principal among these are the necessity to process samples rapidly following their receipt; the limited information which can be gathered concerning the morphology of labelled and unlabelled cells; and the impermanence of the immunofluorescent label.

These disadvantages may be overcome by labelling cell smears rather than cells in suspension (see Table 7.2). Cell smear labelling has not been widely used in the past for the analysis of cellular markers in haematology, principally because of a belief that

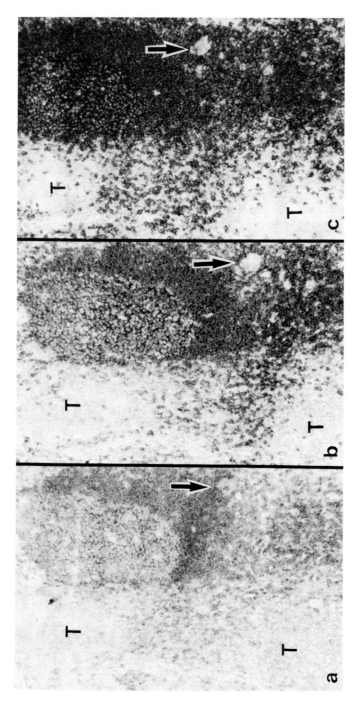

Fig. 7.18 Illustration of the way in which the intensity of APAAP labelling may be enhanced by repeating the second and third steps of the labelling procedure. A cryostat section of normal tonsil has been stained for B-cells (with the monoclonal antibody DAKO-pan-B). In (a) the normal APAAP sequence has been applied, while in (b) and (c) additional incubations with the bridging anti-mouse Ig antibody and the APAAP complexes have been undertaken, either once (b), or twice (c). All incubations were performed before development of the substrate reaction. In (a) a B-cell follicle shows staining of moderate intensity, while adjacent T-cell areas (T) are unstained. The intensity of B-cell labelling is progressively enhanced by the repeated incubations performed in (b) and (c). Note, however, that in even the most strongly labelled section (c), T-cell areas are free of background staining. A transversely sectioned vessel (arrowed in each section) is also clearly unstained, and contrasts strongly in (c) with the adjacent mantle zone B-cells.[1]

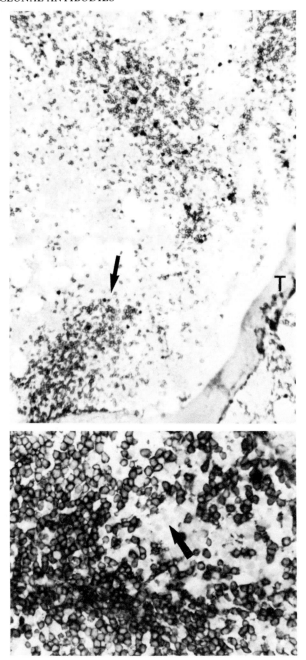

Fig. 7.19 T-cell proliferation involving the bone marrow: Immunoperoxidase staining of a cryostat section for T-cells reveals the presence of nodules scattered through the marrow, one of which (arrowed) is in the paratrabecular area. T indicates a bone trabecula. A higher power view of a neoplastic nodule from this section shows that the majority of cells present are T lymphocytes. A few negative cells (arrowed) are also seen.[8]

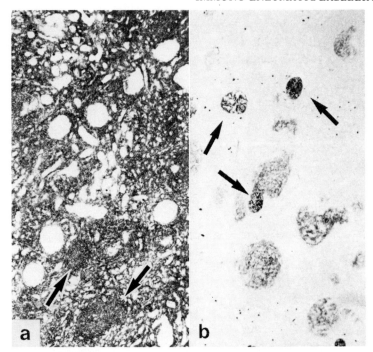

Fig. 7.20 Immunoperoxidase staining of sections from a kidney involved by follicular lymphoma using monoclonal antibodies against B-cells and C3b receptor: (a) The normal elements of the kidney (tubules and glomeruli) can be seen in the section stained for B-cells as negative areas scattered among the dense infiltrate of lymphoma cells. In several areas the tendency of the lymphoma cells to form nodules (arrowed) can be seen; (b) Anti-C3b receptor antibody delineates not only the clusters of DRC but also complement receptor on glomeruli (arrowed).[1]

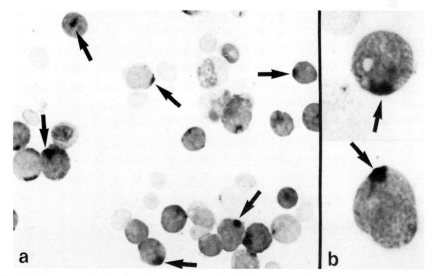

Fig. 7.21 Immuno-alkaline phosphatase staining of bone marrow cells from a case of acute lymphoblastic leukaemia using monoclonal anti-HLA-DR: (a) Many cells are clearly labelled and in several of these a localized clump of reactivity is seen (arrowed). This reaction is more clearly seen in the high power view (b).[6]

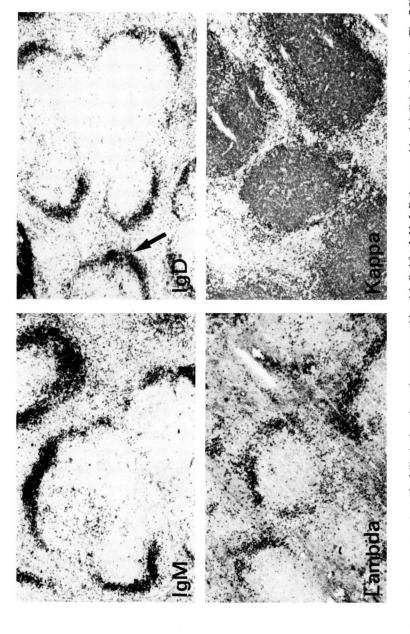

Fig. 7.22 Consecutive cryostat sections of a follicular lymphoma immunoperoxidase labelled for IgM, IgD, kappa and lambda light chains (see Fig. 7.25 for comparison with a reactive follicular hyperplasia). Staining for IgM and IgD shows that the mantle zones, consisting of small lymphoid cells (arrowed), are distorted and breached by the neoplastic germinal centres which express kappa but not lambda light chains. Note that the neoplastic germinal centres lack the normal meshwork of immune complexes (see Fig. 7.25) and that the mantle zones are composed of lymphoid cells showing a polyclonal expression of both kappa and lambda light chains.[13]

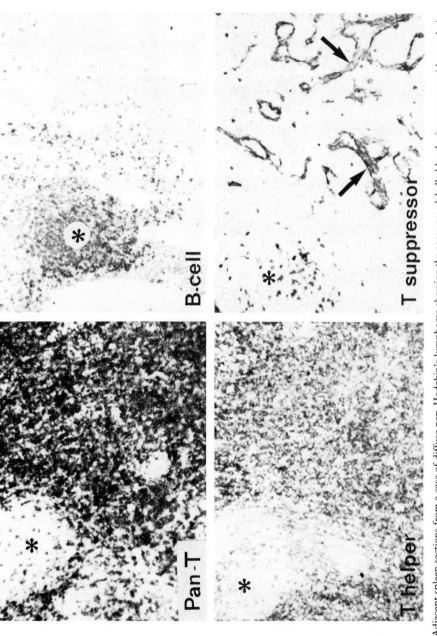

Fig. 7.23 Adjacent spleen sections from a case of diffuse non-Hodgkin's lymphoma showing the same area labelled by the immunoperoxidase technique with monoclonal antibodies reactive with all T-cells (pan T), helper T-cells, suppressor T-cells and B-cells. In each illustration a small residual B-cell follicle (marked by an asterisk) is seen, but the majority of the tissue is diffusely infiltrated by lymphoma cells. These label as T-cells of helper type. This case illustrates the way in which a very marked excess of one or other subclass of T-cells may indicate the presence of a neoplastic T-cell process. Note that the anti-T suppressor cell antibody stains splenic sinusoidal cells, a cross-reaction characteristic of all anti-T suppressor cell antibodies studied to date.[13]

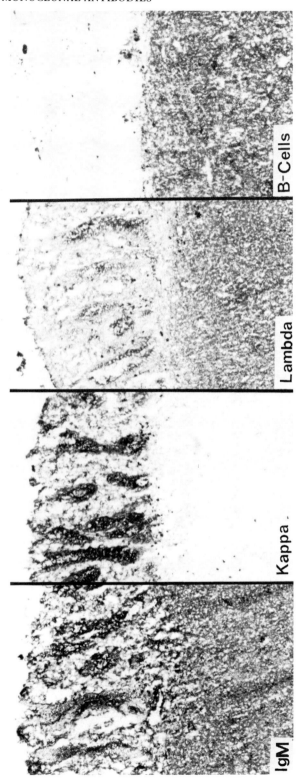

Fig. 7.24 Immunoperoxidase labelling of adjacent cryostat sections of a diffuse intestinal lymphoma stained for IgM, kappa chains, lambda chains and B-cells. The neoplastic cells, which occupy the lower half of each figure, stain for IgM, lambda and the B cell antigen. Staining for kappa chains is negative. The epithelium (in the upper part of each figure) stains for IgM, kappa and lambda, reflecting the presence of polyclonal immunoglobulin. In contrast staining for the B-cell-related antigen is negative within the epithelium, demonstrating the value of using a marker which (unlike immunoglobulin) is not present in the serum at substantial concentration.[14]

Table 7.2 Advantages of labelling antigens on smeared cells rather than in cell suspension

Visualization of cell morphology
Cells are not subjected to preliminary incubation with antibody before smearing, and in consequence morphology is optimally preserved. Furthermore cells are examined by conventional optical microscopy rather than under phase contrast.

Time from sampling to labelling
Once prepared, cell smears can be kept if necessary for prolonged periods (at least 1 year) before staining, without antigenic deterioration. This facilitates batch processing of samples as well as the storage of positive control samples.

Feasibility of labelling whole blood or bone marrow samples
Air dried blood or marrow smears prepared directly after collection are suitable for labelling so that the need for preliminary cell separation and washing is avoided.

Permanence of labelled preparations
The immuno-alkaline phosphatase reaction product is stable on storage of slides, so that it is feasible to examine labelled blood or bone marrow smears at long intervals after staining.

Number of cells required for labelling
Labelling of relatively small numbers of cells is possible, e.g. in CSF samples or finger prick blood smears.

these antigens do not survive smearing, air drying and fixation. However most (and probably all) antigens detectable on human cells in suspension using monoclonal antibodies can also be revealed on air dried cell smears (Figs. 7.2, 7.7, 7.9–7.11)[4,5,6].

Preparation of cell smears
Immuno-alkaline phosphatase labelling may be performed with equally good results on cytospin preparations or conventionally prepared blood or bone marrow smears. White cell rich preparations in which red cells have been depleted by dextran sedimentation (see *Technical Appendix*) may also be analysed by these methods. Smears should be stable for up to a week at room temperature, and we have thus frequently been able to phenotype samples sent by post from other hospitals. However if smears need to be kept for a longer period they should be stored unfixed in the frozen state. The stability of antigens in frozen cell smears facilitates the storage of positive control samples, e.g. smears from known cases of common ALL, T-cell leukaemia, etc.

Interpretation of labelling results
The interpretation of staining results is usually straightforward. As in the case of tissue sections it is important that positive and negative controls are included. It should be remembered that intracytoplasmic antigens are visualised (as well as surface membrane antigens) when cells smears are stained. This is already well documented for μ chains (found within pre-B cells) but has not been widely recognised in the case of other antigenic markers. It is not always possible to distinguish between these two localizations, although in some samples antigens may be seen as small aggregates (Figs. 7.5, 7.21) probably representing newly synthesised antigen in the Golgi apparatus which is destined for insertion into the surface membrane.

The fact that intracellular antigens are visualized in cell smears will probably lead to some revision of the antigenic profiles characteristic for different types of leukaemia, e.g. T-cell antigens may be found earlier in T-cell neoplasms by smear staining than by labelling in suspension.

PRACTICAL APPLICATIONS OF IMMUNO-ENZYMATIC LABELLING

In this section details are given of some of the practical uses to which immuno-enzymatic techniques have been put in the authors' laboratory in the study of haematological samples (see Table 7.3).

Tissue sections

Classification of lymphoid neoplasms
The staining reactions obtained with panels of monoclonal antibodies in the major categories of human non-Hodgkin's lymphoma are now beginning to be documented. A full discussion of this topic is beyond the scope of this chapter, but details may be found in recent reviews. [12-14] Representative examples of labelling reactions in three cases of non-Hodgkin's lymphoma are shown in Figures 7.22–7.24.

Much new data is likely to accumulate in the future. However studies performed to date have been of value in several areas. Firstly, it is now evident that the concept, central to the Kiel classification of non-Hodgkin's lymphomas, that most follicular lymphomas derive from normal lymphoid follicles (Figs. 7.22, 7.25), is amply confirmed.[15] Of value in this context is the availability of monoclonal antibodies directed against antigens on dendritic reticulum cells[9] (a cell type responsible for antigen trapping within B-cell follicles) since these antibodies have revealed the presence of DRC within neoplastic lymphoid follicles (Figs. 7.15, 7.20, 7.22).

A further outcome of immunohistological studies of human lymphomas has been the elucidation of the nature of many diffuse lymphomas.[16] This is still a complex subject since aberrant patterns of antigenic expression may be found in high grade lymphomas. However in many cases it is now possible to distinguish with certainty by immunohistological methods between T-cell and B-cell lymphomas (Figs. 7.23, 7.24), and to sub-divide the latter category into lymphomas which carry surface immunoglobulin and those which are immunoglobulin-negative (although expressing B-cell-associated antigens).

Table 7.3 Haematological applications of immuno-enzymatic labelling

---

Labelling tissue sections
    Classification of lymphoid neoplasms
    Distinction between reactive and neoplastic lymphoproliferative disorders
    Study of bone marrow trephines
    Identification of tumour cell types
    Detection of metastatic neoplasms

Labelling of cell smears
    Classification of leukaemia
    Analysis of normal peripheral white cell populations
    Detection of neoplastic cells in marrow aspirates

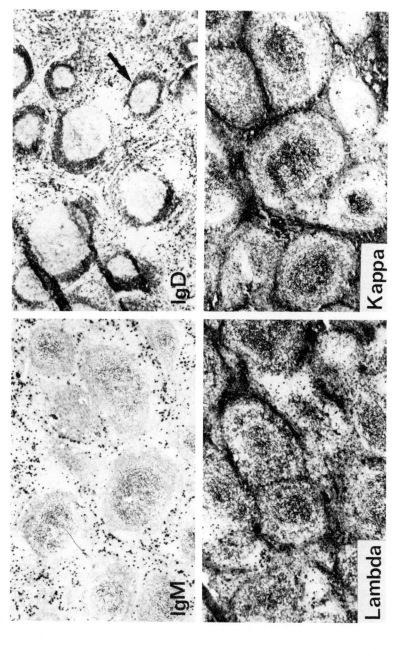

Fig. 7.25 Consecutive cryostat sections from a lymph node showing reactive follicular hyperplasia labelled by the immunoperoxidase technique (as in Fig. 7.22) for IgM, IgD, kappa and lambda light chains. In comparison with the neoplastic follicles seen in Figure 7.22 the reactive germinal centres show a meshwork of immune complexes staining for IgM and for kappa and lambda light chains. Each germinal centre is surrounded by an intact mantle zone of lymphoid cells (revealed most clearly by staining for IgD—arrowed), which contrasts with the irregular and distorted mantle zones seen in the case of follicular lymphoma. The darkly staining cells seen scattered in the interfollicular areas are polymorphs in which endogenous peroxidase has not been suppressed.[13]

There has also been progress in analysing Hodgkin's disease by immuno-histological techniques.[17] There is now evidence that Reed Sternberg cells represent activated lymphoid cells.[18] In most cases of Hodgkin's disease these cells appear to be of T-cell origin, with the interesting exception of lymphocyte predominant disease in which they may be B cell derived. This finding parallels the observation that in the latter subtype of Hodgkin's disease (a rare group with a relatively good prognosis) the infiltrating cells are also predominantly of B-cell origin[17], in contrast to the picture of marked T-cell preponderance in all other categories of the disease.

Distinction between reactive and neoplastic lymphoproliferative states
Histopathologists may on occasion have difficulty in distinguishing between reactive and neoplastic lymphoid disorders. When the differential diagnosis lies between follicular hyperplasia and follicular lymphoma, the distinction is relatively easily made by monoclonal antibody immunohistology (see Figs. 7.22 and 7.25). Diffuse lymphoid infiltrations on the other hand may be more difficult to categorise when their nature is not evident from conventional histological examination. The expression of a single class of immunoglobulin light chain on the surface of neoplastic cells (the traditional hallmark of B-cell monoclonality) is sometimes easily demonstratable (Figs. 7.22 and 7.24) but in other cases is difficult to assess owing to high levels of background immunoglobulin. When an infiltrate contains numerous T-cells, staining for helper and suppressor sub-classes may be of value (Fig. 7.23) but interpretation of these reactions is hampered by our limited knowledge of the degree to which the ratio between these two cell populations may be altered in non-neoplastic conditions. There is thus a requirement for new monoclonal antibodies for use in this area. The fact that lymphoid neoplasms frequently contain a high percentage of infiltrating reactive cells may also complicate the immunohistological differentiation between neoplastic and reactive states.

Study of bone marrow trephines
Immunocytochemical studies of human bone marrow trephines in the past have been restricted almost entirely to paraffin embedded tissue. With the introduction of techniques for staining frozen sections of marrow trephine material (Figs. 7.13–7.16, 7.19), it is now possible to extend the scope of these methods in the diagnosis of haematological disorders.[8] Of particular value is the possibility of analysing samples from patients in whom conventional aspiration yields a 'dry tap'. This may be of value in diagnosing cases of myelofibrosis and acute leukaemia, and secondary malignancy infiltrating the bone marrow (Fig. 7.3). Immunohistological staining of cryostat trephines may also enable neoplastic lymphoid proliferations in the bone marrow to be detected (Fig. 7.19) when they cannot be diagnosed with certainty on conventional histological grounds. Data can also be obtained concerning stromal elements present in normal bone marrow (Fig. 7.14).

Many of the antigens detected by currently available monoclonal antibodies do not survive routine tissue processing. However the epithelial marker detected by antibodies against human milk fat membrane globule antigen (anti-EMA—see Table 7.1) does survive processing of this sort and may be used for the detection of micrometastases of adenocarcinoma in bone marrow trephines. Antibodies reactive with denaturation-resistant determinants on epithelial cytokeratins are also beginning to be produced, and will have an increasingly valuable role in the detection of metastatic carcinoma in routinely processed biopsies.[19]

Identification of tumour cell types

Not infrequently lymphoid tissue biopsies are found on conventional histological examination to contain tumour cells of unknown origin. The differential diagnosis in the majority of these cases lies between lymphoma and secondary carcinoma; the correct diagnosis is hence of obvious clinical importance. Immunohistological labelling with monoclonal antibodies now provides a very effective means of resolving most of these problems[20], as summarized in Table 7.4, (Fig. 7.26). Antibodies of principal value in this context are anti-leucocyte common antigen[22] and anti-milk fat globule membrane antigen, since they both react with paraffin embedded material[23,24], thus making it possible to analyse tumours of unknown origin even when no fresh material is available (Figs. 7.27–7.29).

Detection of metastatic neoplasms

Immuno-enzymatic staining of tissue sections may be used to reveal both extramedullary deposits of haemopoietic neoplasms (e.g. acute lymphoblastic leukaemia infiltrating the testis—see Fig. 7.30) and also non-haemopoietic neoplasms metastasing to the bone marrow (Fig. 7.3).

Cell smears

Classification of acute leukaemia

Immuno-alkaline phosphatase labelling of cell smears or cytocentrifuge preparations allows most cases of leukaemia to be classified.[6] Details of the results obtained are given in Table 7.5, and illustrated in Figures 7.6, 7.9–7.11. These methods may be applied both to peripheral blood and bone marrow samples. In addition the methods are on occasion of value in studying cells in CSF samples from patients with suspected leukaemic relapse. The number of cells in these samples is often too small for conventional suspension labelling, but this does not preclude labelling of cytocentrifuge preparations by immuno-alkaline phosphatase techniques (Fig. 7.6).

Table 7.4 Immuno-enzymatic differentiation between lymphoma and carcinoma

Antigen	Lymphoma	Carcinoma
Leucocyte common	+(−)	−
HLA-DR	+/−	−(+)
Cytokeratin	−	+(−)
Milk fat globule membrane antigen (EMA)	−(+)★	+(−)

+/− = more than 50% of cases positive
+(−) = most cases positive; rare negative cases
−(+) = most cases negative; rare positive cases
★The fact that this antigen is found on a minority of normal and neoplastic human lymphoid cells has been documented recently by Delsol et al.[21]

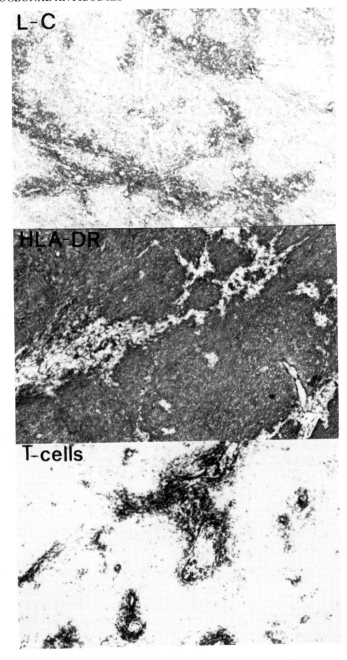

Fig. 7.26 Immunohistological labelling of an anaplastic tumour which was classified on conventional histological grounds as a metastatic carcinoma. However, immunoperoxidase labelling of cryostat sections for leucocyte-common antigen (L-C), HLA-DR, and T-cells revealed that the section contains sheets of HLA-DR-positive white cells interspersed with islands of T-cells. The latter population of lymphocytes stains more strongly for leuococyte-common antigen than do the tumour cells, but is predominantly negative for HLA-DR antigen. These immunohistological staining reactions, together with results obtained (not shown) using other monoclonal antibodies, showed clearly that the tumour was a high grade B-cell lymphoma rather than an anaplastic carcinoma.[13]

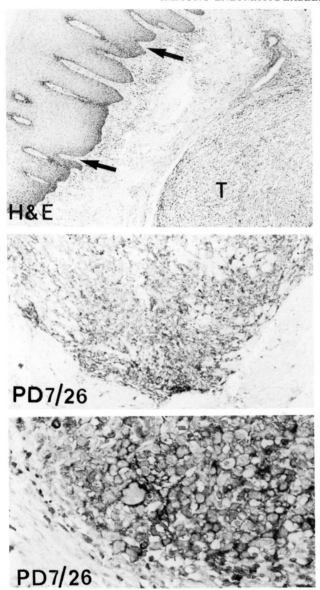

Fig. 7.27 This figure illustrates the case of a 56-year-old male patient who presented with a tumour in the oral cavity. A small biopsy was taken and diagnosed as a poorly differentiated squamous cell carcinoma, which led to the performance of an extensive resection involving hemimandibulectomy and deep neck dissection. However, the oral tumour (T) in the operation specimen in a conventional H & E stained section (top) was found to be deep to the epithelium (arrows) and at no point connected with it. Fresh tissue was not available from either the original biopsy or the operation specimen, so that staining with a full panel of monoclonal antibodies could not be performed. However, it was possible to use the monoclonal anti-leucocyte antibody PD7/26 since this antibody stains white cells in paraffin sections, and in this case (second from top) gave strong tumour cell staining, which at higher power (third from top) can be seen to be mainly confined to the cell membrane. Antibodies against human milk fat globule membrane antigen (EMA) and carcinoembryonic antigen (CEA) gave negative reactions (not shown). The results indicate that the patient had a lymphoma rather than a carcinoma, and systemic chemotherapy was initiated.[13]

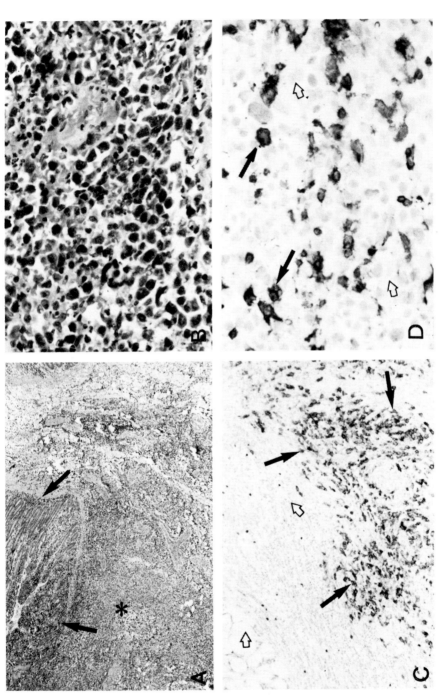

Fig. 7.28 (A) A diffuse tumour (asterisk) is shown at low power, lying beneath the colonic epithelium (arrows). (B) At higher power, the tumour is composed of large anaplastic cells. The differential diagnosis lay between anaplastic carcinoma and a high grade lymphoma; (C and D) The tumour cells (closed arrows) are strongly positive for the human milk fat globule membrane antigen (EMA) recognized by antibody HMFG-2, whereas surrounding lymphoid cells (open arrows) are completely negative. In adjacent sections (not illustrated), the lymphoid cells were strongly positive for the leucocyte common antigen, whereas the tumour cells were not. This case contrasts with that of Figure 7.27 and shows that a positive diagnosis of carcinoma can also be made when the material available has been routinely fixed and paraffin-embedded. In this case, the patient died some weeks after the colonic resection and was found to have widely disseminated secondary disease

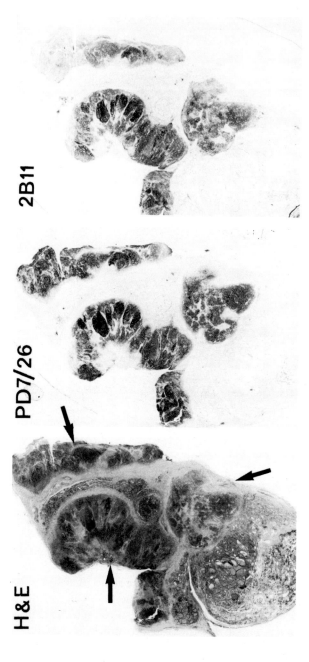

Fig. 7.29 Consecutive paraffin embedded sections of partial thyroidectomy sample from a middle aged man. A tumour is present (arrowed in the H & E stained section) which was initially diagnosed as an anaplastic carcinoma. However, as shown in the two right hand sections, it reacts strongly on immunoperoxidase labelling with monoclonal antibodies directed against the leucocyte common antigen (PD7/26, 2B11). This case illustrates the value of having antibodies which are capable of detecting surface antigens in routinely embedded material. As a result of this staining the patient was reclassified as a case of lymphoma and radiotherapy was initiated. The patient is well, with no evidence of recurrence, after more than twelve months.[13]

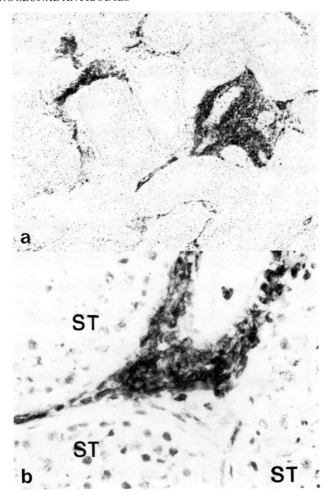

Fig. 7.30 Immunoperoxidase staining of a testicular biopsy (cryostat section) from a case of acute lymphoblastic leukaemia with monoclonal anti-HLA-DR, seen at low (a) and high (b) magnification. Strongly stained leukaemic blast cells are seen infiltrating between the seminiferous tubules (marked ST in the higher magnification view).

Analysis of normal peripheral white cell populations

The major lymphoid cell populations in peripheral blood (T-cells and their subsets, and B cells) may be readily stained by immuno-alkaline phosphatase staining of cell smears (Fig. 7.2). This provides a convenient means of analysing the relative proportions of these cell populations in different disease states.[4] Furthermore the fact that the technique can be applied to very small volumes of blood (i.e. the quantity required to produce a few blood smears) means that samples which are insufficient for analysis by conventional immunofluorescence are suitable for labelling.

Detection of metastatic cells in bone marrow aspirates

The ability of the haematologist to detect metastatic malignant cells of extra-medullary origin in bone marrow aspirates is very much dependent on the number of malignant cells present, samples containing only occasional such cells being almost impossible to diagnose with certainty. Immuno-alkaline phosphatase labelling can reveal these cells with great clarity (Fig. 7.4) and in a recent study from this laboratory it was shown that they can be shown in samples which are not diagnosable on conventional examination.[25] Occasionally immuno-alkaline phosphatase labelling will reveal that what appears to be a marrow derived malignancy is in reality metastatic disease from an extramedullary site—as in the case of rhabdomyosarcoma illustrated in Figure 7.8.

CONCLUSIONS

The immuno-enzymatic techniques described in this Chapter should enable monoclonal antibodies to be used for the analysis of haematological samples on a wider scale than has been possible in the past. In particular the fact that these techniques can be applied to routine blood and bone marrow smears, and that these smears may be stored if necessary for long periods before labelling, should make these methods much more accessible to routine haematology laboratories. It is hoped that in the future, with the availability of new monoclonal antibodies, these labelling procedures will come to have an increasingly important place among the routine diagnostic procedures employed by haematologists.

TECHNICAL APPENDIX: IMMUNO-ENZYMATIC TECHNIQUES FOR STAINING BLOOD, BONE MARROW AND LYMPHOID TISSUE SAMPLES

Reagents

Tris buffered saline (TBS)
Prepare a stock solution of 0.5 M pH 7.6 Tris HCl buffer. Make up TBS by diluting this stock reagent 1 in 10 in isotonic saline (0.15 M).

Fixative for cell smears
Acetone and methanol are mixed in equal volumes. This fixative is suitable for fixing routine blood and bone marrow smears and cytocentrifuge preparations and is the fixative recommended for general use. If it appears that an antigen does not survive this fixative well, acetone alone should be used (although the presevation of cell morphology will be appreciably poorer and red cells tend to lyse). Alternatively, if antigenic preservation is satisfactory but it is desired to obtain the best preservation of cellular morphological detail, concentrated (40%) formalin should be added to the acetone:methanol mixture (one part formalin to 19 parts acetone/methanol).

Immunohistological reagents
The sources of antibodies, immuno-enzyme reagents and enzyme substrates are given in Table 7.6.

Table 7.5 Classification of leukaemia by immuno-enzymatic staining

Antigens	Common ALL	T-cell ALL	AML	CLL
CALLA	+	–	–	–
μ chains	–/+[1]	–	–	+
δ chains	–	–	–	+/–
HLA-DR	+	–	+/–	+
Pan B	+/–	–	–	+
TdT	+	+	–/+[2]	–
T-cell antigen (DAKO T2)	–	+/–	–/(+)	–
T-cell antigen (DAKO T11-like)	–	+	–	–/(+)
T-cell antigen (DAKO T1-like)	–	+/–	–	+/–

1. μ chains are detectable by immuno-enzymatic staining within the cytoplasm of neoplastic cells in many cases of common ALL (representing pre-B-cell leukaemia).
2. Estimates of the frequncy of TdT-positive cases of AML vary (probably reflecting variations in the sensitivity of the labelling procedures).

+	= all cases positive
+(–)	= very occasional negative cases
+/–	= a majority of cases positive
–/+	= a majority of cases negative
–(+)	= very occasional positive cases
–	= all cases negative

Glycerol gelatin mounting medium

This aqueous mounting medium, required for all immuno-alkaline phosphatase stained preparations, is prepared as follows:
Dissolve 10 g gelatin in 60 ml of hot distilled water. Add 0.25 ml phenol and 70 ml glycerol and stir. This solution will solidify on cooling and should be melted (by standing the container in warm water) before using for mounting slides.

Tissue sample preparation

For paraffin embedding

Samples of lymphoid or other biopsy material should be sliced to give a sample no thicker than 2 to 3 mm, fixed in one of the standard histological fixatives and then processed to paraffin. *Neutral buffered formol saline* gives good tissue morphological preservation but denatures or masks most of the antigenic reactivity of the tissue. However many cytoplasmic antigens can be revealed in tissue fixed in this way by treating sections with a proteolytic enzyme (trypsin or pronase—see below). However membrane antigens (e.g. T-cell markers) will usually resist all attempts of this sort to uncover them following formalin fixation. *Formol sublimate* (also known as B5 fixative), *formol acetic, Zenker's* and *Bouin's* fixatives will preserve many cytoplasmic antigens but membrane antigens are usually rendered undetectable. Proteolytic digestion of tissues fixed in these fixatives does not usually improve the staining reactions of cytoplasmic or membrane antigens.

Fixation should not be excessively prolonged, 18 to 24 hours usually being optimal (provided the tissue slice is sufficiently thin—see above).

Marrow trephine samples should be fixed (and simultaneously decalcified) in a 20:1 Zenker's: acetic acid mixture before washing in tap water and processing to paraffin.

Table 7.6 Sources of immunocytochemical reagents for labelling hematological samples

Reagent	Source
Antibodies	
Monoclonal antibodies	see Table 7.1
Peroxidase and alkaline phosphatase reagents	Dakopatts
Unlabelled mouse Ig	Dakopatts
Cytochemical reagents	
Diaminobenzidine tetrahydrochloride	Sigma
Fast Red TR	Sigma
Naphthol AS-MX and AS-BI	Sigma
New Fuchsin	Raymond Lamb
Miscellaneous	
Levamisole	Sigma
Lymphoprep	Nyegaard
Dextran (Lomodex)	Fisons
Plastic tissue storage tubes	Kartell

For cryostat sectioning
Fresh unfixed tissue samples should be rapidly frozen, preferably by immersion in liquid nitrogen. A convenient way to handle samples is to put them in small snap-top flat bottomed tubes made of soft plastic, cover them with a small amount of saline or tissue culture medium and then to immerse the tubes in liquid nitrogen. This facilitates labelling, storage and subsequent sectioning of samples, and tissue morphology is better preserved than in samples which have been stored wrapped in foil.

Bone marrow trephine samples require more careful handling, because of their smaller size. A small cup (about 2 cm deep) should be fashioned from aluminium foil and filled with OCT medium (Ames) or other cryostat freezing medium. The unfixed marrow trephine core is placed in the medium and the foil cup and its contents then frozen by immersion in liquid nitrogen. It is advisable to orientate the trephine core as vertically as possible in the cup so as to facilitate the subsequent cutting of longitudinal sections.

All frozen tissue samples should be stored at $-70°C$ until sectioning.

For preparing cell suspensions
A cell suspension is prepared by teasing the sample in tissue culture medium, visible lumps are allowed to settle and a single cell suspension of viable cells is prepared by density centrifugation on Triosil:Ficoll (as for preparing peripheral blood mononuclear cell suspensions).

Tissue section preparation

Cryostat sections
1. Cut cryostat sections (approximately 5 to 8 mμ) from snap frozen tissue samples.
2. Air dry slides at room temperature for between 2 and 24 hours.

3. If slides are not to be stained immediately, they should be stored at —20°C. It is convenient to put slides back to back in pairs and then to wrap them in aluminium foil before freezing.
4. Shortly before staining, slides should be taken from the freezer and warmed to room temperature and then unwrapped.
5. Sections are fixed in acetone at room temperature for 10 minutes and then allowed to air dry.

Paraffin sections
Sections are prepared for staining by dewaxing, hydrating and washing in Tris buffered saline. Endogenous peroxidase activity may be blocked by exposing sections (either before or after hydration) to methanol containing 1% H_2O_2 for 15 to 30 minutes, but this step is rarely required.

Cell smear preparation

Whole blood smears
1. Smears are prepared as for routine haematological examination and air dried.
2. At this point slides may be stored if necessary for prolonged periods at —20°C without loss of antigenic reactivity. It is convenient to put slides back to back in pairs and then to wrap them in aluminium foil before freezing.
3. Immediately before staining, slides are removed from the freezer, left for a few minutes to reach room temperature, unwrapped and then fixed in methanol:acetone (or methanol:acetone/formalin—see above) for 60 seconds. They are transferred to Tris buffered saline (avoiding drying of the smears).
    If fixing in acetone, rather than an acetone methanol mixture, slides should be immersed in this fixative for 10 minutes and then air dried.

White cell-enriched smears
1. Whole blood is mixed with an approximately equal volume of dextran solution (e.g. 7% Lomodex) and red cells are allowed to sediment.
2. The supernatant white cell-rich plasma is aspirated, centrifuged, and smears are then prepared from the white-cell pellet. These smears will contain numerous white cells with a variable admixture of red cells. The relative proportions of different white cell types will be very close to the values for normal blood.
3. Smears are then stored and fixed as described above.

Mononuclear cell smears
1. Mononuclear cells are isolated from peripheral blood or bone marrow samples by centrifugation on Triosil Ficoll. Defibrinated samples are recommended for this step. Satisfactory results can also be obtained using samples anticoagulated with EDTA or with heparin, although platelets are occasionally plentiful in the final cell smears.
2. The mononuclear cell preparation is washed once or twice in isotonic buffer or in tissue culture medium. Whichever washing solution is used it should contain 1% bovine serum albumin (or other protein) in order to prevent cell damage during cytocentrifugation or smearing. The cells are resuspended in the washing

Table 7.7 Recommended staining techniques for different haematological preparations

Tissue or cell preparation	Recommended staining techniques	
	Peroxidase	Alk Phos
Blood smears	−	+
Mononuclear cell smears	+	+
Bone marrow smears	−	+
Buffy coat smears	(+)	+
Cryostat sections	+	+
Paraffin sections	+	+

solution and cytocentrifuged or smeared onto clean glass slides. When making cytocentrifuge smears the optimal cell concentration is of the order of 1×10^6/ml. When preparing cell smears a much higher concentration is required, to ensure sufficiently thick smears. As a rough guide the final cell suspension should contain approximately equal proportions of cells and suspending medium (i.e. have a 'cellcrit' of roughly 50%).

3. Cell smears are then air dried, stored and fixed as described above.

Choice of immuno-enzymatic labelling technique

Table 7.7 lists the type of staining technique which is recommended for different applications. As will be seen many preparations can be stained by both immunoperoxidase and immuno-alkaline phosphatase methods, but in some instances (e.g. when staining blood smears) immuno-alkaline phosphatase labelling is preferable. The choice between two- and three- stage immunoperoxidase methods should be based on the sensitivity required. For many purposes the two stage technique is suitable but for some applications (e.g. when staining paraffin-embedded material) the three-stage procedure may be required.

Immunoperoxidase staining

Two-stage procedure

1. Apply the primary monoclonal antibody to the slide. When staining *cryostat sections* the antibody is applied directly to dry acetone fixed sections: if sections are hydrated before addition of the antibody the intensity of specific staining will be reduced. When staining *paraffin sections* or *cell smears* excess buffer is removed from around the area to be stained before applying the antibody.

    The antibody should be diluted as required in TBS before use, the optimal dilution having been established by preliminary testing. If the antibody is in the form of tissue culture supernatant (harvested from a hybridoma cell line) the optimal dilution will usually be in the range 1/1 to 1/50. Ascitic fluid (or purified immunoglobulin) from a hybridoma bearing mouse will usually require dilution between 1/500 and 1/50 000. The antibody should be left on the slide for 30 to 60 minutes.

2. Wash briefly in TBS. Several brief immersions should be sufficient to remove unbound monoclonal antibody. Washing for longer than 1 minute is rarely necessary, especially if the antibody is in the form of tissue culture supernatant.

3. Incubate with peroxidase-conjugated rabbit anti-mouse Ig. This reagent should be diluted between 1 in 10 and 1 in 50 in TBS (the optimal dilution to be determined in individual laboratories). It is usually necessary to add normal human serum (at a final dilution of 1/25) to the solution in order to block cross-reactivity against human Ig. Incubation is continued for 30 minutes.
4. Wash in TBS (as above).
5. Add diaminobenzidine/H_2O_2 substrate to slides and incubate for approximately 8 minutes.
6. Wash in tap water and counterstain with haematoxylin.
7. Mount directly in aqueous mountant or dehydrate and mount in a medium such as DPX.

Three-stage procedure

1. Perform steps 1 to 4 as detailed above for the two-stage technique.
2. Incubate with peroxidase-conjugated swine anti-rabbit Ig. This reagent should be diluted between 1 in 10 and 1 in 50 in TBS and normal human serum should be added at a final concentration of 1/25. Incubation is continued for 30 minutes.
3. Wash in TBS (as above).
4. Add diaminobenzidine/H_2O_2 substrate to slides and incubate for approximately 8 minutes.
5. Wash in tap water, counterstain with haematoxylin and mount as for the two-stage procedure.

Immunoperoxidase substrate

Substrate is prepared shortly before use by dissolving diaminobenzidine tetrahydrochloride in Tris buffered saline at a concentration of 0.6 mg/ml. Add hydrogen peroxide to this solution to give a final concentration of 0.01% and apply immediately to slides. This concentration of hydrogen peroxide may be achieved by adding 10 μl of stock (10%) solution to 10 ml of diaminobenzidine solution.

Immuno-alkaline phosphatase staining techniques

APAAP method

1. Add 100 μl of monoclonal antibody to fixed cell smears and incubate for 30 to 60 minutes. The same considerations concerning the dilution of this reagent apply as for the immunoperoxidase procedure (see step 1 in the two-stage technique).
2. Wash briefly in Tris buffered saline (TBS).
3. Add anti-mouse Ig antiserum. The optimal working concentration should be determined in individual laboratories but will be of the order of 1 in 25. Note that it is impossible to use this reagent at too high concentration and that one can therefore afford to err on the generous side. It may be necessary to add normal human serum (at between 1 in 5 and 1 in 20) to block cross-reactivity against human immunoglobulin. Incubation is carried out for 30 minutes.
4. Wash briefly in TBS.
5. Add APAAP complexes and incubate for 30 minutes.
6. Wash briefly in TBS.

7. Add alkaline phosphatase substrate and incubate for 15 minutes.
8. Wash in tap water to terminate reaction.
9. Counterstain with haematoxylin.
10. Wash in tap water, transfer to distilled water and mount in an aqueous mounting medium (e.g. Apathy's). N.B. Do not dehydrate and mount in non-aqueous mountant since the reaction product will be dissolved.

'Enhanced' APAAP method

This technique may be of value if labelling by the standard APAAP technique is relatively weak. It is analogous to the 'double-bridge' PAP immunoperoxidase procedures described by other authors.
1. Perform the incubation steps 1–6 as detailed above for the APAAP method.
2. Repeat stages 3–6, but shorten the incubation period for steps 3 and 5 to 10 minutes each.
3. Perform steps 7–10 as detailed above under 'APAAP method'.

Indirect immuno-alkaline phosphatase technique

1. Perform the steps 1 and 2 of the APAAP method.
2. Incubate with alkaline phosphatase-conjugated rabbit anti-mouse Ig. The optimal dilution of this reagent should be determined by preliminary titration, but should be in the region of 1:10 to 1:30. Continue incubation for 30 minutes.
3. Wash briefly in TBS.
4. Incubate with alkaline phosphatase-conjugated swine anti-rabbit Ig. The optimal dilution of this reagent should be determined in individual laboratories, but will be in the region of 1:10 to 1:30. Continue incubation for 30 minutes.
5. Wash briefly in TBS.
6. Perform steps 6–10 of the APAAP method.

Alkaline phosphatase substrate

Fast red technique. Dissolve 2 mg naphthol-AS-MX phosphate in 0.2 ml of dimethylformamide in a glass tube. Add 9.8 ml of 0.1 M tris buffer, pH 8.2. This solution is made up fresh each time. Immediately before staining dissolve Fast Red TR salt at a concentration of 1 mg/ml and filter directly onto slide. If it is required to block endogenous alkaline phosphatase activity levamisole should be added to the substrate solution at a final concentration of 1 mM.

New fuchsin technique. Add 0.5 ml of a 5% solution of New Fuchsin in 2 N HCl to 1.25 ml of a freshly prepared 4% solution of sodium nitrite. When the nitrite has entered solution add it to 150 ml of 0.05 M Tris HCl (pH 8.7) containing 90 mg of levamisole, followed by 125 mg of naphthol AS-BI which has been freshly dissolved in dimethylformamide at 10 mg/ml. This solution is then filtered and used immediately for staining. Incubation with the substrate is continued up to 30 minutes with continual agitation.

REFERENCES

1. Cordell J L, Falini B, Erber W N, Ghosh A K, Abdulaziz Z, MacDonald S, Pulford K A F, Stein H, Mason D Y 1984 Immunoenzymatic labelling of monoclonal antibodies using immune complexes of alkaline phosphatase and monoclonal anti-alkaline phosphatase (APAAP complexes). Journal of Histochemistry and Cytochemistry 32: 219–229

2. Gatter K C, Falini B, Mason D Y 1984 The use of monoclonal antibodies in histopathological diagnosis. In: Anthony P, MacSween R (eds) Recent advances in histopathology. Churchill Livingstone, Edinburgh p 35–67

3. Erber W N, Falini B, Ghosh A K, Moir D J, Mason D Y 1983 Immuno-alkaline phosphatase labelling of haematological samples with monoclonal antibodies. In: Feldmann G (ed) Proceedings of the 2nd international symposium on immunoenzymatic techniques. Elsevier/ North Holland, p 29–40

4. Erber W N, Pinching A J, Mason D Y 1984 Immunocytochemical detection of T and B cell populations in routine blood smears. Lancet i: 1042–1046

5. Falini B, Schwarting R, Erber W N, Posnett D N, Martelli M F, Grignani F, Zuccaccia M, Gatter K C, Cernetti C, Stein H, Mason D Y 1985 The differential diagnosis of hairy cell leukaemia with a panel of monoclonal antibodies. American Journal of Clinical Pathology 83: 289–300

6. Moir D J, Ghosh A K, Abdulaziz Z, Knight P M, Mason D Y 1983 Immunoenzymatic staining of haematological samples with monoclonal antibodies. British Journal of Haematology 55: 395–410

7. Ponder B A, Wilkinson M M 1981 Inhibition of endogenous tissue alkaline phosphatase with the use of alkaline phosphatase conjugates in immunohistochemistry. Journal of Histochemistry and Cytochemistry 29: 981–984

8. Falini B, Martelli M F, Tarallo F, Moir D J, Cordell J L, Gatter K C, Loreti G, Stein H, Mason D Y 1984 Immunohistological analysis of human bone marrow trephine biopsies using monoclonal antibodies. British Journal of Haematology 56: 365–386

9. Naiem M, Gerdes J, Abdulaziz Z, Stein H, Mason D Y 1983 Production of a monoclonal antibody reactive with human dendritic reticulum cells and its use in the immunohistological analysis of human lymphoid tissue. Journal of Clinical Pathology 36: 167–175

10. Stein H, Gatter K C, Heryet A, Mason D Y 1984 Freeze-dried paraffin-embedded human tissue for antigen-labelling with monoclonal antibodies. Lancet 2: 71–73

11. Stein H, Gatter K C, Asbahr H, Mason D Y 1985 The use of freeze-dried paraffin embedded sections for immunohistological staining with monoclonal antibodies. Laboratory Investigation (In press)

12. Stein H, Mason D Y 1985 Immunological analysis of tissue sections in diagnosis of lymphoma. In: Hoffbrand A V (ed) Recent Advances in Haematology. Churchill Livingstone Vol 4 pp 127–169

13. Gatter K C, Cordell J L, Falini B, Ghosh A K, Heryet A, Nash J R G, Pulford K A, Moir D J, Erber W N, Stein H, Mason D Y 1983 Monoclonal antibodies in diagnostic pathology: techniques and applications. Journal of Biological Response Modifiers 2: 369–395

14. Mason D Y, Naiem M, Abdulaziz Z, Nash J R G, Gatter K C, Stein H 1982 Immunohistological applications of monoclonal antibodies. In: McMichael A J, Fabre J W (eds) Monoclonal antibodies in clinical medicine. Academic Press, p 585–635

15. Stein H, Gerdes J, Mason D Y 1982 The normal and malignant germinal centre. Clinics in Haematology 11: 531–559

16. Pallesen G, Beverley P C L, Lane E B, Madsen M, Mason D Y, Stein H 1984 Nature of non-B, non-T lymphomas: an immunohistological study on frozen tissues using monoclonal antibodies. Journal of Clinical Pathology 37: 911–918

17. Abdulaziz Z, Mason D Y, Stein H, Gatter K C, Nash J R G 1984 An immunohistological study of the cellular constituents present in Hodgkin's disease samples detected by a monoclonal antibody panel. Histopathology 8: 1–25

18. Stein H, Mason D Y, Gerdes J, O'Connor N, Wainscoat J, Pallesen G, Gatter K, Falini B, Delsol G, Lemke H, Lennert K 1985 The expression of the Hodgkin's disease associated antigen Ki-1 in reactive and neoplastic lymphoid tissue. Evidence for a relationship between Reed-Sternberg cells and polymorphic large cell lymphomas Blood (In Press)

19. Wells C A, Heryet A, Gatter K C, Mason D Y 1984 The immunohistological detection of axillary lymph node micrometastases in breast cancer. British Journal of Cancer 50: 193–197

20. Gatter K C, Abdulaziz Z, Beverley P, Corvalan J R F, Ford C, Lane E B, Mota M, Nash J R G, Pulford K, Stein H, Taylor Papadimitriou J, Woodhouse C, Mason D Y 1982 Use of monoclonal antibodies for the histopathological diagnosis of human malignancy. Journal of Clinical Pathology 35: 1253–1267

21. Delsol G, Gatter K C, Stein H, Erber W N, Pulford K A F, Zinne K, Mason D Y 1984 Human lymphoid cells express epithelial membrane antigen. Lancet ii: 1124–1128

22. Warnke R A, Gatter K C, Falini B, Hildreth P, Woolston R E, Pulford K A F, Cohen B, De Wolf-Peeters C, Mason D Y 1983 The diagnosis of human lymphoma using monoclonal

anti-leucocyte antibodies. New England Journal of Medicine 309: 1275–1281

23. Gatter K C, Alcock C, Heryet A, Pulford K A, Taylor-Papadimitriou J, Stein H, Mason D Y 1984 The differential diagnosis of routinely processed anaplastic tumours using monoclonal antibodies. American Journal of Clinical Pathology 82: 33–43

24. Gatter K C, Alcock C, Heryet A, Mason D Y 1985 Clinical importance of analysing malignant tumours of uncertain origin with immunohistological techniques. Lancet i: 1302–1305

25. Ghosh A K, Erber W N, Hatton C, Falini B, O'Connor N J, Osborn M, Mason D Y 1984 Detection of metastatic tumour cells in routine bone marrow smears by immuno-alkaline phosphatase labelling with monoclonal antibodies. British Journal of Haematology (In press)

8

Monoclonal antibodies to murine haematopoietic cells

H. S. Micklem

INTRODUCTION

During the last decade monoclonal antibodies have added impressively to our understanding of the murine haematopoietic system. The reason for this is not so much that numerous new antigenic specificities have been discovered (although that is true too) as that existing specificities have been studied and characterized in much greater detail than was previously possible. Even the best allo-antisera, such as those produced between lines of mice supposedly congenic for the character in question, frequently contained unwanted antibodies directed against unknown cell membrane or viral determinants. Moreover, they commonly recognized more than one epitope on a single antigenic molecule. I have written in the past tense as if alloantisera no longer existed. Of course this would be an exaggeration; such antisera are still made and used, and for some purposes they may even be superior in practice to monoclonal reagents; but the more important point is that monoclonal reagents directed against cell surface antigens perform better than conventional antisera in almost every context (see, for example, Shortman et al[1]). Moreover they make possible many studies that cannot be entertained with antisera. Monoclonal antibody technology does not, however, escape all the problems associated with specific antibody production. A strong immunogen is still a strong immunogen and a weak one weak. This means that when immunized with a mixture of cells (say mouse lymphocytes) a mouse or rat will tend to produce many cells that make antibody to antigens such as Thy-1 and the T-200 family, and relatively few to more sparsely expressed or less immunogenic molecules; these frequencies are reflected in the hybridomas obtained from fusion of the cells. It is no accident that Mabs directed against certain membrane glycoproteins of murine haematopoietic cells have been reported repeatedly from several laboratories, while Mabs to the B-lymphocyte differentiation antigens Lyb-3 and Lyb-5, for example, have yet to be obtained. One strategy to overcome this problem is to make membrane protein preparations and absorb out the immunodominant molecules on antibody columns before using the residual material for immunization. Many more interesting and desirable reagents undoubtedly remain to be discovered and will be obtained in due course.

USES OF MONOCLONAL ANTIBODIES FOR STUDYING THE HAEMATOPOIETIC SYSTEM

What constitutes an interesting and desirable reagent? Almost any new reagent will be useful in some context. The problem is to identify those that should be saved for any particular study. The main uses of Mabs in haematopoietology are twofold. (1) What one may call the functional taxonomy of cells. This includes such things as attempts to demarcate cell lineages, and the relationship of cell function to lineage, to differentiation and maturation within the lineage, and to morphology. An antigenic map of a population of cells can be built up, and Mabs can then be used preparatively to isolate or remove particular subsets and thus study their function; (2) The study of molecular function. This includes the physicochemical characterization of cell surface molecules and the analysis of their function. Although many membrane glycoproteins have been characterized as to molecular weight, electrophoretic mobility, polypeptide chain composition and (in a few cases) amino acid sequence, the functions of most of them remain obscure. This is certainly an area where important developments can be expected before long. The converse approach may also be used: monoclonal antibodies are raised against a characterized macromolecule and then used to study cells. Examples are the widespread use of anti-immunoglobulin reagents to study B-lymphocytes and recently the identification of spectrin in non-erythroid cells[2].

ASSOCIATED TECHNIQUES

The traditional method of identifying the effect of antibodies on a cell population, complement-mediated lysis, has several disadvantages. It provides a rather crude measure of cell frequency, may be insensitive, and destroys those cells that carry the antigen(s) in sufficiently high concentration. With Mabs, there is the further problem that not all fix complement efficiently. A hybridoma secretes molecules of uniform heavy-chain class (isotype), and this isotype may not fix complement. In the rat, for example, only IgM and IgG_{2b} fix complement and effect lysis at all reliably. Even for applications where it is very commonly used, such as the elimination of T-lymphocytes from a bone marrow or spleen cell suspension with anti-Thy-1 Mab, care has to be taken lest cells that carry low concentrations of Thy-1 escape the massacre. Cells may also show a paradoxical resistance to lysis. For example, some cells that carry high concentrations of Ly-1 antigen may be more resistant to lysis than cells that carry less[3], and anti-T200 Mabs may selectively lyse T-lymphocytes while B-lymphocytes, which bind as much of the antibody, are spared. It is possible to overcome the problem of unsatisfactory isotype by selecting for isotypic variants of a hybridoma with a fluorescence-activated cell sorter (review[4]).

Other widely used methods include (1) rosetting with antibody-coated erythrocytes[5]; (2) panning on antibody-coated plastic surfaces[6,7] and (3) flow cytofluorometry (with or without electronic sorting of selected cells) after staining with fluorochrome-labelled antibodies[8]. Each of these has its advantages and disadvantages and often it is desirable to use more than one. Generally, panning is useful where large numbers of cells have to be processed, where recovery of antibody-bound cells is desired, and where some degree of cross-contamination is tolerable. Flow cytofluorometry/sorting has the unique advantages of measuring relative *quantities* of an antigen on the surface of cells and of providing highly purified cell populations for study. Its powers of discrimination can be further widened by the use of two- and three-colour fluorescence[9]. Its disadvantages are expense and, for preparative purposes, slowness: the necessary instruments are costly to buy and maintain and they can process no more than about 10 million cells per hour; thus, to obtain sufficient cells of a minority subpopulation for functional or other studies may take an impracticable amount of sorting time. Despite these shortcomings, Mabs and cell sorters are natural and synergistic partners.

Cell membrane antigens

Most of the antigenic molecules in the cell membrane that have been characterized so far are glycoproteins, although glycolipid and nonglycosylated protein antigens have also been reported. In distribution, they vary between those that are found on all haematopoietic cells and on other cells besides (notably Class I MHC molecules), to those such as PC2[10] that appear to be restricted to a single cell type. These variations in distribution provide some clues as to the function of the molecules concerned, although definite associations with function have been identified for only a few molecules such as immunoglobulin on B-lymphocytes and receptors for immunoglobulin Fc[11,12], complement[13] and transferrin[14,15].

'Lineage' antigens. Of particular interest are those molecules whose expression may be limited to particular cell lineages. However, appearances have several times proved to be deceptive and this has led to some confusion in the literature. For example, the Ly-1 antigen was believed for several years to be confined to the T-lymphocyte lineage and hence was re-named Lyt-1; but it is now known to be present on a subset of B-cells as well[16,17]. Similarly, the antigenic molecule controlled by the Ly-5 locus was briefly re-named Lyt-4 when it was (wrongly) concluded on the basis of cytotoxicity to be confined to T-cells. In fact, there seems to be no known example of an antigen that is both confined to a single lineage and present on all stages of that lineage. Lyb-2 seems to be confined to B-cells, but is absent from some later (secretory) maturational stages[18]; this would be logical in view of Lyb-2's proposed role as a transducer of proliferative signals[19,20]. Possibly the nearest approach to a cell lineage marker corresponding to Berridge's[21] definition is the epitope present on the B-220 molecule and recognized by the Mabs RA3-2C2 and RA3-6B2[22]. B-220 has usually been considered to be absent from haematopoietic stem cells as detected by the spleen colony assay (CFU-S), but Ralph & Berridge[23] have recently reported that a proportion of anti-B220 Mabs do bind to CFU-S. If it can be shown that these antibodies, unlike some other anti-B220 Mabs[22], do not bind to a subset of T-cells and do bind to all B-cells and plasma cells, they may identify an antigenic marker of the B-lymphocyte lineage that is both exclusive and comprehensive. Antibodies to the Lyt-2 and Lyt-3 antigens may also be lineage specific, though in a more restricted way. The macromolecule that carries both Lyt-2 and Lyt-3 is generally believed to be confined to a line of T lymphocytes (the mediators of cytotoxic and suppressor functions) that is distinct from other T lymphocytes from an early intrathymic stage. However, recent evidence that Lyt-2 occurs on many intraepithelial lymphocytes in the intestine of mice, including congenitally athymic nude mice largely lacking in T cells as defined by other markers[24] throws doubt on Lyt-2 as a lineage-specific marker. These cells lack Lyt-3, however[24], so the credentials of this antigen may still stand. Most commonly, Mabs react with a range of cell types; sometimes (as with the complex of Ly-6-associated antigens: see below) the range includes cells for which no functional relationship is immediately apparent.

NOMENCLATURE OF MEMBRANE ANTIGENS AND ANTIBODIES

Three forms of nomenclature are in common use. (1) Nomenclature based on the genetic locus coding for, or controlling expression of, the antigen. Such antigens are defined on the basis of mouse inter-strain immunizations, i.e. they are allo-antigens. Linkage studies often enable the controlling locus to be mapped in relation to other known loci. In the case of lymphocyte alloantigens, the prefix Ly is used, followed by a number. Unfortunately, as noted above, this simple procedure has been complicated by attempts to incorporate further information into the name. Thus Lyt and Lyb are used to designate loci controlling the expression of antigens supposedly restricted to T and B-lymphocytes respectively. The numbering overlaps in some cases, so that Lyb-2, Lyb-3 and Lyb-5 are distinct from Lyt-2, Lyt-3 and Ly-5. More recently 'Lym' has come into use to designate new specificities originally defined by monoclonal antibodies as opposed to allo-antisera. Antigens encoded by loci belonging to the major histocompatibility complex (MHC) are an exception to the above generalization. These are designated by the name of the appropriate locus: I-A, Qa etc.. The Thy-1 locus and its associated antigen (originally called theta) is a further exception: only historical reasons prevent it being called an Ly locus. There is no general agreement as to how Ly antigens should be numbered. For example, new specificities controlled by the Ly-6 region have recently been labelled Ly-6A, B, C etc. by one group[25] and Ly-27 and Ly-28 by another[26]. Newly described specificities may turn out later to be similar or identical to others already described; similarities are easily masked by the use of different assay methods. It has been suggested, for example, that Ly-17, Ly-m20 and Ly-m22 may in fact be the same[27]; (2) Nomenclature based on the characteristics of the molecule detected. For example, LGP-100 defines a glycoprotein expressed on lymphocytes with an apparent molecular weight of 100 kilodaltons (kDa)[28]. This is commonly used for molecules that are initially identified by means of xenogeneic (e.g. rat anti-mouse) immunizations. Subsequently the molecule concerned may be identified with the product of a polymorphic Ly locus, as LGP-100 has been with Ly-9[29]. In such cases the Ly terminology is sometimes used loosely to describe the molecule even when it is being identified by a xeno-antibody to a non-polymorphic or 'framework' epitope. Such names are sometimes misleading since the full distribution range of the antigen may not be apparent when it is first described; (3) Nomenclature based on the laboratory name for the particular Mab concerned. This has the advantage of making no assumptions about the distribution of the antigen. On the other hand, it conveys no information and it means that several antibodies with distinct names may recognize the same molecule or even the same epitope. Conversely, similar-sounding antibodies may detect different antigens: many laboratories name their Mabs after the particular well of a microplate in which the hybridoma arose and it takes a fine memory to distinguish between one antibody and another.

In the remainder of this chapter, I shall attempt to review some of the contributions that Mabs have made to our understanding of the murine haematopoietic system. A few paragraphs will also be spared for the rat. By 'haematopoietic system' I understand haematopoietic stem cells and all those cells that are believed to be descended from them. This of course includes lymphocytes and indeed these cells have received far more attention than any others. Any complete review of work done on rodent cell antigens with Mabs must cover practically the whole of experimental immunology. Some limits are therefore necessary. I propose, with a mixture of regret and relief, virtually to ignore several important categories of Mab: those to MHC determinants and to idiotypic and clonotypic structures on B and T-lymphocytes. Otherwise I shall attempt to catalogue many of the reagents that are available for studying haematopoietic differentiation, and to indicate on a selective (and probably idiosyncratic) basis some of the contexts in which they are of value. Much of the material has been reduced to tabular form, with all the dangers of over-simplification and omission that this entails. Some antibodies appear in more than one table, with emphasis on different attributes. The reactivity and other characteristics of many of the antibodies have not been fully worked out.

B-LYMPHOCYTE DIFFERENTIATION

Table 8.1 lists monoclonal reagents that have proved valuable or offer scope for the study of B-lymphocytes and their precursors. These include antibodies to immunoglobulins, especially IgM and IgD, Lyb-2, Lym-10 and a variety of reagents that recognize antigens on subsets of B-cells, pre-B-cells and/or plasmacytes.

The definition of B-cell subsets has in general lagged behind that of T-cells. However, it has become clear from studies in normal and various immunologically abnormal mouse strains (CBA/N, NZB, nude etc) that both phenotypic and functional subsets do exist, although the correlations between the two are often unclear. That such correlations exist seems probable a priori. The proposal is supported experimentally by the absence from X-linked immunodeficient (*xid*) and athymic nude mice of certain B cell subsets defined by varying concentrations of surface IgM and IgD[30], the BLA-1 and BLA-2 antigens[31] and the presence or absence of Ly-1[17]. *Xid* mice are specifically deficient in the capacity to synthesize IgG$_3$ and to respond to so-called TI-2 ('T-independent') antigens, including pneumococcal capsular polysaccharides and various haptenated polysaccharides[32]; this has led to the suggestion that cells with the surface phenotype that is missing in *xid* mice (high-D, low-M, Lyb-3,5-positive) make these responses. However, recent work with an X-linked alloenzyme marker suggests that the *xid* gene also affects the development of other B-lymphocyte subsets to some extent[33,34]. Experiments in which mice were treated repeatedly with anti-delta serum from birth cast some doubt on the relevance of the surface Ig phenotype to function. Such animals were found to have virtually no IgD-positive cells, yet they responded normally to a range of antigens, including TI-2 antigens[35]. Unlike *xid* mice, anti-delta-treated animals possessed Lyb-3,5-positive cells[36], and it may be that this feature is more closely related to function than the surface Ig phenotype. Lyb-3 has been associated with the initiation of secretory differentiation[37].

The antibodies to BLA-(=B lymphocyte antigen) 1 and 2 referred to above, appear to have considerable potential as probes for B-cells. At least four apparent subsets have been identified, the presence of which differs in relation to age and genotype[31]. However, the functions of the subsets and of the molecules concerned are still unknown.

Table 8.1 Monoclonal antibodies for the study of B-lymphocytes

Name	Locus/antigen		Distribution on cells	Comments	Refs.
	Igh-6	IgM	Most B	Variable density	30
	Igh-5	IgD	Most B	Variable density	30
	Lyb-2		All B and B-prec. not Ig secretors.	Ab stimulates proliferation	155
14.8					39
RA3-2C2	Ly-5	B220	All B & pre-B	Most react also	40
14D10				with Lyt-2+ T, but	137
DNL1.9				not RA3-6B2	158
RA3-6B2					
	Ly-6 group		See details in Table 8.6.		
	Lym 10		T & some B: expression correl with 30-E2	Linked to Ly-1 on chromosome 19.	156
		PC2	PC only		10
30-E2		BLA2	All neonatal B most		31
14G8			*xid* B. <50% normal adult B.		137
53-10.1		BLA1	All neonatal B. <50% adult B, including blasts & GC. E. Not T or thy.		31
4B9			B, most thy, E, most		138
J11d			BM. Not T.		139
NIMR-2			Most BM, pre-B, some B. Not T.	Conc identifies B subsets.	49
NIMR-3			Most BM, some B. Not in neonate up to 3 weeks.	B cells differ from NIMR-2+ set.	49
19B5			Thy, pre-B, some B, some T, 35% BM.	Anti-mouse brain	153 154
	Qa-M2		All T. B subset and some PC in some strains		47
	Ly-1		B subset, T.	B may make auto-Ab	16 17
R17 208			Proliferating cells,	Transferrin receptor	15
YE1 9.9			incl GC.		14

For abbreviations, see p. 199

Membrane glycoproteins controlled by the Ly-5 and Ly-6 loci

The Ly-5 locus controls the expression of a family of large transmembrane glycoproteins that are confined to the haematopoietic system and present on nearly all haematopoietic cell types. When tested by immunofluorescence, antibodies to the 200 kDa form found on thymocytes (T-200) bind to all haematopoietic cells with the exception of erythrocytes and the later erythroid precursor stages in bone marrow[38]. B-cells have been found to carry a larger (220 kDa) form of the molecule, to which monoclonal antibodies have been raised[39-41]. Mabs to determinants that are confined to the B-220 form, which consequently do not react with T-200, have proved useful in the study of B cell differentiation. They react with all identified cells of the B lineage, including pre-B-cells that lack surface Ig but have μ-chains in the cytoplasm[42,43]. Used in conjunction with anti-Ig reagents, they allowed the positive identification and study of the pre-B-compartment, defined as surface Ig-negative,

B-220-positive and possessing surface μ-chains. Such cells were either large proliferating or small resting cells, distinct from CFU-S (which were reported to be B-220-negative[42]) and all carried cytoplasmic μ-chains.

The use of Mabs to the ThB antigen (controlled by a gene in the Ly-6 region[44] allowed the large and small pre-B-cells to be separated, since only the latter were ThB-positive[43]. Since mature B-cells all carry ThB, while CFU-S do not, this suggested that the small cells were probably the most mature of the pre-B compartment. Coffman & Weissman[43] studied the rearrangement of immuno-globulin heavy- and light-chain genes[45] in these cells and concluded that the H-chain genes were rearranged, at latest, very soon after the initial expression of B-220; this was consistent with the synthesis of μ-chains in most B-220$^+$ cells). L-chain rearrangements, however, were present only in the small pre-B-cells. Thus L-chain gene rearrangements probably do not occur until very shortly before the synthesis of L-chains and the expression of whole IgM molecules on the cell surface.

It should be noted here that many, but not all, anti-B-220 Mabs react also with the Lyt-2$^+$ subset of T-lymphocytes[22]; fluorescent staining is relatively weak. Bright fluorescent staining of T-cells, comparable to that seen with B-cells, is only observed in MLR/1pr autoimmune mice[46]. The dominant type of lymphocyte in these mice appears to be an aberrant T cell which is Ly-1$^+$2$^-$ and which, unlike normal T-cells of this phenotype, carries B-220.

Further discussion of ThB and other Ly-6-related antigens is deferred to a later section.

Of the MHC antigens, both Class I and Class II (Ia) antigens are found on all B-cells and Ia molecules function as recognition targets for T-helper cells. Qa-M2, however, is reported to show a rather complex distribution pattern which varies between strains of mice. Some strains carry it on Lyb-3,5-negative B-cells, while in others it appears to be restricted to T-cells. It has also been reported to distinguish between IgM- and IgG-synthesizing plasma cells, only the latter being positive[47,48].

The quantitative expression of a molecule recognized by the NIMR-2 Mab has been reported to differentiate between virgin and memory B-cells to the antigen dinitrophenylated Keyhole Limpet hemocyanin[49,50].

T-LYMPHOCYTE DIFFERENTIATION

Since the demonstration, initially by means of allo-antisera, that functionally distinct T-cells could be distinguished by the presence of different antigenic macromolecules on their surface[51], many groups have exploited such differences to analyse T-cell subsets and dissect their complex interactions with each other and with other cell types such as B-cells and macrophages. Rather fortunately, monoclonal antibodies arrived at an early stage in this process and have enabled it to advance with enhanced speed and precision. Whereas allo-antisera were only capable of detecting macromolecules that happened to carry polymorphic determinants, the production of Mabs from immunized rats removed this restriction. (However, interestingly enough, it has turned out that a substantial proportion of the molecules recognized by the rat are in fact polymorphic and capable of being detected by alloantibodies.) Early hybridizations produced a range of reagents reactive with various haematopoietic subsets and in particular with thymocytes, T-cells and subsets of these[52]. These included antibodies to Thy-1, Ly-1, Ly-2, Lyt-3 and others. A few individual Mabs were found to react in a strain-restricted manner. It is worth noting that strain-specificity of rat reagents is not always an all-or-nothing matter. For example, the anti-Lyt-3 Mab 53-5.8[53] binds to both Lyt-3.1 and Lyt-3.2 molecules, but much more avidly to the latter. In practice this means that it is useless for FACS analysis of AKR (Lyt-3.1) cells, while working excellently for most other (Lyt-3.2) strains (unpublished data). A range of monoclonal alloantibodies is now commercially available to allotopes of Ly-1, Ly-2 and Lyt-3, so that such problems can be circumvented. Rat Mabs to Thy-1 are perhaps a special case, because rats possess a 'Thy-1' molecule that is structurally very similar to murine Thy-1.1. Thus many rat anti-Thy-1 reagents are specific for murine Thy-1.2, while others react with determinants common to both allotypes[52]. Allotype-specific reagents, whether monoclonal or conventional, can be used to follow the fate of allotransplanted cells. Thy-1 has been the most widely used marker for this purpose, although since it can produce false-positives[54,55] and other anomalies of fluorescent staining[56], its use demands an element of caution. Some other unresolved questions concerning Thy-1 are discussed below.

In general, T-subset analysis with Mabs has upheld the initial conclusions of Cantor & Boyse[51], namely that antibodies to Ly-1 and Ly-2 were capable of distinguishing between functionally different cells. These showed predominately helper activity (Ly-1$^+$, Ly-2$^-$) or cytotoxic or suppressor activity (Ly-1$^-$, Ly-2$^+$) respectively. However, monoclonal antibodies detected Ly-1 on all T-cells, although in variable quantity, so that this marker can no longer be regarded as specific for T-helper or inducer cells[57]. T-helper-specific markers were identified in the rat[58] and man some years before the mouse, but the recently described 'L3T4' molecule (so named to identify it with the human helper-associated molecule carrying Leu-3 and T4 markers) is the murine equivalent[59]. The situation has become more complicated than originally envisaged. Firstly, these markers do not invariably correlate with a cell's function, but rather with the type of molecule that it can interact with on other cells[60,61]. Thus, Ly-2$^+$ cell usually interact with targets expressing MHC Class I antigens, and a plausible view is that they serve to stabilize low-avidity interaction between such cells[62]. L3T4, on the other hand, is involved in interactions with MHC Class II-expressing cells[63,64]. Secondly, relatively simple ideas about help and suppression have now been replaced by a complex series of regulatory T-cell circuits in which the net effect of a cell on the outcome of an immune response is not deducible simply from its Ly phenotype[65].

Some disagreement exists concerning the stability of Ly-phenotypes in defined cell populations. Originally Huber et al[66] reported that there was little or no interconversion of Ly-2$^+$ (Ly-1$^-$) and Ly-2$^-$ T-cells, but it was subsequently stated that T helper cells could acquire Ly-2 during the course of an immune response, after adoptive transfer to irradiated recipients[67,68]. The concentration of Ly-2 per cell as revealed by FACS analysis was unusually heterogeneous and lower on average than in normal mice[68]. Experiments in the rat, using the Mab OX-8, which detects a molecule that appears to be equivalent in many respects to the murine Ly-2 molecule, failed to confirm this phenotypic shift[69].

Many groups[70-77] have used Mabs to Thy-1 and the Ly-1, Ly-2 and recently L3T4 antigens in conjunction with FACS analysis to study the differentiation and maturation of T-lineage cells. Many other cell surface molecules associated with murine thymocytes and/or T-cells have been identified by monoclonal antibodies, and some of these are listed and annotated in Table 8.2. None has so far proved of such value as the antibodies to Ly-1, 2 & 3 in the delineation of T-cell subsets, but Ly-m22 appears promising as it is said to differentiate between cytotoxic and suppressor T-cells[78].

Thy-1 maintains its position as the pre-eminent pan-T marker in the mouse, but only by virtue of its absence from B-cells; it is present on various other cell types and tissues, including epithelial cells, fibroblasts and brain. Recently it has been reported to be present, in very small quantities, on murine CFU-S[79], and in larger amounts on various cultured bone marrow progenitor cells[80]. This would not be particularly surprising since bone marrow stem cells in the rat are known to carry Thy-1[81,82]. The cell distribution of Thy-1 in the rat is in fact quite different from that in the mouse, B-cells rather than T-cells being positive[81]. Considering how extensively Thy-1 has been studied, it is surprising that the function of the molecule, which is a membrane glycoprotein showing some homology with an Ig domain, is still unknown. It has recently been reported that one anti-Thy-1 Mab, G7, has a mitogenic effect on resting T cells and induces the synthesis of interleukin-2 (IL-2) and the expression of IL-2 receptors[83]. In these respects it differs from other Thy-1 Mabs, but resembles Mabs directed against human T3 (Leu-4) molecules; these molecules are believed to be associated with antigen-specific receptor molecules on human T-cells and antibodies to them are mitogenic. Gunter et al[83] have proposed the hypothesis that the Thy-1 and T3 molecules are in some way related both structurally and functionally. It is curious that only one of several anti-Thy-1 Mabs behaved as a mitogen and the possibility should be considered that G7 does not bind to Thy-1, but to another molecule of similar molecular weight such as T-30[52]. However, pre-clearing experiments showed that G7 removed all protein reactive with 30-H12 (probably the most widely used rat anti-mouse-Thy-1 reagent) but 30-H12 did not remove all the material reactive with G7[83]; thus it remains possible that G7 reacts not only with the 'classical' Thy-1 molecule, but also with another molecule sharing one or more epitopes with Thy-1. Sidman et al[84] also discuss the possible relationship between Thy-1 and Leu-4 in the context of their Mab B14-2-14 which reacts with a Thy-1-like molecule detected on thymocytes, but only a small minority of peripheral T-cells. Again, it is not clear whether this antibody is reacting with Thy-1 itself (possibly an epitope which becomes masked during T-cell maturation) or another associated or structurally related molecule. Other authors, too, have described anomalies of various kinds in the expression of Thy-1[85-87] or of specific determinants on it. Particularly curious is the different pattern of expression of Thy-1.1 and Thy-1.2 products on T-cells, even in 1.1/1.2 heterozygotes[87].

Other interesting reagents listed in Table 8.2 include those recognizing antigens associated with the Ly-6 locus, which will be discussed separately below, antigens present on fetal thymus and T-lymphomas but absent on most or all normal adult thymocytes and T-cells[88,89], and the group of antigens, identified by Owen and colleagues[90-93], encoded by genes closely linked to the immunoglobulin heavy chain (Igh) region on murine chromosome 12. The FT-1 antigen[88] identifies a receptor for *Dolichos biflorus* lectin and appears to behave as an oncofetal antigen. It appears to be distinct on the grounds of molecular weight from the YE1/7.1[89] and

Table 8.2 Monoclonal antibodies for the study of murine thymocytes and T-lymphocytes

Name	Locus/antigen		Distribution on cells	Comments	Refs.
Many available Thy-1	Thy-1	28kDa	All thy & T	Conc variable; poss ± on CFU-S	52 70–72
Ly-1	Ly-1	67 kDa	All thy, T & subset B	Conc variable	17, 51, 57
Lyt-2	Lyt-2	30+35 kDa	Ts, Tc, most thy, most non-T IEL. Not Th	Interact with MHC class I. Ab may block killing by Tc	74–77 53 24
Lyt-3	Lyt-3		As Lyt-2, but absent from non-T IEL		151
GK1.5 H.129.19	L3T4	55 kDa	Thy & Th	Interaction with MHC-II	63, 152 64
G7	Thy-1			Mitogenic Ab.	83
B14-2-14	Thy-1?		25–85% thy. Few T	Freq & conc vary with strain; cf refs 85 & 86	84
	Ly-6		T & B, ConA blasts. Not thy	(See Table 8.6)	
49h4 53-9.1 17C9	ThB	16 kDa	Cortical thy, B. Not T	Linked to Ly-6. Strains vary in quantitative expression	44 134 137
T28.45	Ly-m22		Ts, not Tc or Th	Linked to Mls on chro-1. May = Lym20 & Ly17	78 27
4B9 J11d M1/69			Most BM, thy, B, E. Not T		137 138 139
19B5			Thy, 35% BM, T & B subsets	Anti-mouse brain Ab	153 154
M7/14 H35-89.9	LFA-1	180 + 95 kDa	T & B, most BM	See Table 8.5. Ab blocks Th & Tc functions	130, 131 132
34-10-7			B & abnormal T of MLR/lpr mice.	Linked to Ly-6	143, 144
9F3			Lpr T & most thy. Most normal T, but 10–50x lower Ag conc		135
YE1/19.1		115 + 115 kDa	MLR/lpr T		160
100C5		220 kDa	B & proliferating T of MLR/lpr mice	Prob=B220, cf Table 8.1	46
YE1/9.9 R17 208	TfR	2 × 100 kDa	Proliferating cells	Transferrin receptor	14 15
YE1/48.10		2 × 50 kDa	Transformed T & ? a few normal T, not ConA blasts		14
B2A2			Thy T, B, some BM.	Can distinguish cortical thy, medullary thy & T	75
YE1/7.1		60 kDa	Subset of fetal thy & ConA-activ adult thy. Some T-lymphoma lines. MLR/lpr T		89 160
FT-1		130 kDa	Fetal thy, decreasing thru gestation. Some T lymphomas. Not adult T	Receptor for *Dolichos biflorus* lectin. Onco-fetal antigen	88

Table 8.2—Cont.

Name	Locus/antigen	Distribution on cells	Comments	Refs.
	Tpre	Thy & prec	Group of antigens linked	93
	Tthy	Thymocytes	to Igh locus; suggested	
	Tind	Inducer T subset	to represent isotypes of	
	Tsu	Suppressor T subset	T receptor for Ag	
	Ly-25.1	Thy, T subset & B	Strain-distribution of alleles like Ly-1	157
ER-TR4, 5, 6, 7		Four thymic stromal cell types	See text	97
ART-18		T blasts (rat)	Receptor for IL-2	125

For abbreviations, see p. 199

YE1/48.10[16] antigens which show some similarities in cellular distribution. Further studies with these reagents seem likely to be very interesting.

The Mabs that detect the Owen antigens (review[93]) are allo-antibodies, being the products of mice immunized with T-cells from Igh-congenic donors. In addition to being closely linked to *Igh* (between the alpha-C and the prealbumin gene, *Pre-1*), their presence on thymocytes and T-cells appears to correlate with the production and functional differentiation of specific subsets. On these and other grounds, Owen suggested that the antigens might mark different isotypes of a constant region of the T-cell receptor for foreign antigens. This interpretation was strengthened by data of Tokuhisa et al[94]. They used similar congenic immunizations to produce Mabs that reacted with antigen-specific T-cell factors (suppressive or augmenting) thought to represent free forms of the T-cell membrane receptors for antigen. They too suggested that their Mabs recognized constant region isotypes of the receptors. Moreover Mab to Tind, the antigen found on inducer cells, was found to react with a determinant on an antigen-specific T-augmenting factor and the determinant appeared to be located on an antigen-specific, not on the I-A carrying chain of the factor (review[93]). All these data are consistent with the idea of a two-chain T-cell receptor for antigen, one chain carrying I-region determinants and the other having constant and variable regions encoded by genes linked to *Igh* on chromosome 12. It has recently been reported, however, that the T-cell receptor β-chain, which has a variable region, is located on murine chromosome 6 near Ig-kappa[95]. Still more recently the α-chain locus (review[96]) has been reported to reside on chromosome 14. Thus the status of the *Igh*-linked antigens remains unclear.

Antibodies to thymic stromal cells. Van Vliet et al[97] have produced a potentially useful series of Mabs directed against various components of murine thymic stroma. These antibodies reacted respectively with cortical epithelial cells (ER-TR4), medullary epithelial cells (ER-TR5), medullary interdigitating cells and macrophages (ER-TR6) and reticular fibroblasts (ER-TR7).

T-CELL ANTIGENS IN THE RAT

Although the rat has received relatively little attention by students of T-cell differentiation, it offers several advantages, not least the fact that a particularly well-characterized set of reagents for delineating basic subsets has been developed[58,

[98-101]. These are summarized in Table 8.3 and probable human and murine equivalents of the antigens are indicated. It is noteworthy that MRC OX-22 appears to distinguish two subpopulations of helper T-cells, which is something that no antibody has yet been reported to do in mouse or man. The molecule involved is a high molecular weight form of the 'leukocyte common' antigen, possibly equivalent to murine B-220. As noted earlier, however, the latter is not present on any T-helpers.

Table 8.3 Monoclonal antibodies for the study of rat thymocytes and T lymphocytes[58, 100]

Name	Mol weight of antigen	Distribution on cells	Comments	Refs.
W3/13	95 kDa	All T, thy, N, PC, some NK; not B	Similar to glycophorin	101
MRC OX-19	69 kDa	All T, thy, prob a few B	Prob = mouse Lyl & human Leu1/T1	100
MRC OX-8	39+35 kDa	Ts, Tc, 90% thy, most NK, granular IEL. Not Th	Prob = mouse Ly2 & human Leu2/T5	98, 101 149, 150
W3/25	48–53 kDa	Th, 90% thy, M. Not Ts or Tc	Prob = mouse L3T4 & human Leu3/T4	98, 150
MRC OX-22	220 kDa	B, few thy, all OX8+ T, 70% W3/25+ T	High Mw form of 'leukocyte common' antigen	99

For abbreviations, see p. 199

THE USE OF ANTI-T-CELL MABS FOR DISEASE PREVENTION AND THERAPY

Avoidance of graft-versus-host disease after transplantation of bone marrow

The occurrence of 'secondary disease' in mice that had been saved from the immediate effects of lethal X-irradiation by a transfusion of allogeneic bone marrow cells, was described many years ago[102]. Many lines of experiment indicated that it was in the main due to a reaction by grafted cells against the host, although under some circumstances a similar syndrome appeared in the absence of a graft-versus-host (GvH) reaction and was attributed to inadequate lymphocyte regeneration[103,104]. Although T and B-cells had not been distinguished at that time, it seems probable in retrospect that lack of T-cells or an imbalance of T-cell subsets was the main problem. More recently, the occurrence of severe GvH disease after bone marrow transplantation in man has reawakened interest in the pathogenesis of the syndrome and in possible ways of avoiding or curing it. Korngold & Sprent[105] focussed attention on the early role of mature T-cells in inducing the disease. They reported that in some circumstances as few as 0.3% of such cells present in a bone marrow suspension were sufficient to induce lethal GvH disease. Several groups have subsequently sought to prevent the development of GvH disease by selectively eliminating T-cells from bone marrow suspensions with monoclonal antibodies to Thy-1, Ly-1 and Ly-2 before injection into the host. Destruction of the cells may be effected by complement[105,106] or by attachment of a toxin such as ricin, ricin α-chain or gelonin to the antibody[107-109]. This approach has produced encouraging results in the mouse. It appears that the removal of Ly-2$^+$ cells alone may be insufficient, while removal of Thy-1 or Ly-1 cells is effective[116]. This parallels another report suggesting that Ly-2⁺ cells are not important in allogeneic skin graft rejection[110]. Since anti-Thy-1 and anti-Ly-1 may both be expected to remove all T-cell subsets, it will be interesting to see whether the recently available L3T4 reagent is effective. The key to all these experiments is the specificity of the antibodies for T-cells and, in particular, their lack of effect on haematopoietic stem cells and T-cell progenitors.

Many hybridomas derived from fusion with commonly used myelomas such as NS1 produce monovalent as well as bivalent IgG antibodies; the former carry one non-specific light chain derived from the myeloma parent. Using Sepharose-coupled antibody to a rat kappa allotypic determinant present on the myeloma-derived light chain, but absent from the specific spleen cell-derived light chain, Cobbold & Waldmann[111] were able to adsorb and elute monovalent antibodies, separating them from bivalent molecules. They found that the monovalent antibodies had an enhanced capacity to mediate complement lysis under the conditions employed (including incubation at room temperature or at 37°C in the absence of azide). This may have been due to their inability to cross-link and 'cap off' cell surface molecules or to increased complement fixation. Such an approach seems to be worth further investigation in the context of toxin targeting as well as complement lysis. However, the absence of murine kappa allotypes restricts its use to hybridomas where at least one parent is rat.

Therapy of autoimmune disease: the MLR/1pr mouse model

Because they can be obtained in pure form and large amounts, Mabs lend themselves to in vivo therapeutic applications. For example, Seaman et al[112] treated MRL/1pr mice with a single dose of 6 mg of rat anti-Thy-1.2 antibody (30-H12). Untreated mice spontaneously develop a lupus-like autoimmune disease characterized by anti-DNA antibodies, immune complex glomerulonephritis and extensive proliferation of an abnormal set of T-cells. Treatment at 8 weeks of age, before the onset of overt disease, reduced the number of circulating T-cells substantially over a period of three months. It also resulted in better renal function, although anti-DNA antibodies were not reduced significantly. Long-term therapy with multiple repeated injections of antibody would probably be impossible with heterologous Mabs, owing to development of antibodies by the recipient. These experiments also suggest that requirements for successful therapy may include large amounts of antibody (in this case 10-times more than was needed to clear circulating T-cells completely from normal mice) and careful selection of antigen specificity: anti-T200 antibody of the same isotype was almost completely ineffective, despite the presence of the antigen on the cells. It is of interest that much smaller amounts of anti-Ly-1.1 monoclonal alloantibody suppressed various T-cell functions in vivo[113]. In these experiments, mice received up to 1.25 ml of hybridoma culture supernatant intraperitoneally. The quantity of antibody was not stated, but was presumably not greater than about 50 μg.

MACROPHAGES, GRANULOCYTES AND THEIR RELATIVES

Study of macrophages and putatively related cells such as Langerhans and other antigen-presenting cells has benefited greatly from the development of Mabs.

Several such reagents are summarized in Table 8.4. F4/80[114] appears to be the nearest thing to a universal and specific macrophage label available, and it is tempting to consider it as a touchstone of authentic macrophagy. Its absence on osteoclasts[115] is interesting since these cells are thought to be derived from fused macrophages[116]. It is present on Langerhans cells, but not detected on the interdigitating cells of lymph nodes[117], cells widely believed to be close relatives of Langerhans cells. The significance of this pattern of occurrence may become clearer when the function of the macromolecule recognized by F4/80 is ascertained. Macrophage-like cells form a substantial and functionally important part of bone marrow stroma, and the F4/80 antigen was found on them, including the cells at the centre of haematopoietic islands (foci of proliferating erythrocyte and granulocyte precursors)[117]. The M1/70 and 2.4G2 antibodies are somewhat ususual in identifying cell surface molecules of known function (Table 8.4), but they are not macrophage-specific. The other antibodies in the series recognize antigens with fairly wide cell distributions and without established functions.

Table 8.4 Monoclonal antibodies for the study of macrophages & granulocytes

Name	Antigen	Cell distribution	Comments	Refs.
F4/80	160 kDa	All M and related cells except osteoclasts. LC. Not ID, B, T, fibroblasts or other cells		114 115 116 147
M1/70	Mac-1 170 + 95 kDa	Most M, but not Kupffer. 50% BM incl N precs; NK. Not B, T or LC	Type 3 complement receptor. β-chain like β-chain of LFA-1 (Table 8.2); α-chain distinct. Chain linkage non-covalent.	139 148
M3/38	Mac-2 32 kDa	M, LC, epithel. cells. Not B or T	Concentration increased on thioglycollate-stimulated macrophages.	141
M3/84	Mac-3 110–170 kDa	M, LC, epithel & endothel cells. Not T or B	Mw variation probably related to glycosylation; precursor = 76 kDa	141 148
146	On Fc-binding part of Clq	M (only?)	Can function as surface Fc-receptor.	12
2.4G2	47 + 60–70 kDa	M, T & B	Trypsin-resistant FcR for IgG_{2b} & IgG_1	13
7/4		N. Not T, B, M, mast cells eosinophils, E, E-prec	Strain differences in quantiative expression	142
YBM 6.1		N, monocytes, eosinophils. Not T or B		120

For abbreviations, see p. 199

USE OF MONOCLONAL ANTIBODIES TO SEPARATE HAEMATOPOIETIC PROGENITOR CELLS

The presence of many membrane glycoproteins on haematopoietic stem and progenitor cells is at present a matter of some speculation. It has been suggested that pluripotent cells may carry on their surface a wide variety of macromolecules that characterize the descendant cell lineages to which they are capable of giving rise. Commitment to one lineage would be accompanied by loss of many of these molecules and enhanced expression of those specific to the lineage concerned[21,118]. Some support for this idea comes from the claim that Thy-1 is present on murine CFU-S[79]. However, Thy-1 is not an ideal example since, as mentioned elsewhere, it is present on several murine cell types and is, moreover, quite differently distributed among haematopoietic cells of the rat. It would be unsafe to infer that other T-related antigens are present or to regard the hypothesis as substantially strengthened. A general problem is that the hypothesis predicts small amounts of lineage-specific molecules on stem cells. The smaller the quantity of a molecule, the greater is the difficulty of establishing that it is really there. The problem is compounded by the fact that stem cells are rare and it is only recently that substantial progress has been made towards isolating them. In the case of Thy-1, it was necessary to use highly amplified fluorescence methods to demonstrate its presence on CFU-S by cell sorting[79] and it is difficult to be certain that the positive result was really due to specific binding of anti-Thy-1 Mab by membrane Thy-1.

Notwithstanding these uncertainties, there is no doubt that certain antigens are carried by at least some mouse stem cells and can be demonstrated by negative or positive selection for CFU-S[38,119-120].

Watt et al[38] exploited the fact that the leukocyte common antigen (LCA) is absent from nucleated erythroid cells to enrich for early progenitors in suspensions of mouse fetal liver. Using the anti-LCA Mab YBM 42, they were able to separate relatively mature ('day 2 CFU-E') and immature erythroid colony-forming cells, since the latter had not lost the antigen. Quantitatively, the expression of this antigen is very heterogeneous on bone marrow cells, and FACS separation on the basis of brightness enabled these workers to make some (incomplete) distinctions between progenitors of different lineages. Another Mab (YBM 10.14.9) was found by the same group to be strongly expressed on progenitors, including day 2 CFU-E, but absent from more mature erythroid cells[121]. By using these two Mabs in combination (negative selection with YBM 42 and positive selection with YBM 10) they achieved cell suspensions containing up to 60% day 2 CFU-E. A similar approach was followed by Hoang et al[122] with two other Mabs, YBM 34.3 and YBM 6.1. YBM 34.3 bound to a heat-stable antigen expressed on B-lymphocytes, neutrophils and erythroid cells, while YBM 6.1 bound to cells of the neutrophil, eosinophil and monocyte series but not to colony-forming progenitors. The combinations of these reagents, using panning and/or FACS separation, made possible a substantial enrichment of immature cells from mouse bone marrow. Differential binding of YBM 34.3 allowed the separation of erythroid clonogenic cells of different stages of maturity (day 7 BFU-E, day 5 BFU-E and day 2 CFU-E).

These studies illustrate what can be achieved with reagents that, individually, show relatively little specificity for particular cell types. The approach should prove to be generally applicable and open to refinement through the use of further cell sorting parameters (including multiple colours and wide-angle scatter).

Despite our general policy of omitting anti-MHC Mabs, the anti-QaM2 antibody described by Hogarth et al[123] deserves brief mention since it is claimed to distinguish between stem cells (assayed as CFU-S) with different powers of self-renewal. If so, this will be a valuable tool: heterogeneity of self-renewal has long been known to characterize the CFU-S compartment, but no satisfactory means of separating those with high self-renewal (i.e. those most like real stem cells) from the rest has hitherto been available. However the concentration of antigen on bone marrow cells appears to be very low and it is too early to say whether the reagent will prove easy to use in practice.

MISCELLANEOUS REAGENTS FOR THE STUDY OF HAEMATOPOIESES

A selection of such reagents is listed in Table 8.5.

Reagents for receptors for IL-2 and transferrin

An antibody (ART-18) to receptors for interleukin-2 on rat T-cells has been described by Osawa & Diamantstein[124,125]. Like anti-Tac antibodies in man[126], ART 18 precipitated a major glycoprotein of 50 kDa, but also a minor component of 36 kDa under reducing conditions. Antibodies to the murine Il-2 receptor have also been obtained[159]. A murine transferrin receptor has been identified by several Mabs[14,15]. YE1/9.9 precipitates two covalently linked 100 kDa polypeptide chains[14]. Both of these reagents are of special interest in recognizing macromolecules of known function, and hold out the hope that antibodies recognizing other cell surface molecules involved in the control of cell proliferation will be obtained in due course.

Table 8.5 Miscellaneous monoclonal antibodies for the study of haematopoiesis

Name	Antigen	Comments	Refs.
MEL-14		Lymphocyte receptor for HEV of LN	127
ART-18	50+36 kDa	Receptor for interleukin 2 (rat)	125
3C7 7D4 2E4	50–60 kDa also 20–25 kDa and 110–120 kDa	Receptors for murine interleukin 2	159
R17 208 YE1/9.9	2×95 kDa 2×100 kDa	Receptor for transferrin Receptor for transferrin	15 14
60.3	95+130+150 kDa	Blocks CTL & NK lysis & in vitro mitogen responses	129
M7/14 H35–89.9	LFA. 180+95 kDa	'Lymphocyte function antigen' β-chain like Mac-1 β-chain	130, 131 132
ER-TR4, 5, 6, 7		Identify four thymic stromal cell populations	97
	Qa-m2	Distinguishes CFU-S with differing self-renewal	123
30-H11 55–7.2	Glycolipid	On some CFU-S. Varied conc on BM. On T	52 120
(Many)	Ly-5, T-200	Varied conc on BM (high on T & B). On CFU-S	38, 120

Control of lymphocyte migration

The Mab MEL-14[127] blocks the recirculation pathway of lymphocytes across the high-endothelial venules of lymph nodes and is thought to react with a recognition structure on the lymphocytes for the venule endothelium. Since this Mab does not block passage across the endothelium of Peyers patches, distinct recognition events are postulated to account for migration in the nodes and the patches. Germinal center cells, believed to non-recirculating, do not carry the MEL-14 antigen[128].

Lymphocyte activation

Several groups have described Mabs that interfere with the activation of lymphocytes and precipitate complexes of noncovalently linked polypeptides. Mab 60.3[129] precipitates components of 95, 130 and 150 kDa. These molecules were found on most nucleated cells in peripheral blood and bone marrow. The Mab blocked lysis by cytotoxic T-cells and NK-cells and inhibited in vitro blastogenesis by antigens and mitogens. In addition it blocked chemotactic migration of neutrophils across a millipore membrane. These molecule bear some similarity to the 'lymphocyte function antigen' (LFA-1) previously described by Sanchez-Madrid et al[130]. LFA-1 appears as a molecule composed of two non-covalently linked components 180 kDa and 95 kDa, the smaller of which is homologous with the β-chain of Mac-1[131] (see Table 8.4). Other workers[132] have described a Mab, H35-89.9, which precipitates what is probably an identical molecule to LFA-1. This macromolecular complex has been suggested to form a part of a 'membrane-dependent cell activation pathway', but its precise function remains to be elucidated.

The Ly-6 complex

Tada et al[133] have pointed out that several lymphocyte antigens are encoded or controlled by clusters of genes and that clustering might imply both an evolutionary and a functional relationship. The most notable such cluster is, of course, the major histocompatibility complex (MHC), including the Qa and Tla regions, on Chromosome 17 in the mouse. Others that they discuss include Ly-1/Lym10 on chromosome 19 and the Ly-6 complex on chromosome 9. The latter seems particularly interesting insofar as it controls the expression of several distinct macromolecules with distinct distributions on haematopoietic (and some non-haematopoietic) cells. Ly-6 was extensively studied (under that name or others: DAG, ALA-1, Ly-8) with conventional antisera, but progress has been accelerated by the arrival of monoclonal antibodies. The main features of several such reagents are shown in Table 8.6. Since different groups employed different methods of assay (cytotoxicity, rosetting, FACS analysis), it is difficult to make comparisons between some of these reagents, monoclonal though they are. FACs analysis emphasises the importance of variation in quantitative antigen expression between different cell types[44,134]. It may turn out that there are fewer distinct antigens than Table 8.6 implies. For example, Ly-28.2 appears similar to the Ly-6.2C and/or H9/25 antigen(s). Conversely, it is conceivable that some other existing Mabs may prove to be associated with Ly-6. These include 9F3[135], which reacts strongly with the abnormal T-cells of autoimmune MRL/1pr mice; Y3/19 ('MALA-1'), which binds to ConA-and LPS-induced blasts and precipitates a 14-18 kDa protein[136]; and

Table 8.6 Monoclonal antibodies to antigens of the murine Ly-6 group

Antigen	Cell distribution etc.	Refs.
Ly-6 ⎫ Ly-m6.2A ⎬	Most T, M, N & ConA blasts Mw = 33.5 kDa	25, 134, 140, 143, 144
Ly-m6.2B	Most BM	25
Ly-m6.2C H9/25	Most BM, some LN & spl. Some ConA blasts. Tc, Tcp, PFC, Mw=12–15 kDa	25 145, 146
Ly-m6.2D	Thy	25
Ly-m6.2E	ConA blasts (=ALA-1)	25
ThB	B & cortical thy Mw = 16 kDa	44, 134 140
Ly-27.2	All thy, T & B	26
Ly-28.2	Most BM, subsets of T & B	26
34-10-7	BM, abnormal T of MLR/lpr	143

ABBREVIATIONS USED IN TABLES

T	= T lymphocyte (Th=helper; Ts=suppressor; Tc=cytotoxic)
B	= B-lymphocyte
PC	= plasmacyte
Thy	= thymocyte
E	= erythrocyte
NK	= natural killer cell
M	= macrophage
ID	= interdigitating cell
N	= neutrophil
LC	= Langerhans cell
IEL	= intraepithelial lymphocyte (of intestine)
BM	= bone marrow
Spl	= spleen
LN	= lymph node
GC	= germinal center
HEV	= high-endothelial venule
ConA	= concanavalin A
IL-2	= interleukin-2
Ab	= antibody
Ag	= antigen
Conc	= concentration
Freq	= frequency
Prob	= probably
Chr	= chromosome
Correl	= correlations

several other antibodies which recognize antigens with 'patchy' cell distributions— 4B9[137], NIMR-2[49], J11d[138], M1/69[139] and YBM 34.3[122].

M1/69 was thought to recognize a glycolipid, since it precipitated no detectable radiolabelled protein, but detection of some Ly-6-related proteins by surface labelling and immunoprecipitation seems to be troublesome and subject to false negatives[26,44,140].

There is much about the Ly-6 complex that remains obscure. It is not yet known whether the different-sized molecules precipitated by some of the Mabs are distinct proteins or a single protein modified post-translationally (e.g. glycosylated) in various ways. More important, the functions of these molecules and the significance of their varied cell distributions are unknown. However, their differential expression on lymphocyte and other haematopoietic cell subsets, and particularly the specific association of some of them with activated lymphoblasts, identify the Ly-6 complex as an important area for further study.

REFERENCES

1. Shortman K, Linthicum D S, Battye F L, Goldschneider I, Liabeuf A, Golstein P et al 1979 Cytotoxic and fluorescent assays for thymocyte subpopulations differing in surface Thy-1 level. Cell Biophysics 3: 255
2. Kasturi K, Fleming J, Harrison P 1983 A monoclonal antibody against erythrocyte spectrin reacts with both α and β-subunits and detects spectrin-like molecules in non-erythroid cells. Experimental Cell Research 144: 241–246
3. Ledbetter J A, Rouse R V, Micklem H S, Herzenberg L A 1980 T cell subsets defined by expression of Lyt-1,2,3 and Thy-1 antigens. Journal of Experimental Medicine 152: 280–295
4. Dangl J L, Herzenberg L A 1982 Selection of hybridomas and hybridoma variants using the fluorescence-activated cell sorter. Journal of Immunological Methods 52: 1–14
5. Parish C R, Hayward J A 1974 The lymphocyte surface. II Separation of Fc receptor, C3 receptor and surface immunoglobulin bearing lymphocytes. Proceedings of the Royal Society, Series B 187: 65–81
6. Mage M G, McHugh L L, Rothstein T L 1977 Mouse lymphocytes with and without surface immunoglobulin: preparative scale separation in polystyrene tissue culture dishes. Journal of Immunological Methods 15: 47–56
7. Wysocki L J, Sato V L 1978 'Panning' for lymphocytes; a method for cell selection. Proceedings of the National Academy of Sciences of the USA 75: 2844–2848
8. Herzenberg L A, Herzenberg L A 1978 Analysis and separation using the fluorescence activated cell sorter (FACS). In: Weir D M (ed) Handbook of Experimental Immunology, 3rd edn. Blackwells, Oxford, ch 22
9. Parks D R, Hardy R R, Herzenberg L A 1984 Three-color immunofluorescence analysis of mouse B lymphocyte subpopulations. Cytometry 5: 159–167
10. Tada N, Kimura S, Hoffman M, Hämmerling U 1980 A new surface antigen (PC.2) expressed exclusively on plasma cells. Immunogenetics 11: 351–362
11. Mellman I S Unkeless J C 1980 Purification of a functional mouse Fc receptor through the use of a monoclonal antibody. Journal of Experimental Medicine 152: 1048–1069
12. Heinz H-P, Dlugonska H, Rude E, Loos M 1984 Monoclonal anti-mouse macrophage antibodies recognize the globular portions of C1q, a sub-component of the first component of complement. Journal of Immunology 133: 400–404
13. Beller D I, Springer T A, Schreiber R D 1982 Anti-Mac-1 selectively inhibits the mouse and human type three complement receptor. Journal of Experimental Medicine 156: 1000–1009
14. Takei F 1983 Two surface antigens expressed on proliferating mouse T lymphocytes defined by rat monoclonal antibodies. Journal of Immunology 130: 2794–2797
15. Trowbridge I S, Lesley J, Schulte R 1982 Murine cell surface transferrin receptor: studies with an anti-receptor monoclonal antibody. Journal of Cellular Physiology 112: 403–410
16. Manohar V, Brown E, Leiserson W M, Chused T M 1982 Expression of Lyt-1 on a subset of B lymphocytes. Journal of Immunology 129: 532–538
17. Hayakawa K, Hardy R R, Parks D R, Herzenberg L A 1983 The "Ly-1 B" cell subpopulation in normal, immunodefective and autoimmune mice. Journal of Experimental Medicine 157: 202–218
18. Subbarao B, Mosier D 1982 Lyb antigens and their role in B lymphocyte activation. Immunological Reviews 69: 81–97
19. Scheid M P, Landreth K S, Tung J-S, Kincade P W 1982 Preferential but nonexclusive expression of macromolecular antigens on B-lineage cells. Immunological Reviews 69: 141–159
20. Shen F-W, Yakura H, Tung J-S 1982 Some compartments of B cell differentiation. Immunological Reviews 69: 69–80
21. Berridge M V 1979 A new class of cell surface antigens. Quantitative absorption studies defining cell-lineage-specific antigens on hemopoietic cells. Journal of Experimental Medicine 150: 977–986
22. Morse H C, Davidson W F, Yetter R A, Coffman R L 1982 A cell surface antigen shared by B cells and Ly2$^+$ peripheral T cells. Cellular Immunology 70: 311–320

23. Ralph S J, Berridge M V 1984 Expression of antigens of the 'T200' family of glycoproteins on hemopoietic stem cells: evidence that thymocyte cell lineage antigens are represented on 'T200'. Journal of Immunology 132: 2510–2514

24. Parrott D M V, Tait C, MacKenzie S, Mowat A M, Davies M D J, Micklem H S 1983 Analysis of the effector functions of different populations of mucosal lymphocytes. Annals of the New York Academy of Sciences 409: 307–319

25. Kimura S, Tada N, Liu-Lam Y, Hämmerling U 1984 Studies of the mouse Ly-6 alloantigen system. II. Complexities of the Ly-6 region. Immunogenetics 20: 47–56

26. Hogarth P M, Houlden B A, Latham S E, Sutton V R, McKenzie I F C 1984 Definition of new alloantigens encoded by genes in the *Ly-6* complex. Immunogenetics 20: 57–69

27. Kozak C A, Davidson W E, Morse H C 1984 Genetic and functional relationships of the retroviral and alloantigen loci on mouse chromosome 1. Immunogenetics 19: 163–168

28. Ledbetter J A, Goding J W, Tsu T, Herzenberg L A 1979 A new mouse lymphoid alloantigen (Lgp100) recognized by a monoclonal rat antibody. Immunogenetics 8: 347–360

29. Hogarth P M, Craig J, McKenzie I F C 1980 A monoclonal antibody detecting the Ly-9.2 (Lgp 100) cell-membrane alloantigen. Immunogenetics 11: 65–74

30. Hardy R R, Hayakawa K, Haaijman J J, Herzenberg L A, Herzenberg L A 1982 B cell subpopulations identified by two-color fluorescence analysis. Nature 297: 589–591

31. Hardy R R, Hayakawa K, Parks D R, Herzenberg L A, Herzenberg L A 1984 Murine B cell differentiation lineages. Journal of Experimental Medicine 159: 1169–1188

32. Scher I 1982 The CBA/N mouse: an experimental model illustrating the influence of the X chromosome on immunity. Advances in Immunology 33: 1–71

33. Nahm M H, Paslay J W, Davie J M 1983 Unbalanced X chromosome mosaicism in B cells of mice with X-linked immunodeficiency. Journal of Experimental Medicine 158: 920–931

34. Witkowski J, Forrester L M, Ansell J D, Micklem H S 1984 Influence of the *xid* mutation on B lymphocyte development in adult mice. In: Germinal Centers in Immune Responses: Proceedings of the Tenth International Conference (In press)

35. Metcalf E S, Mond J J, Finkleman F D 1983 Effects of neonatal anti-δ antibody on the murine immune system. II. Functional capacity of a stable sIg⁺Ia⁺sIgD⁻ B cell population. Journal of Immunology 131: 601–605

36. Skelly R R, Baine Y, Ahmed A, Xue B, Thorbecke G J 1983 Cell surface phenotype of lymphoid cells from normal mice and mice treated with monoclonal anti-IgD from birth. Journal of Immunology 130: 15–18

37. Kemp J D, Rohrer J W, Huber B T 1982 Lyb3; a B cell surface antigen associated with triggering secretory differentiation. Immunological Reviews 69: 127–140

38. Watt S M, Gilmore D J, Metcalf D, Cobbold S P, Hoang T K, Waldmann H 1983 Segregation of mouse hemopoietic progenitor cells using the monoclonal antibody YBM/42. Journal of Cellular Physiology 115: 37–45

39. Kincade P W, Lee G, Watanabe T, Sun I, Scheid M P 1981 Antigens displayed on murine B lymphocyte precursors. Journal of Immunology 127: 2262–2265

40. Coffman R L, Weissman I L 1981 A monoclonal antibody that recognizes B cells and B cell precursors in mice. Journal of Experimental Medicine 153: 269–279

41. Coffman R L 1982 Surface antigen expression and immunoglobulin gene rearrangement during mouse pre-B cell development. Immunological Reviews 69: 5–23

42. Landreth K S, Kincade P W, Lee G, Medlock E S 1983 Phenotypic and functional characterization of murine B lymphocyte precursors isolated from fetal and adult tissues. Journal of Immunology 131: 572–580

43. Coffman R L, Weissman I L 1983 Immunoglobulin gene rearrangement during pre-B cell differentiation. Molecular and Cellular Immunology 1: 31–38

44. Eckhardt L A, Herzenberg L A 1980 Monoclonal antibodies to ThB detect close linkage of *Ly-6* and a gene regulating ThB expression. Immunogenetics 11: 275–291

45. Honjo T 1983 Immunoglobulin genes. Annual Review of Immunology 1: 499–528

46. Dumont F J, Habbersett R C, Nichols E A, Treffinger J A, Tung A S 1983 A monoclonal antibody (100C5) to the Lyt-2⁻ T cell population expanding in MRL/Mp-1pr/1pr mice. European Journal of Immunology 13: 455–459

47. Hogarth P M, Crewther P E, McKenzie I F C 1982 Description of a Qa-2 like alloantigen (Qa-m2). European Journal of Immunology 12: 374–379

48. Rucker J, Horowitz M, Lerner E A, Murphy D B 1983 Monoclonal antibody reveals *H-2*-linked quantitative and qualitative variation in the expression of a Qa-2 region determinant. Immunogenetics 17: 303–316

49. Chayen A, Parkhouse R M E 1982 B cell subpopulations in the mouse: analysis with monoclonal antibodies NIM-R2 and NIM-R3. European Journal of Immunology 12: 725–732

50.   Marshall-Clarke S, Chayen A, Parkhouse R M E Monoclonal antibody NIM-R2 shows differential reactivity with virgin and memory B cells. European Journal of Immunology 12: 733–738

51.   Cantor H, Boyse E A 1975 Functional classes of T lymphocytes bearing different Ly antigens. Journal of Experimental Medicine 141: 1376–1389

52.   Ledbetter J A, Herzenberg L A 1979 Xenogeneic monoclonal antibodies to mouse lymphoid differentiation antigens. Immunological Reviews 47: 63

53.   Ledbetter J A, Seaman W E 1982 The Lyt-2, Lyt-3 macromolecules: structural and functional studies. Immunological Reviews 68: 197–218

54.   Micklem H S, Ledbetter J A, Eckhardt L A, Herzenberg L A 1980 Analysis of lymphocyte subpopulations with monoclonal antibodies to Thy-1, Lyt-1, Lyt-2 and ThB antigens. In: Pernis B, Vogel H J (eds) Regulatory T lymphocytes. Academic, New York, p 119–132

55.   Lepault F, Weissman I L 1981 An in vivo assay for thymus-homing bone marrow cells. Nature 293: 151–154

56.   Scollay R 1982 Inconsistencies detected by flow cytometry following immunofluorescence staining with anti-Thy-1 antibodies. Journal of Immunological Methods 52: 15–23

57.   Ledbetter J A, Rouse R V, Micklem H S, Herzenberg L A 1980 T cell subsets defined by expression of Lyt-1,2,3 and Thy-1 antigens. Journal of Experimental Medicine 152: 280–295

58.   Mason D W, Arthur R P, Dallman M J, Green J R, Spickett G P, Thomas M L 1983 Function of rat T-lymphocyte subsets isolated by means of monoclonal antibodies. Immunological Reviews 74: 57–82

59.   Dialynas D P, Quan Z S, Wall K A, Pierres A, Quintans J, Loken M R et al 1983 Characterization of the murine T cell surface molecule, designated L3T4, identified by monoclonal antibody GK1.5. Journal of Immunology 131: 2445–2451

60.   Swain S L 1983 T cell subsets and the recognition of MHC class. Immunological Reviews 74: 129–142

61.   Swain S L, Dennert G, Wormsley S, Dutton R W 1981 The Lyt phenotype of a long-term allospecific T cell line. Both helper and killer activities to IA are mediated by Ly-1 cells. European Journal of Immunology 11: 175–180

62.   Glasebrook A L, Kelso A, MacDonald H R 1983 Cytolytic T lymphocyte clones that proliferate autonomously to specific alloantigenic stimulation II. Journal of Immunology 130: 1545–1551

63.   Wilde D B, Marrack P, Kappler J, Dialynas D, Fitch F W 1983 Evidence implicating L3T4 in class II MHC antigen reactivity. Journal of Immunology 131: 2178–2183

64.   Pierres A, Naquet P, van Agthoven A, Bekkhoucha F, Denizot F, Mishal Z et al 1984. A rat anti-mouse T4 monoclonal antibody (H129.19) inhibits the proliferation of Ia-reactive T cell clones. Journal of Immunology 132: 2775–2782

65.   Green D R, Flood P M, Gershon R K 1983 Immunoregulatory T cell pathways. Annual Review of Immunology 1: 439–463

66.   Huber B, Cantor H, Shen F-W, Boyse E A 1976 Independent differentiative pathways of Ly-1 and Ly-23 subclasses of T cells. Journal of Experimental Medicine 144: 1128–1133

67.   Thomas D B, Calderon R A 1982 T helper cells change their Ly1,2 phenotype during an immune response. European Journal of Immunology 12: 16–23

68.   Thomas D B, Keeler K D 1984 Flip-flop in the Lyt 2 phenotype of T cells from radiation chimaeras between Thy 1 congenic donor and recipient mice. Immunology 51: 563–570

69.   Spickett G P, Mason D W 1983 Demonstration of the stability of the membrane phenotype of T helper cells after priming and boosting with a hapten-carrier conjugate. European Journal of Immunology 13: 785–788

70.   Boersma W J A, Kokenber E, Westen G v d, Haaijman J J 1982 Postirradiation thymocyte regeneration after bone marrow transplantation. III. European Journal of Immunology 12: 615–619

71.   Van Ewijk W, Jenkinson E J, Owen J J T 1982 Detection of Thy-1, T-200, Lyt-1 and Lyt-2-bearing cells in the developing lymphoid organs of the mouse embryo in vivo and in vitro. European Journal of Immunology 12: 262–271

72.   Van Ewijk W, van Soest P L, van den Engh G 1981 Fluorescence analysis and anatomic distribution of mouse T lymphocyte subsets defined by monoclonal antibodies to the antigens Thy-1, Lyt-1, Lyt-2 and T-200. Journal of Immunology 127: 2594–2604

73.   Ceredig R, Dialynas D, Fitch F W, MacDonald H R 1983 Precursors of T cell growth factor producing cells in the thymus. Journal of Experimental Medicine 158: 1654–1671

74.   Ceredig R, MacDonald H R, Jenkinson E J 1983 Flow microfluorometric analysis of mouse thymus development in vivo and in vitro. European Journal of Immunology 13: 185–190

75.   Scollay R, Wilson, Shortman K 1984 Thymus cell migration: analysis of thymus emigrants with markers that distinguish medullary thymocytes from peripheral T cells. Journal of Immunology 132: 1089–1094

76. Haaijman J J, Micklem H S, Ledbetter J A, Dangl J L, Herzenberg L A, Herzenberg L A 1981 T cell ontogeny. Organ location of maturing populations as defined by surface markers is similar in neonates and adults. Journal of Experimental Medicine 153: 605–614

77. Mathieson B J, Sharrow S O, Campbell P S, Asofsky R 1979 An Lyt differentiated subpopulation of thymocytes detected by flow microfluorometry. Nature 277: 478–480

78. Chan M M, Tada N, Kimura S, Hoffman N K, Miller R A, Stutman O, Hämmerling U 1983 Characterization of T lymphocyte subsets with monoclonal antibodies: discovery of a distinct marker, Ly-m22, of T suppressor cells. Journal of Immunology 130: 2075–2078

79. Basch R S, Berman J W 1982 Thy-1 determinants are present on many murine hematopoietic cells other than T cells. European Journal of Immunology 12: 359–364

80. Schrader J W, Battye F, Scollay R 1982 Expression of Thy-1 antigen is not limited to T cells in cultures of mouse hemopoietic cells. Proceedings of the National Academy of Sciences of the USA 79: 4161–4165

81. Hunt S V, Mason D W, Williams A F 1977 In rat bone marrow Thy-1 antigen is present on cells with membrane immunoglobulin and on precursors of peripheral B lymphocytes. European Journal of Immunology 7: 817–823

82. Goldschneider I, Gordon L K, Morris R J 1978 Demonstration of the Thy-1 antigen on pluripotent hemopoietic stem cells in the rat. Journal of Experimental Medicine 148: 1351–1366

83. Gunter K C, Malek T R, Shevach E M 1984 T cell-activating properties of an anti-Thy-1 monoclonal antibody. Possible analogy to OKT3/Leu-4. Journal of Experimental Medicine 159: 716–730

84. Sidman C L, Forni L, Köhler G, Langhorne J, Fischer-Lindahl K 1983 A monoclonal antibody against a new differentiation antibody of thymocytes. European Journal of Immunology 13: 481–488

85. Thomas D B, Calderson R A, Blaxland L J 1978 A new Thy-1 alloantigen as a temporal marker of T lymphocyte differentiation. Nature 275: 711–715

86. Del Guercio P, Motta I, Metezeau P, Brugere S, Perret R, Truffa-Bachi P 1982 Heterogeneity of mouse Thy 1.2 antigen expression revealed by monoclonal antibodies. Cellular Immunology 73: 72–82

87. Abehsira O, Edwards A, Simpson E 1981 Functional and binding activity of monoclonal anti-Thy-1 antibodies: evidence for different expression of the two alleles. European Journal of Immunology 11: 275–281

88. Kasai M, Takashi T, Takahashi T, Tokunaga T 1984 A new differentiation antigen (FT-1) shared with fetal thymocytes and leukemic cells in the mouse. Journal of Experimental Medicine 159: 971–980

89. Takei F 1984 A novel differentiation antigen of proliferating murine thymocytes identified by a rat monoclonal antibody. Journal of Immunology 132: 766–771

90. Owen F L 1982 Products of the IgT-C region of chromosome 12 and maturational markers for T cells. Journal of Experimental Medicine 156: 703–718

91. Owen F L 1983 Tpre, a new alloantigen encoded in the IgT-C region of chromosome 12, is expressed on bone marrow of nude mice, fetal T cell hybrids and fetal thymus. Journal of Experimental Medicine 157: 419–432

92. Keesee S K, Owen F L 1983 Modulation of Tthy alloantigen expression in the neonatal mouse. The Tthy bearing thymocyte is a precursor for the peripheral cells expressing Tind and Tsu. Journal of Experimental Medicine 157: 86–97

93. Owen F L 1983 T cell alloantigens encoded by the IgT-C region of chromosome 12 in the mouse. Advances in Immunology 34: 1–39

94. Tokuhisa T, Komatsu Y, Uchida Y, Taniguchi M 1982 Monoclonal alloantibodies specific for the constant region of T cell antigen receptors. Journal of Experimental Medicine 156: 888–897

95. Lee N E, d'Eustachio P, Pravtcheva D, Ruddle F H, Hedrick S M, Davis M M 1984 Murine T cell receptor beta chain is encoded on chromosome 6. Journal of Experimental Medicine 160: 905–913

96. Robertson M 1984 T cell antigen receptor. The capture of the snark. Nature 312: 16–17

97. Van Vliet E, Melis M, van Ewijk W 1984 Monoclonal antibodies to stromal cell types of the mouse thymus. European Journal of Immunology 14: 524–529

98. Thomas M L, Green J R 1983 Molecular nature of the W3/25 and MRC OX-8 marker antigens for rat T lymphocytes: comparisons with mouse and human antigens. European Journal of Immunology 13: 855–858

99. Spickett G P, Brandon M R, Mason D W, Williams A F, Woollett G R 1983 MRC OX-22, a monoclonal antibody that labels a new subset of T lymphocytes. Journal of Experimental Medicine 158: 795–810

100. Dallman M J, Thomas M L, Green J R 1984 MRC OX-19: a monoclonal antibody that labels

rat T lymphocytes and augments in vitro proliferative responses. European Journal of Immunology 14: 260–267

101. Cantrell D A, Robins R A, Baldwin R W 1983 A comparison of membrane markers on rat cytotoxic cells. Immunology 49: 139–146

102. Micklem H S, Loutit J F 1966 Tissue Grafting and Radiation. Academic, New York, p 134–164

103. Barnes D W H, Loutit J F, Micklem H S 1962 "Secondary disease" of radiation chimeras: a syndrome due to lymphoid aplasia. Annals of the New York Academy of Sciences 99: 374–385

104. Loutit J F, Micklem H S 1962 "Secondary disease" among lethally irradiated mice restored with haemopoietic tissues from normal or iso-immunized foreign mice. British Journal of Experimental Pathology 43: 77–87

105. Korngold R, Sprent J 1978 Lethal graft-versus-host disease after bone marrow transplantation across minor histocompatibility barriers in mice. Prevention by removing mature T cells from marrow. Journal of Experimental Medicine 148: 1687–1698

106. Vallera D A, Soderling C C B, Kersey J H 1982 Bone marrow transplantation across major histocompatibility barriers in mice. III. Treatment of donor grafts with monoclonal antibodies directed against Lyt determinants. Journal of Immunology 128: 871–875

107. Vitetta E S, Krolick K A, Miyama-Inaba M, Cushley W, Uhr J 1983 Immunotoxins: a new approach to cancer therapy. Science 219: 644

108. Vallera D A, Youle R J, Neville D M, Soderling C C B, Kersey J H 1983 Monoclonal antibody toxin conjugates for experimental graft-versus-host disease prophylaxis. Transplantation 36: 73–80

109. Colombatti M, Nabholz M, Gros O, Bron C 1983 Selective killing of target cells by antibody-ricin A chain or antibody-gelonin hybrid molecules: comparison of cytotoxic potency and use in immunoselection procedures. Journal of Immunology 131: 3091–3095

110. Loveland B E, Hogarth P M, Ceredig R, McKenzie I F C 1981 Cells mediating graft rejection in the mouse. I. Lyt-1 cells mediate skin graft rejection. Journal of Experimental Medicine 153: 1044–1057

111. Cobbold S P, Waldmann H 1984 Therapeutic potential of monovalent monoclonal antibodies. Nature 308: 460–462

112. Seaman W E, Wofsy D, Greenspan J S, Ledbetter J A 1983 Treatment of autoimmune MLR/1pr mice with monoclonal antibody to Thy-1.2. Journal of Immunology 130: 1713–1718

113. Michaelides M, Hogarth P M, McKenzie I F C 1981 The immunosuppressive effect of monoclonal anti-Lyt-1.1 antibodies in vivo. European Journal of Immunology 11: 1005–1012

114. Austyn J M, Gordon S 1981 F4/80, a monoclonal antibody directed specifically against the mouse macrophage. European Journal of Immunology 11: 805–815

115. Hume D A, Loutit J F, Gordon S 1984 The mononuclear phagocyte system of the mouse defined by immunohistochemical localization of antigen F4/80: macrophages of bone and associated connective tissue. Journal of Cell Science 66: 189–201

116. Loutit J F, Nisbet N W 1982 The origin of osteoclasts. Immunobiology 161: 193–203

117. Hume D A, Robinson A P, Macpherson D G, Gordon S 1983 The mononuclear phagocyte system of the mouse defined by immunohistochemical localization of antigen F4/80. Journal of Experimental Medicine 158: 1522–1536

118. Till J E 1976 Regulation of hemopoietic stem cells. In: Cairnie A B, Lala P K, Osmond D G (eds) Stem cells of renewing cell populations. Academic, New York p 143–145

119. Ralph S J, Tan S A, Berridge M V 1982 Monoclonal antibodies detect subpopulations of bone marrow stem cells. Stem Cells 2: 88–107

120. Van den Engh G, Bauman J, Mulder D, Visser J 1983 Measurement of antigen expression of hemopoietic stem cells and progenitor cells by fluorescence-activated cell sorting. In: Killmann S A, Cronkite E P, Muller-Berat C N (eds) Stem cells, characterization, proliferation, regulation. Munksgaard, Copenhagen, p 59–71

121. Watt S M, Metcalf D, Gilmore D J, Stenning G M, Clark M R, Waldmann H 1983 Selective isolation of murine erythropoietin-responsive progenitor cells (CFU-E) with monoclonal antibodies. Molecular Biology & Medicine 1: in press

122. Hoang T, Gilmore D, Metcalf D, Cobbold S, Watt S, Clark M et al 1983 Separation of hemopoietic cells from adult mouse marrow by use of monoclonal antibodies. Blood 61: 580–588

123. Harris R À, Hogarth P M, Wadeson L J, Collins P, McKenzie I F C, Penington D G 1984 An antigenic difference between cells forming early and late haematopoietic spleen colonies (CFU-S). Nature 307: 638–641

124. Osawa H, Diamantstein T 1983 Studies on T lymphocyte activation II. Monoclonal antibody inhibiting the capacity of rat T lymphoblasts to absorb and to respond to IL-2: an anti-IL-2 receptor antibody? Immunology 48: 617–621

125. Osawa H, Diamantstein T 1984 Partial characterization of the putative rat interleukin 2 receptor. European Journal of Immunology 14: 374–376
126. Leonard W J, Depper J M, Uchiyama T, Smith K A, Waldmann T A, Greene W C 1982 A monoclonal antibody that appears to recognize the receptor for human T cell growth factor; partial characterization of the receptor. Nature 300: 267–269
127. Gallatin W M, Weissman I L, Butcher E C 1983 A cell surface molecule involved in organ-specific homing of lymphocytes. Nature 304: 30–34
128. Reichert R A, Gallatin W M, Weissman I L, Butcher E C 1983 Germinal center B cells lack homing receptors necessary for normal lymphocyte recirculation. Journal of Experimental Medicine 157: 813–827
129. Beatty P G, Ledbetter J A, Martin P J, Price T H, Hansen J A 1983 Definition of a common leukocyte cell-surface antigen (Lp95-150) associated with diverse cell-mediated immune functions. Journal of Immunology 131: 2913–2918
130. Sanchez-Madrid F, Davignon D, Martz E, Springer T A 1982 Antigens involved in mouse cytolytic T-lymphocyte (CTL)-mediated killing: functional screening and topographic relationship. Cellular Immunology 73: 1–11
131. Sanchez-Madrid F, Simon P, Thompson S, Springer T A 1983 Mapping of antigenic and functional epitopes on the α and β-subunits of two related mouse glycoproteins involved in cell interactions, LFA-1 & Mac-1 Journal of Experimental Medicine 158: 586–602
132. Pierres M, Goridis C, Golstein P 1982 Inhibition of murine T cell-mediated cytolysis and T cell proliferation by a rat monoclonal antibody. European Journal of Immunology 12: 60–69
133. Tada N, Kimura S, Hämmerling U 1982 Immunogenetics of mouse B cell alloantigen systems defined by monoclonal antibodies and gene-cluster formation of these loci. Immunological Reviews 69: 99–125
134. Matossian-Rogers A, Rogers P, Herzenberg L A 1982 Analysis of Ly-6.2-bearing murine lymphocyte subpopulations in relation to the T-lymphocyte markers, Thy-1, Lyt-1 and Lyt-2. Cellular Immunology 69: 91–100
135. Dumont F J, Habbersett R C, Nichols E A 1984 A new lymphocyte surface antigen defined by a monoclonal antibody (9F3) to the T cell population expanding in MRL/Mp-lpr/lpr mice. Journal of Immunology 133: 809–815
136. Takei F 1984 MALA-1: a surface antigen expressed on activated murine T and B lymphocytes. Journal of Immunology 133: 345–350
137. Kung J T, Sharrow S O, Thomas C A, Paul W E 1982 Analysis of B lymphocyte differentiation antigens by flow microfluorometry. Immunological Reviews 69: 51–68
138. Bruce J, Symington F W, McKearn T J, Sprent J 1981 A monoclonal antibody discriminating between subsets of T and B cells. Journal of Immunology 127: 2496–2501
139. Springer T, Galfré G, Secher D S, Milstein C 1979 Mac-1: a macrophage differentiation antigen identified by monoclonal antibody. European Journal of Immunology 9: 301–306
140. Matossian-Rogers A, Rogers P, Ledbetter J A, Herzenberg L A 1982 Molecular weight determination of the genetically linked cell surface murine antigens: ThB and Ly-6. Immunogenetics 15: 591–599
141. Ralph P, Ho M-K, Litcofsky P B, Springer T A 1983 Expression and induction in vitro of macrophage differentiation antigens on murine cell lines. Journal of Immunology 130: 108–114
142. Hirsch S, Gordon S 1983 Polymorphic expression of a neutrophil differentiation antigen revealed by monoclonal antibody 7/4. Immunogenetics 18: 229–239
143. Melino M R, Dumont F J, Habersett R C, Hansen T H 1983 Expression of a bone marrow-associated Ly-6 determinant on the T cell population expanding in the lymph nodes of the autoimmune mouse strain MRL/Mp-1pr/1pr. Journal of Immunology 130: 1843–1847
144. Auchincloss H, Ozato K, Sachs D H 1981 Two distinct murine differentiation antigens determined by genes linked to the Ly-6 locus. Journal of Immunology 127: 1839–1843
145. Takei F, Galfré G, Alderson T, Lennox E S, Milstein C 1980 H9/25 monoclonal antibody recognizes a new allospecificity of mouse lymphocyte subpopulations. European Journal of Immunology 10: 241–246
146. Takei F, Waldmann H, Lennox E S, Milstein C 1980 Monoclonal antibody H9/25 reacts with functional subsets of T and B cells: killer, killer precursor and plaque-forming cells. European Journal of Immunology 10: 503–509
147. Hume D A, Halpin D, Charlton H, Gordon S 1984 The mononuclear phagocyte system of the mouse defined by immunohistochemical localization of antigen F4/80: macrophages of endocrine organs. Proceedings of the National Academy of the USA 81: 4174–4177
148. Haines K A, Flotte T J, Springer T A, Gigli I, Thorbecke G J 1983 Staining of Langerhans cells with monoclonal antibodies to macrophages and lymphoid cells. Proceedings of the National Academy of Sciences of the USA 80: 3448–3450

149. Woda B A, McFadden M L, Welsh R M, Bain K M 1984 Separation and isolation of rat natural killer (NK) cells from T cells with monoclonal antibodies. Journal of Immunology 132: 2183-2184

150. Lyscom N, Brueton M J 1982 Intraepithelial, lamina propria and Peyers Patch lymphocytes of the rat small intestine. Immunology 45: 775-783

151. Schrader J W, Scollay R, Battye F 1983 Intramucosal lymphocytes of the gut: Lyt-2 and Thy-1 phenotype of the granulated cells and evidence for the presence of both T cells and mast cell precursors. Journal of Immunology 130: 558-564

152. Dialynas D P, Wilde D B, Marrack P, Pierres A, Wall K, Havran W et al 1983 Characterization of the murine antigenic determinant, designated L3T4a, recognized by monoclonal antibody GK1.5. Immunological Reviews 74: 29-56

153. Shinefield L A, Sato V L, Rosenberg N E 1980 Monoclonal rat anti-mouse brain antibody detects Abelson murine leukemia virus target cells in mouse bone marrow. Cell 20: 11-17

154. Paige C J, Kincade P W, Shinefield L A, Sato V L 1981 Precursors of murine B lymphocytes. Physical and functional characterization and distinctions from myeloid stem cells. Journal of Experimental Medicine 153: 154-165

155. Subbarao B, Mosier D 1983 Induction of B lymphocyte proliferation by monoclonal anti-Lyb2 antibody. The Journal of Immunology 130: 2033-2037

156. Kimura S, Tada N, Hämmerling U 1980 A new lymphocyte alloantigen (Ly-10) controlled by a gene linked to the Lyt-1 locus. Immunogenetics 10: 363-372

157. Hogarth P M, Rigby A, Sutton V R, McKenzie I F C, Hilgers J 1984 The Ly-25.1 specificity: definition with a monoclonal antibody. Immunogenetics 19: 83-86

158. Dessner D L, Loken M R 1981 DNL1.9: a monoclonal antibody which specifically detects all murine B lineage cells. European Journal of Immunology 11: 282-285

159. Ortega R, Robb R J, Shevach E M, Malek T R 1984 The murine IL-2 receptor. I. Monoclonal antibodies that define distinct functional epitopes on activated T cells and react with activated B cells. Journal of Immunology 133: 1970-1975

160. Takei F 1984 Unique surface phenotype of T cells in lymphoproliferative autoimmune MRL/Mp-lpr/lpr mice. Journal of Immunology 133: 1951-1954

9

Monoclonal antibodies to human lymphocytes

Lewis L. Lanier Joseph H. Phillips Noel L. Warner

INTRODUCTION

The elegant concept originated by Kohler & Milstein[1] of immortalization of antigen-specific antibody producing cells using somatic cell hybridization has revolutionized basic and clinical medical research. Perhaps one of the most visible impacts of this technology has been in the use of monoclonal antibodies to identify human lymphoid cell subsets that possess defined functional abilities. The terms 'helper' T-cell and 'suppressor' T-cell, a few years ago recognized only by research immunologists primarily studying murine model systems, are now commonplace in clinical laboratories. These concepts and terms are gaining the attention even of the media and general public. However as the intensity of research has grown in the past few years in this field, so has the recognition of the complexity of human lymphocyte subpopulations. Cell populations that were first recognized as 'subsets', are now in themselves major populations that are quite heterogeneous and composed of distinct further subsets. In this review, we will illustrate some of the significant advances which have been made in the identification of human lymphocyte subsets primarily as a consequence of the use of monoclonal antibodies, and particularly when used in concert with flow cytometry.

MAJOR SUBSETS OF MATURE HUMAN LYMPHOCYTES

Human peripheral blood is the most readily available source of lymphocytes and for this reason has been the most intensively studied population of hematopoietic cells. In early hematological studies, this population of cells was identified exclusively on the basis of morphological criteria. In general, lymphocytes are easily identified in Wright's or Giemsa stained blood smears, in that they comprise a group of small (5-7 μm) mononuclear cells with little cytoplasm and few granules. The recognition of the existence of cell surface components that were controlled by genes preferentially expressed at certain stages of differentiation provided a new approach to identification and characterization of leukocyte populations. Experimental studies in the mouse first indicated that mature T-lymphocytes, identified by the presence of the Thy-1 alloantigen[2], could be subdivided on the basis of cell surface expression of the Ly-1 and Ly-2,3 alloantigens.[3-5] Cytotoxic and suppressor cell function was correlated with the phenotype, LY-1,2+,3+; whereas helper cell function generally was found within the Ly-1+,2-,3- population.[3-5] Based on the prediction that this subdivision of lymphocyte populations would also exist in man, several laboratories undertook studies to define functional subsets of human T lymphocytes. As a result of these investigations, the TH1 and TH2 subsets of human T cells, which contained helper and cytotoxic/suppressor cell function, respectively, were established.[6] However, the xenogeneic antisera used to identify and define the human T-cell subsets were difficult to prepare and render specific by absorption. This proved a major impediment to the study of human lymphocyte subsets and discouraged many investigators who were interested in pursuing the functional and phenotypic diversity of these hematopoietic cells.

The key event which further promoted research development of this area was the discovery of hybridoma technology. The ability to produce unlimited quantities of true monoclonal antibodies in xenogeneic animals permitted experiments that were previously feasible only in limited experimental systems where allotypic markers and congenic strains of mice were available.

In the late 1960's and early 1970's, it became apparent that human lymphoid cells could be divided into three major groups: B-cells, a population which expressed surface immunoglobulin; T-cells, a population initially identified by its ability to form rosettes with sheep erthrocytes; and a third group, simply referred to as 'null' cells which lacked surface Ig or avid receptors for sheep erythrocytes. The development and use of mouse monoclonal antibodies against human cell surface antigens facilitated a refinement of the establishment of the three major groups, with several key reagents being defined as the hallmark of these populations (Table 9.1).

T-lymphocytes are derived initially from a precursor pool in the bone marrow, and then mature in the thymus. T-cells are responsible for antigen specific cell-mediated immunity and helper cell function in Ig secretion. Although initially identified by the presence of sheep erythrocyte binding receptor, it is now appreciated that leukocytes other than T-lymphocytes may possess this receptor.[7] A more definitive 'pan' T-cell marker is the Leu 4 (or T3) antigen on the cell surface of mature T-lymphocytes.[8-9] Hence, there is presently some confusion about what precisely constitutes the T-cell population. Monoclonal antibodies such as anti-Leu 5 and T11 which react with

Table 9.1 Major subsets of mature human lymphocytes

T-lymphocytes	Major subsets	Associated functions
	LEU 2 (T8)	Cytotoxic and suppressor cells
LEU 4		
	LEU 3 (T4)	Helper and amplifier cells
B-lymphocytes		
	LEU 1 Negative	Ig secretion
SURFACE IG		
	LEU 1 Positive	Ig secretion
NK (K)-cells		
	LEU 7 Negative	NK cytotoxicity
LEU 11		
	LEU 7 Positive	NK cytotoxicity

determinants associated with the E receptor molecule, certainly define a population of cells which includes the majority of cells with T-cell function.[10] However, to the 'basic cellular immunologists', the definition of T-cells requires a thymic dependent maturation and the development of a recognitive repertoire. This has NOT been demonstrated for some of the E rosette positive cells. Hence, the 'T-cell' status of Leu 4-,Leu 5+ cells must still be questioned.

B-lymphocytes, the cells responsible for humoral immunity, arise from precursors in the bone marrow (pre-B-cells), which are identified by the expression of cytoplasmic Ig heavy chains. After passing through a stage of membrane Ig expression B-cells differentiate into plasma cells and secrete large quantities of Ig. Recent experiments employing recombinant DNA techniques have demonstrated that gene rearrangement of both heavy and light chains occurs in pre-B cells prior to heavy or light chain protein synthesis.[11-13] Rearrangement of Ig genes and synthesis of Ig proteins are the most reliable and characteristic marker of B-lymphocytes.

The function of the 'null' cell is less well understood. These cells were defined on the basis of 'what they are not', (i.e. non-T, non-B-cells), rather than because of any specific function or expression of a unique surface antigen. However, within this subset certain lymphocytes possessed the ability to mediate lysis of certain tumour cell lines or xenogeneic erythrocytes in the presence of antibody specific for the target cell (a process referred to as antibody dependent cellular cytotoxicity, ADCC).[14,15] Furthermore, the 'null' cell subset also contains lymphocytes which are cytotoxic for certain tumour cell lines in the absence of antibody or any deliberate prior immunization. Lymphocytes with this function became known, as 'natural killer' cells.[16] Within the last few years, we[17,18], as well as others[19-25], have developed several monoclonal antibodies which react with NK-cells in human peripheral blood. In particular, the anti-Leu 11 antibody serves as a 'pan' NK-cell marker and is useful in isolating highly purified populations of these cells for further studies.[17,18,26]

SUBSETS OF HUMAN T-CELLS: CORRELATION WITH FUNCTIONAL ABILITIES

T-lymphocytes are known to mediate a broad range of immunological functions, including delayed-type hypersensitivity, specific cytotoxicity, specific and non-specific suppression of the immune response, helper activity in immunoglobulin production, and amplification of the cytotoxic T-cell response. A major question raised early in these studies was whether or not all mature T-cells were endowed with the capacity to mediate all functions. Alternatively, it was possible that functionally discrete subsets of cells existed. In the latter case it would be ideal if it were possible to identify a unique cell surface antigen which was exclusively associated with each functionally defined cell. Several approaches have been used to achieve this goal. Heterogeneous populations of T-cells have been used to immunize mice, and monoclonal antibodies were selected which bound only to a proportion of the T-cell population. Those monoclonal antibodies which reacted with a subset of T-cells could then be used to separate antigen positive and negative cells for use in functional assays. By this approach, the two major functionally defined subsets of T-cells, i.e. the suppressor/cytotoxic and helper/amplifier subsets, were identified by the Leu 2 (T8) and Leu 3 (T4) monoclonal antibodies, respectively.[8,9,27-29] However, this initial subdivision has turned out not to be absolute, but rather should be considered a useful generalization. For example, cells with cytotoxic function have now been found within both the Leu 2(T5/T8) and Leu 3 (T4) subsets.[30-36] A further distinction has been made between these subsets. Cytotoxic cells directed against Class I (HLA-A,B,C) major histocompatibility antigens express Leu 2.[32-36] Cytotoxic cells against Class II (HLA-D) antigens express Leu 3[32-36], although exceptions to this already have been noted.[37-38] In addition, it has become evident that the particular function associated with these cell surface antigens is likely NOT dependent on these molecules, since often cell types of quite dissimilar lineage and function have been shown to express these molecules. For example, Leu 3 antigen expression is not exclusively restricted to T-lymphocytes in that it is present in low density on human monocytes.[39] Similarly, Leu 2 is present on a subset of human NK cells, which do not express pan T-cell antigens such as Leu 1 or Leu 4.[26,40] Moreover, these cells do not show MHC restriction in their cytotoxic function. Attempts to generate single monoclonal antibodies which discriminate between cytotoxic versus suppressor cells, or monoclonal antibodies which demonstrate an absolute correlation with functional ability have not as yet succeeded, nor need they theoretically be successful. Some of these existing monoclonal antibodies may actually identify a particular stage of maturation. Hence, the most precise identification of a cell subset may require the use of two markers, one for lineage (e.g. T-cells) and the other for maturation stage (e.g. activation). Thus, one alternative is to identify functional subsets not by the presence of a single antigen, but rather by the correlated presence or absence of a number of different antigens.[41]

SUBSETS OF SUBSETS

Use of multiparameter analysis to define populations of lymphocytes based on correlation of two or more cell surface antigens

Recent developments in both fluorochrome dye technology[42] and flow cytometry instrumentation have permitted the identification and isolation (sorting) of small subsets of cells in a heterogeneous population. This can now be achieved by identifying individual cells on the basis of both biophysical properties (i.e. cell size or light scattering properties) and immunological properties using a combination of several fluorochrome conjugated monoclonal antibodies.[41,43-45] To illustrate the potential application of this approach, peripheral blood mononuclear cells were stained with both FITC (green emitting fluorochrome) conjugated anti-Leu 8 and phycoerythrin (orange/red emitting fluorochrome) conjugated anti-Leu 3 monoclonal antibodies. This cell preparation was analyzed using a single argon laser (488 nm excitation) FACS 440 system.[26] On the basis of the characteristic low forward and 90° angle light scatter profiles, lymphocytes were discriminated from monocytes, and the specific fluorescence of only the lymphocytes was examined. Although the Leu 8 antigen has a broad pattern of reactivity, including granulocytes, monocytes, most T-cells and some B-cells, expression of this marker was capable of subdividing the Leu 3 positive lymphocytes into two discrete populations, i.e. Leu

3+,8– and Leu 3+,8+. Studies by Gatenby and co-workers[46] have demonstrated that helper T-cell function for Ig secretion is encompassed within the few cells of the Leu 3+,8– subset. Similarly, another broadly distributed cell surface antigen, Leu 15 (present on monocytes, granulocytes, NK-cells, and some T-cells), can be used to identify subsets of Leu 2 positive lymphocytes (Fig. 9.1). Of particular importance, is that Landay and co-workers[47] have shown that the Leu 2+,15– subset is largely

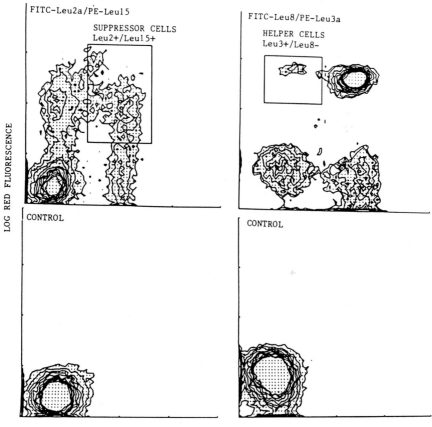

Fig. 9.1 Subpopulations of human peripheral blood T-lymphocytes with defined functional abilities.
Human peripheral blood mononuclear cells were isolated from the interface of a Ficoll/Hypaque gradient and were stained with FITC anti-Leu 2a and PE anti-Leu 15 (upper left); FITC anti-Leu 8 and PE anti-Leu 3a (upper right); or FITC isotype matched control myeloma proteins (lower left and right). Samples were prepared and analyzed with a FACS 440 system as described elsewhere.[26] The lymphocytes were discriminated from the monocytes by their characteristic low forward and 90° light scatter profiles. The red (y axis, log scale) and green (x axis, log scale) fluorescence of the lymphocyte population are presented in the contour plots. Approximately 20 000 cells were analyzed for each sample. Plots shown were obtained from two different individuals.
The Leu 2+,15+ and Leu 3+,8– lymphocyte subsets are indicated in the enclosed areas in the contour plots. Landy and co-workers[47] have shown that the Leu 2+,15+ population contains suppressor cell function, whereas Gatenby et al[46] have demonstrated that the Leu 3+,8– cells possess the majority of helper cell activity. Integration of the subsets incidated the following: Upper left: Leu 2+,15+ 17.9%; Leu 2+,15– 11.8%; Leu 2–,15+ 18.3%. Upper right: Leu 3+,8+ 31.0%; Leu 3+,8– 4.8%; Leu 3–8+ 34.1%.

responsible for T-cell mediated cytotoxicity including both cytotoxic precursors and effector cells. Other examples of using two or more monoclonal antibodies in combination to identify functionally discrete subsets of T-lymphocytes and T subsets with unknown function are summarized in Table 9.2. More recently we[48,49] and others[50,51] have used simultaneous three colour FACS analysis using three different fluorochrome conjugated monoclonal antibodies to identify lymphocyte subsets. Hence, cell separation on the basis of multiple biophysical and immunological properties provides a powerful tool to examine directly the relationship between antigenic phenotype and function.

SUBSETS OF HUMAN B-LYMPHOCYTES

The study of B-lymphocyte subsets is a relatively new field of investigation. Although a variety of non-Ig 'pan' B-cell antigens have been discovered on mature peripheral B-cells such as Leu 12, Leu 14, and B1[52], there has been little evidence for functionally distinct subsets defined by antigens recognized by monoclonal antibodies. However, in both mouse[53,54] and man[55], it has been shown that adult B-cells can be divided into two subsets based on expression of surface Ly-1 or Leu 1 antigens, respectively. In early studies, Leu 1 and Ly-1 were considered T-cell specific, however this has subsequently been shown incorrect.[53-56] The Leu 1/Ly-1 B-cells appear in low frequency in lymphoid organs of adults. As shown in Figure 9.2, this cell can be identified in two-colour immunofluorescence studies by co-expression of Leu 1 and surface Ig, or by the presence of Leu 1+, Leu 4– cells in an E-enriched cell population. In mice, elegant studies by Hawakawi et al.[53] have demonstrated that the Ly-1 positive B-cells arise early in ontogeny, can be distinquished on the basis of surface IgD and IgM levels, and may possess unique functional activities. Furthermore, in both mouse B-lymphomas[56] and human B-

Table 9.2 Subsets of human lymphocytes expressing T-cell associated antigens

Subsets which encompass defined functions

	Phenotype	Function	Reference
LEU 2	LEU 2+, 15+	Suppressor cell	Landy et al[47]
	LEU 2+, 15–	Cytotoxic cell Cytotoxic precursor	Landy et al[47]
	LEU 2+, DR+	Activated suppressor cell	Gatenby et al[72]
	LEU 2+, 9.3–	Suppressor cell precursor	Damle & Engleman[74]
	LEU 2+, 9.3+	Cytotoxic cell precursor	Damle & Engleman[74]
LEU 3	LEU 3+, 8–	Helper cell	Gatenby et al[46]

Newly defined subsets with unknown functional significance

	Phenotype	Function	Reference
LEU 2	LEU 2+, 3+	Recent thymic migrants?	
	LEU 2+, 8+ ⎫	Co-operate to yield	Gatenby et al[46]
	LEU 2+, 8– ⎭	suppression	
	LEU 3+, 8+	Suppressor inducer?	Gatenby et al[46]

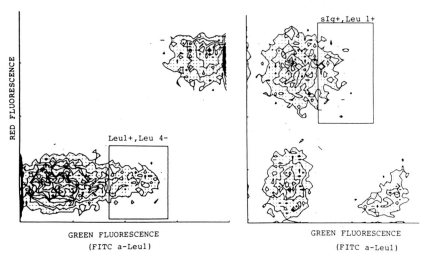

Fig. 9.2 Subsets of human peripheral blood B-lymphocytes identified by expression of the Leu 1 antigen.

Human peripheral blood mononuclear cells were separated into E+ and E– populations by the sheep erythrocyte rosette method. The E– enriched fraction was stained with: FITC anti-Leu 1 and PE anti-Leu 4 (left) FITC anti-Leu 1 and PE anti-human kappa + lambda light chain monoclonal antibodies (right, or FITC isotype matched myeloma proteins. Analysis was performed as described in Figure 9.1. Plots shown were obtained from two different individuals. The unique Leu 1+ B-cell subset is indicated in the enclosed area of the contour plots. Integration of the subsets indicated: Leu 1+,4– 12.2%; Leu 1–,4+ <1%; Leu 1+,4+ 24.1%; Leu 1+,sIg+ 14.4%; Leu 1+,sIg– 17.2%; Leu 1–,sIg+ 40.9%. **Note** that the B-cell subset expressing Leu 1 possesses low cell surface density of this antigen, compared to the T-cells.

CLL malignancies[57] the Leu 1/Ly-1 B-cell is apparently a major target for transformation.

SUBSETS OF HUMAN NATURAL KILLER CELLS: CORRELATION OF PHENOTYPE WITH CYTOTOXIC ACTIVITY

Early studies investigating the immune mechanisms of T-cell-mediated anti-tumour cytotoxicity indicated that many non-tumour bearing control individuals possessed substantial 'background' cell-mediated cytotoxicity to various tumour cell targets. It was first believed that this persistent 'background cytotoxicity' was an artifact of the in vitro assay conditions. It is now clear, however, that a cell population distinct from the T-lymphocyte can manifest anti-tumour cytotoxicity. Lymphoid cells from many mammalian species including humans and rodents exhibit spontaneous cell-mediated cytotoxicity against a variety of syngeneic, allogeneic, and xenogeneic tumour cell targets. The effector cells mediating spontaneous cytotoxicity have been designated natural killer (NK) cells. This phenomenon of natural cell-mediated cytotoxicity may be an important functional component of the normal immune armamentarium.[58-61]

With the development of human NK cell purification procedures employing discontinuous gradients of Percoll[62], it has been demonstrated that the majority of human NK cells display the light microscopic morphology of large lymphocytes with prominent azurophilic granules (LGL).[63-65] Human NK cells do not appear to possess cytoplasmic immunoglobulins or B-cell associated complement receptors and are thus not believed to be of the B-cell lineage.[61] The majority of the human NK cells do not adhere to plastic or nylon wool, however, they do display Fc-receptors and low affinity receptors for sheep red blood cells.[7,66] Several recent studies have investigated the cell surface phenotypes of purified human NK cells using a panel of well characterized monoclonal antibodies.[19-26,67-69] These studies have demonstrated that some, but not all human NK cells express several T-cell antigens (Leu 2 (T8), OKT-10, Leu 5 (T11), Leu 9 (3A1), 5A12,[22,65-68] as well as several myelomonocytic associated antigens (M-1, Mac-1, and M522). Comparison of the cell surface phenotype of Percoll purified NK-cells with that of T-cells, B-cells, granulocytes and monocytes has generated a great deal of controversy as to the cellular lineage of these particular effector cells. All evidence would appear to indicate that human NK-cells are a heterogeneous population of effector cells both with respect to phenotype and also functional cytolytic activity.

The recent development of monoclonal antibodies that react with NK-cells has enabled the more precise delineation of these potentially important effector cells. The monoclonal antibody, anti-Leu 7 (HNK-1), which was generated against the human lymphoblastoid tumour line HSB-2, has been shown to react with an antigen found on a large percentage of the peripheral blood NK-cells[24] and on neuroectodermal tissues.[70,71] The Leu 7 positive lymphoid cells purified by fluorescent activated cell (FACS) sorting were shown to be a homogenous population of LGL, which accounted for some, but not all NK-cell activity in the peripheral blood.[20,24,26] Recently, the monoclonal antibody, anti-Leu 11 (NKP-15) was produced by immunizing mice with highly purified LGL.[11] The anti-Leu 11 monoclonal antibody was shown to react with approximately 15% of the peripheral blood lymphocytes and 90% of the granulocytes.[17,18] The Leu 11 epitope is associated with the Fc-receptor on NK-cells and neutrophils.[17,26] This antigen is not expressed on monocytes or B-lymphocytes.[18] FACS cell sorting of Leu 11 positive cells demonstrated that the Leu 11 antigen is expressed on essentially all peripheral blood NK-cells.[18,26]

The recent development of simultaneous two-colour flow cytometry has enabled us to precisely define discrete subsets within the human NK-cell population. Figure 3 demonstrates several of these NK-cell subsets as revealed by the co-expression of Leu 11 and Leu 7; Leu 11 and Leu 2a; and B73.1[20] and Leu 8. (The anti-B73.1 antibody has been demonstrated to be essentially equivalent to anti-Leu 11 in its reactivity with large granular lymphocytes in peripheral blood[75]). By using two-colour immunofluorescence and correlated multiparameter flow cytometric analysis, four lymphocyte subpopulations can be delineated by the expression of Leu 11 and Leu 7 antigens (i.e., Leu 7–,11+, Leu 7+,11+, Leu 7+,11–, and Leu 7–,11–; Fig. 9.3). Using FACS sorting of each lymphocyte subpopulation, it was determined that the Leu 7–,11+ population was the most cytotoxic NK-cell subset.[26] However, NK-cell activity also was observed in the Leu 7+,11+ subset and in the Leu 7+, 11– subset of some individuals[26] (Fig. 9.4). We do not know whether the various NK-cell subsets defined by Leu 11 and Leu 7, reflect differentiation or lineage related

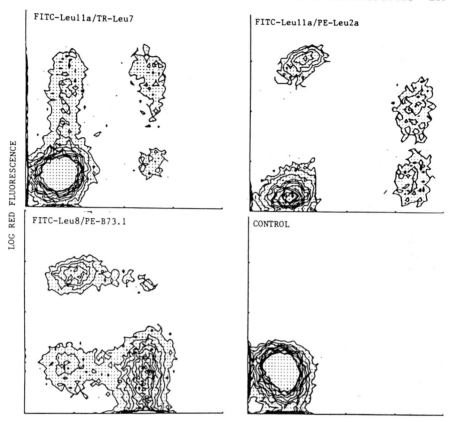

Fig. 9.3 Subsets of human peripheral blood NK-cells identified by two-colour immunofluorescence analysis.

Human peripheral blood mononuclear cells were isolated from the interface of a Ficoll/Hypaque gradient and were stained with: FITC anti-Leu 11a and Texas Red avidin/biotin anti-Leu 7 (upper left), FITC anti-Leu 11a and PE anti-Leu 2a (upper right), FITC anti-Leu 8 and PE anti-B73.1 or FITC isotype matched myeloma protein (lower right). Analysis was performed as described in Figure 9.1. Plots shown were obtained from three different individuals. Note that all three combinations of antibodies revealed distinct subsets of Leu 11 positive cells. Also observe that the Leu 11 positive lymphocytes which express the Leu 2a antigen possess relatively low density of this antigen. Integration of the subsets indicated: Upper left: Leu 7+,11+ 9.8%; Leu 7+,11– 12.9%; and Leu 7–,11+ 6.1%; Upper right: Leu 2+,11+ 11.8%; Leu 2+,11– 14.1%; and Leu 2–11+ 11.6; Lower left: Leu 8+,B73.1+7.2%; Leu 8+B73.1– 60.6%; and Leu 8–B73.1+ 16.0%.

differences. However, it is possible to isolate these subsets and address these questions.

Our studies[26] and others[69] have demonstrated that a large percentage of the Leu 7 positive cells co-express the T-cell associated antigens Leu 1 (T1), Leu 4 (T3), and Leu 2a (T8) antigens. In some individuals as much as 40% of the Leu 7 positive cells co-expressed the T-cell antigen Leu 4. In these same individuals, Leu 11 positive cells showed no co-expression with the T-cell antigens Leu 1 and Leu 4.[26] However, in some individuals a significant percentage of Leu 11 positive cells demonstrated the

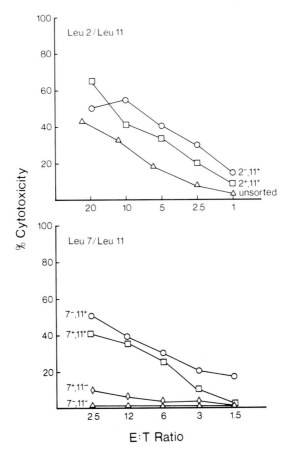

Fig. 9.4 Cytotoxic activity of NK subsets identified by two-colour FACS cell sorting.
Peripheral blood mononuclear cells isolated from a Ficoll/Hypaque gradient were depleted of monocytes and Leu 3+ cells by adherence and panning procedures using the anti-Leu 3 monoclonal antibody, respectively. These cells were stained with: FITC anti-Leu 11a and Texas Red avidin/biotin anti-Leu 7 (bottom panel) or FITC anti-Leu 11a and PE anti-Leu 2a (top panel). The resulting phenotypic subsets were separated using a FACS 440 cell sorter as described in detail elsewhere.[26] The sorted populations were re-analyzed and were determined to be >90% pure. These cells were placed into a 4-hour 51 Cr release NK cytotoxicity assay using K562 target cells, as described in detail elsewhere.[26] Cells stained with antibody and not sorted were also tested. The results are displayed as the percentage of specific 51 Cr release versus effector to target ratio.

co-expression of low density Leu 2a antigen (Fig. 9.3).[26] Recently using FACS sorting, we determined that the Leu 2+,11+ NK-cell subset is an extremely efficient cytotoxic cell and as efficient as the Leu 2-,11+ population (Fig. 9.4). Similarly, the Leu 8-,11+ and Leu 8+,11+ populations have been isolated by two-colour FACS sorting and examined for cytotoxic activity against K562. As shown in Figure 9.5, both the Leu 8-,11+ and Leu 8+,11+ cells mediated potent cytotoxicity compared to unsorted cells.

The use of two-colour flow cytometery has now made it possible to identify by phenotypic characteristics several subsets of human NK-cells. Table 9.3 summarises some of the presently identified subsets of human NK-cells. Although the functional

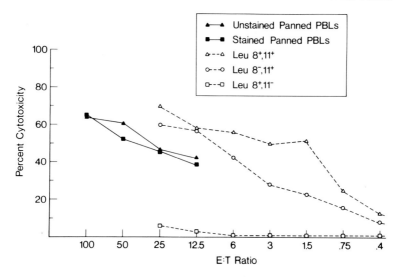

Fig. 9.5 NK cytotoxicity mediated by Leu 8–,11+ and Leu 8+,11+ subsets.

Peripheral blood mononuclear cells isolated form a Ficoll/Hypaque gradient were depleted of monocytes and Leu 3+ cells by adherence and panning procedures using the anti-Leu 3 monoclonal antibody, respectively. These cells were stained with: FITC anti-Leu 11a and PE anti-Leu 8. The subsets were separated using a FACS 440 cell sorter as described in detail elsewhere.[26] The sorted populations were re-analyzed and were determined to be >90% pure. These cells were placed into a 4 hour 51 Cr release NK cytotoxicity assay using K562 target cells, as described in detail elsewhere.[26] Cells stained with antibody and not sorted were also tested. The results are displayed as the percentage of specific 51 Cr release versus effector to target ratio.

Table 9.3 Subsets of human large granular lymphocytes: correlation with function

Phenotype	Function	Reference
Subsets with defined function		
LEU 11+, LEU 7–	High cytotoxicity	Lanier et al[26]
LEU 11+, LEU 7+	Variable cytotoxicity	Lanier et al[26]
LEU 11+, LEU 2–	High cytotoxicity	Lanier et al*
LEU 11+, LEU 2+	High cytotoxicity	Lanier et al*
(Low density LEU 2)		
LEU 11–, LEU 7+	Low cytotoxicity	Lanier et al[26]
LEU 11+, LEU 8+	High cytotoxicity	Lanier et al*
LEU 11+, LEU 8–	High cytotoxicity	Lanier et al*
LEU 7+, LEU 4– (T3–)	High cytotoxicity	Abo et al[69]
	Ig complex activated suppressor cell	Tilden et al[73]
LEU 7+, M1+	High cytotoxicity	Abo et al[69]

Newly defined subsets with unknown functional significance			
LEU 11+, LEU 5+	Lanier et al*	LEU 7+, LEU 1+ (T1+)	Abo et al[69]
LEU 11+, LEU 5–	Lanier et al*	LEU 7+, LEU 1– (T1–)	Abo et al[69]
LEU 11+, DR–	Lanier et al[26]	LEU 7+, LEU 3+ (T4+)	Abo et al[69]
LEU 11+, DR+	Lanier et al*	LEU 7+, LEU 4+ (T3+)	Abo et al[69]
LEU 7+, M1–	Abo et al[69]	LEU 7+, LEU 2+ (T8+)	Abo et al[69]
		LEU 7+, LEU 2– (T8–)	Abo et al[69]
		LEU 7+, DR+	Abo et al[69]
		LEU 7+, DR–	Abo et al[69]

*This chapter

significance of most these NK-cell subsets is at present unknown, the expression of various specific antigens on NK-cells may help to delineate the cellular lineage(s) of these effector cells and to clarify their differentiation sequence. The existence of NK-cell subsets may also be of major importance in understanding the immune response during disease.

SUMMARY

It is becoming increasingly clear that the immune system involves an elaborate and diverse network of cells with specific functional capabilities. As more reagents and more sensitive methods of detection have been developed the ability to dissect the components of the system and understand its workings is being achieved. One of the most successful approaches has been the identification of cell subpopulations by multiparameter analysis based on the presence or absence of combinations of several antigens and/or biophysical properties. The next phase of investigation is to determine whether these human subsets whose functions have been identified by in vitro assays are representative of the in vivo role of these cells. In this regard it is encouraging to observe that the use of monoclonal antibodies has progressed rapidly from basic research applications to the clinical research laboratory.

ACKNOWLEDGEMENTS

We thank Mr Bryan Woodhouse for expert assistance with the flow cytometry and Ms An My Le and Ms Jane Gross Pelose for excellent technical assistance.

REFERENCES
1. Kohler G, Milstein C 1975 Continuous cultures of fused cells secreting antibody of predefined specificity. Nature 256: 495–497
2. Reif A E, Allen J M V 1964 The AKR thymic antigen and its distribution in leukemias and nervous tissue. Journal of Experimental Medicine 120: 413–422
3. Cantor H, Boyse E A 1975 Functional subclasses of T-lymphocytes bearing different Ly antigens. I. The generation of functionally distinct T-cell subclasses in a differentiative process independent of antigen. Journal of Experimental Medicine 141: 1376–1388
4. Shiku H, Kisielow P, Bean M A, Takahashi T, Boyse E A, Oettgen H F, Old L J 1975 Expression of T-cell differentiation antigens on effector cells in cell-mediated cytotoxicity in vitro. Evidence for functional heterogeneity related to the surface phenotype of T-cells. Journal of Experimental Medicine 141: 227–241
5. Cantor H, Shen F W, Boyse E A 1976 Separation of helper from suppressor T-cells expressing Ly components. II. Activation of antigen: after immunization, antigen-specific suppressor and helper activities are mediated by distinct T-cell subclasses. Journal of Experimental Medicine 143: 1391–1403
6. Evans R L, Breard J M, Lazarus H, Schlossman S F, Chess L 1977 Detection, isolation, and functional characterization of two human T-cell subclasses bearing unique differentiation antigens. Journal of Experimental Medicine 145: 221–230
7. West W H, Boozer R B, Herberman R B 1978 Low affinity E rosette formation by the human K cell. Journal of Immunology 120: 90–96
8. Kung P C, Goldstein G, Reinherz E, Schlossman S F 1979 Monoclonal antibodies defining distinctive human T-cell surface antigens. Science 206: 347–351
9. Ledbetter J A, Evans R L, Lipinski M, Cunninghan-Rundles C, Good R A, Herzenberg L A 1981 Evolutionary conservation of surface molecules that distinguish T-lymphocyte helper/inducer and cytotoxic/suppressor subpopulations in mouse and man. Journal of Experimental Medicine 153: 310–321

10. Howard F D, Ledbetter J A, Wong J, Bieber C P, Stinson E B, Herzenberg L A 1981 A human T-lymphocyte differentiation marker defined by monoclonal antibodies that block E rosette formation. Journal of Immunology 126: 2117–2122

11. Honjo T, Nakai S,Nishida Y, Kataoka T, Yamawaki-Kataoka Y, Takahashi N, Obata M, Shimizua A, Yaoita Y, Nikaido T, Ishida N 1981 Rearrangements of immunoglobulin genes during differentiation and evolution. Immunological Reviews 59: 33–67

12. Korsmeyer S J, Arnold A, Bakshi A, Ravetch J V, Siebenlist U, Kieter P A, Sharrow S O, Le Bien T W, Kersey J H, Poplack D G, Leder P, Waldmann T A 1983 Immunoglobulin gene rearrangement and cell surface antigen expression in acute lymphocytic leukemias of T-cell and B-cell precursor origins. Journal of Clinical Investigation 71: 301–316

13. Ravetch J V, Siebenlist U, Korsmeyer S J, Poplack D G, Waldmann T A, Leder P 1981 Developmental hierarchy of immunoglobulin mu locus: characterization of embryonic and rearranged J and D genes. Cell 27: 583–590

14. Perlmann P, Perlmann H, Wigzell H 1972 Lymphocyte mediated cytotoxicity in vitro induction and inhibition by humoral antibody and nature of effector cells. Transplantation Reviews 13: 91–123

15. Maclennan I C M 1972 Antibody in the induction and inhibition of lymphocyte cytotoxicity. Transplantation Reviews 13: 67–90

16. Herberman R B, Gaylord C E 1973 Conference and Workshop on cellular immune reactions to human tumour associated antigens. National Cancer Institute Monograph 37: 1–9

17. Phillips J H, Babcock G F 1983 NKP-15: a monoclonal antibody reactive against purified human natural killer cells and granulocytes. Immunology Letters 6: 143–147

18. Lanier L L, Phillips J H, Warner N L, Babcock G F 1984 A human natural killer cell associated antigen defined by monoclonal antibody anti-Leu 11 (NKP-15): Functional and two-colour flow cytometry analysis. Journal of Leukocyte Biology (In press)

19. Griffin J D, Hercent T, Beveridge R, Schlossman S F 1983 Characterization of an antigen expressed by human natural killer cells. Journal of Immunology 130: 2947–2952

20. Perussia B, Starr S, Abraham S, Fanning V, Grinchieri G 1983 Human natural killer cells analyzed by B73.1, a monoclonal antibody blocking Fc receptor functions I. Characterization of the lymphocyte subset reactive with B73.1. Journal of Immunology 130: 2133–2138

21. Rumpold H, Kraft D, Obexer G, Bock G, Gebhart W 1982 A monoclonal antibody against a surface antigen shared by human large granular lymphocytes and granulocytes. Journal of Immunology 129: 1458–1463

22. Lohmeyer J, Rieber P, Feucht H, Johnson J, Hadam M, Riethmuller G 1981 A subset of human natural killer cells isolated and characterized by monoclonal antibodies. European Journal of Immunology 11: 997–908

23. Mieminen P, Paasivuo R, Saksela E 1982 Effect of a monoclonal anti-large granular lymphocyte antibody on the human NK activity. Journal of Immunology 128: 1097–1107

24. Abo T, Balch C M 1981 A differentiation antigen of human NK and K cells identified by a monoclonal antibody (HNK-1). Journal of Immunology 127: 1024–1030

25. Ault K A, Springer T A 1981 Cross-reaction of rat anti-mouse phagocyte-specific monoclonal antibody (anti-Mac 1) with human monocytes and natural killer cells. Journal of Immunology 126: 359–365

26. Lanier L L, Le A M, Phillips J H, Warner N L, Babcock G F 1983 Subpopulations of human natural killer cells defined by expression of the Leu 7 (HNK-1) and Leu 11 (NKP-15) antigens. Journal of Immunology 131: 1789–1795

27. Evans R L, Wall D W, Platsouca C D, Siegal F P, Fikrig S M, Testa C M, Good R A 1981 Thymus dependent membrane antigens in man: inhibition of cell mediated lympholysis by monoclonal antibodies to the TH2 antigen. Proceedings of the National Academy of Sciences 78: 544–549

28. Reinherz E L, Kung P C, Goldstein G, Schlossman S F 1979 Separation of functional subsets of human T-cells by a monoclonal antibody. Proceedings of the National Academy of Sciences 76: 4061–4067

29. Reinherz E, Schlossman S F 1980 The differentiation and function of human T-lymphocytes. Cell 19: 821–824

30. Reinherz E L, Kung P C, Goldstein G, Schlossman S F 1980 A monoclonal antibody reactive with the human cytotoxic/suppressor T-cell subset previously defined by a heteroantiserum termed TH2. Journal of Immunology 124: 1301–1306

31. Moretta L, Mingari M C, Sekaly P R, Moretta A, Chapius B, Cerotinni J C 1981 Surface markers of cloned human T-cells with various cytolytic activities. Journal of Experimental Medicine 154: 569–581

32. Biddison W E, Rao P E, Talle G, Goldstein G, Shaw S J 1982 Possible involvement of the

OKT4 molecule in T-cell recognition of class I antigens. Evidence from studies of cytotoxic T-lymphocytes specific for SB antigen. Journal of Experimental Medicine 156: 1065–1072

33. Engleman E G, Benike C, Grument F C, Evans R L 1981 Activation of human T-lymphocyte subsets: Helper and suppressor/cytotoxic T-cells recognize and respond to distinct histocompatibility antigens. Journal of Immunology 127: 2124–2129

34. Krensky A M, Reiss C S, Mier J W, Strominger J L, Burakoff S J 1982 Long term cytotoxic T-cell lines allospecific for HLA-DR 6 antigen are OKT4+. Proceedings of the National Academy of Sciences 79: 2365–2370

35. Heuer S C, Schlossman S F, Reinherz E L 1982 Clonal analysis of human cytotoxic T-lymphocytes: T4+ and T8+ effector T-cells recognize products of major histocompatibility complex regions. Proceedings of the National Academy of Sciences 79: 4395–4400

36. Meuer S C, Hussey R E, Hodgdon J C, Hercend T, Schlossman S F 1982 Surface structures involved in target recognition by human T-lymphocytes. Science 218: 471–474

36. Ball E J, Stastny P 1982 Cell-mediated cytotoxicity against HLA-D region products expressed in monocytes and B-lymphocytes. IV. Characterization of effector cells using monoclonal antibodies against human T-cell subsets. Immunogenetics 16: 157–163

38. Spits H, Ijssel H, Thompson A, and deVries J E 1983 Human T4+ and T8+ cytotoxic T-lymphocyte clones directed at products of different class II major histocompatibility complex loci. Journal of Immunology 131: 678–684

39. Wood G S, Warner N L, Warnke R A 1983 Anti-Leu 3/T4 antibodies react with cells of monote/macrophage and Langerhans lineage. Journal of Immunology 131: 212–217

40. Perussia B, Fanning V, Trinchieri G 1983 A human NK and K cell subset shares with cytotoxic T-cells expression of the antigen recognized by antibody OKT8. Journal of Immunology 131: 223–229

41. Lanier L L, Engleman E G, Gatenby P, Babcock G F, Warner N L, Herzenberg L A 1983 Correlation of functional properties of human lymphoid cell subsets and surface marker phenotypes using multiparameter analysis and flow cytometry. Immunological Reviews 74: 143–162

42. Oi V T, Glazer A N, Stryer L 1982 Fluorescent phycobiliprotein conjugates for analysis of cells and molecules. Journal of Cell Biology 93: 981–990

43. Herzenberg L A, Herzenberg L A 1978 Analysis and separation using the fluorescence activated cell sorter. In: Weir D W (ed) Handbook of experimental immunology. Blackwell Scientific Publications, London, p 22.1

44. Miller R G, Lalande M E, McCutcheon M J, Steward S S, Price G B 1981 Usage of the flow cytometer-cell sorter. Journal of Immunological Methods 47: 13–22

45. Loken M R, Stall A M 1982 Flow cytometry as an analytical and preparative tool in immunology. Journal of Immunological Methods 50: 85–112

46. Gatenby P A, Kansas G, Xian C, Evans R, Engleman E G 1982 Dissection of immunoregulatory subpopulations of T-lymphocytes within the helper and suppressor sublineages in man. Journal of Immunology 129: 1997–2003

47. Landay A, Gartland G L, Clement L T 1983 Characterization of a phenotypically distinct subpopulation of Leu 2+ cells that suppress T-cell proliferative responses. Journal of Immunology 131: 2757–2762

48. Lanier L L, Loken M R 1984 Human lymphocyte subpopulations identified by using three-colour immunofluorescence and flow cytometry analysis: Correlation of Leu 2, Leu 3, Leu 7, Leu 8, and Leu 11 cell surface antigen expression. Journal of Immunology (In press)

49. Loken M R, Lanier L L 1984 Three-colour immunofluorescence analysis of Leu antigens on human peripheral blood using two lasers on a Fluorescence Activated Cell Sorter. Cytometry 5: 151–158

50. Parks D R, Hardy R R, Herzenberg L A 1984 Three-colour immunofluorescence analysis of mouse B-lymphocyte subpopulations. Cytometry 5: 159–168

51. Hardy R R, Hayakawa K, Parks D R, Herzenberg L A 1983 Demonstration of B-cell maturation in X-linked immunodeficient mice by simultaneous three-colour immunofluorescence. Nature 306: 270–273

52. Stashenko P, Nadler L M, Hardy R, Schlossman S F 1980 Characterization of a human B-lymphocyte specific antigen. Journal of Immunology 125: 1506–1511

53. Hayakawa K, Hardy R R, Parks D R, Herzenberg L A 1983 The 'Ly-1 B'-cell subpopulation in normal, immunodefective, and autoimmune mice. Journal of Experimental Medicine 157: 202–214

54. Manohar V, Brown E, Leiberson W M, Chused T M 1982 Expression of Lyt-1 by a subset of B-lymphocytes. Journal of Immunology 129: 532–538

55. Caligaris-Cappio F, Gobbi M, Bofill M, Janossy G 1982 Infrequent normal B-lymphocytes

express features of B-chronic lymphocytic leukemia. Journal of Experimental Medicine 155: 623–636

56. Lanier L L, Warner N L, Ledbetter J A, Herzenberg L A 1981 Expression of Lyt-1 antigen on certain murine B-lymphomas. Journal of Experimental Medicine 153: 998–1009

57. Wang C Y, Good R A, Ammirati P, Dymbort G, Evans R L 1980 Identification of a P69,71 complex expressed on human T-cells sharing determinants with B-type chronic lymphatic leukemia cells. Journal of Experimental Medicine 151: 1539–1550

58. Herberman R B (ed) 1982 NK-cells and other natural effector cells. Academic Press, New York

59. Oldham R K Natural killer cells: History and significance. Journal of Biological Response Modifiers 1: 217–228

60 Roder J C, Pross H F 1982 The biology of the human natural killer cell. Journal of Clinical Immunology 2: 249–258

61. Herberman R B, Djeu J Y, Kay H D, Ortaldo J R, Riccardi C, Bonnard G D, Holden H T, Fagnani R, Santoni A, Puccetti P 1979 Natural killer cells: characteristics and regulation of activity. Immunological Reviews 44: 43–62

62. Timonen T, Saksela E 1980 Isolation of human NK-cells by density gradient centrifugation. Journal of Immunological Methods 36: 285–292

63. Timonen T, Ortaldo J R, Herberman R B 1981 Characterization of human large granular lymphocytes and relationship to natural killer and K cells. Journal of Experimental Medicine 153: 569–581

64. Babcock G F, Phillips J H 1983 NK-cells: light and electron microscope characteristics. Surveys of Immunological Research 2: 88–303

65. Huhn D, Huber C, Gastl J 1982 Large granular lymphocytes: morphological studies. European Journal of Immunology 12: 985:995

66. West W H, Cannon G B, Kay H D, Bonnard G D, Herberman R B 1977 Natural cytotoxic reactivity of human lymphocytes against a myeloid cell line: characterization of effector cells. Journal of Immunology 118: 555–561

67. Kay H D, Howitz D A 1980 Evidence by reactivity with hybridoma antibodies for a probably myeloid origin of peripheral blood cells active in natural cytotoxicity and antibody-dependent cell-mediated cytotoxicity. Journal of Clinical Investigation 66: 847–856

68. Ortaldo J R, Sharrow S O, Timonen T, Herberman R B 1981 Determination of surface antigens on highly purified human NK cells by flow cytometry with monoclonal antibodies. Journal of Immunology 127: 2401–2407

69. Abo T, Cooper M D, Balch C M 1982 Characterization of HNK-1 (Leu 7) human lymphocytes I. Two distinct phenotypes of human NK-cells with different cytotoxic capacities. Journal of Immunology 129: 1752–1757

70. McGarry R C, Helfand S L, Quarles R H, Roder J C Recognition of myelin-associated clycoprotein by the monoclonal antibody HNK-1. Nature 306: 376–379

71. Lipinski M, Braham K, Caillaud J M, Carlu C, Tursz T 1983 HNK-1 antibody detects an antigen expressed on neuroectodermal cells. Journal of Experimental Medicine 158: 1775–1790

72. Gatenby P A, Kotzin B L, Kansas G S, Engleman E G 1982 Immunoglobulin secretion in the human autologous mixed leukocyte reaction. Definition of a suppressor-amplifier circuit using monoclonal antibodies. Journal of Experimental Medicine 156: 55–67

73. Tilden A B, Abo T, Balch C M 1983 Suppressor cell function of human granular lymphocytes identified by the HNK-1 (Leu 7) monoclonal antibody. Journal of Immunology 130: 1171–1177

74. Damle N K, Engleman E G 1983 Immunoregulatory T-cell circuits in man: Alloantigen-primed inducer T-cells activate alloantigen-specific suppressor T-cells in the absence of the initial antigenic stimulus. Journal of Experimental Medicine 158: 159–170

75. Perussia B, Trinchieri G, Jackson A, Warner N L, Faust J, Rumpold H, Kraft D, Lanier L L 1984 The Fc receptor for IgG on human natural killer cells: Phenotypic, functional and comparative studies with monoclonal antiobodies. Journal of Immunology 133: 180–189

10
Monoclonal antibodies reactive with myeloid associated antigens

D. C. Linch J. D. Griffin

REVIEW OF MYELOID DIFFERENTIATION

Granulocytes and monocytes in the blood are derived from bone marrow *precursor cells* which can be identified by morphological examination of the marrow. In the granulocyte lineage, for instance, there is a progression from the myeloblast to the promyelocyte, myelocyte, metamyelocyte and then polymorphonuclear cell. This morphological differentiation is linked to the acquisition of cell receptors such as that for the Fc portion of IgG and C3b and cell functions such as chemotaxis and phagocytosis[1]. Such morphological analysis reveals information about the terminal five or six divisions in the differentiation pathway. A greater number of divisions have already occurred however, between the haematopoietic stem cells and the earliest recognizable precursor cells, and it is at this level that many regulatory cell interactions take effect, and many haematological disorders arise.

In 1961 Till & McCulloch described an assay for haematopoietic *stem cells* capable of forming colonies in the spleens of irradiated syngeneic mice[2]. These stem cell derived colonies (CFU-S) are derived from single cells and contain red cells, granulocytes, megakaryocytes and further colony forming cells[3]. The cells giving rise to CFU-S are thus multipotential and capable of self replication, the traditional hallmarks of stem cells. No equivalent assay exists in man, but chromosomal and G6PD isoenzyme studies in patients with chronic granulocytic leukaemia indicate that such multipotential cells do exist[4].

Myeloid colonies (> 40 cells) and clusters (4–40 cells) can be grown in vitro from human marrow[5]. Cluster forming cells are partially separable from colony forming cells (GM-CFC) by physical means and cluster forming cells represent the immediate progeny of the GM-CFC[6]. Although GM-CFC may have large proliferative potential they do not self replicate in vitro and are therefore *progenitor cells* and not stem cells. Individual myeloid colonies (CFU-C) may consist of neutrophils, monocytes or eosinophils. Mixed colonies of neutrophils and monocytes are frequently seen, whereas mixed neutrophil and eosinophil colonies are not[7]. This indicates that monocytes and neutrophils have a close common ancestor and that these cell types are more closely related than is either cell type to the eosinophil lineage (Fig. 10.1). To grow CFU-C it is necessary to provide a source of 'colony stimulating activity' (CSA). The major physiological sources of CSA are probably the marrow monocytic cells and T-cells and the production of CSA appears to be regulated by a wide range of cellular interactions and soluble factors[8].

Committed human erythroid progenitor cells can also be grown in vitro using

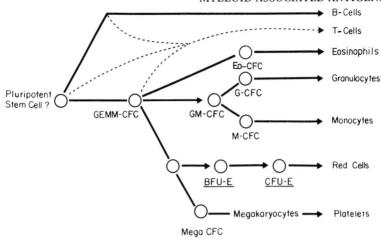

Fig. 10.1 Schematic representation of haemopoietic differentiation.

erythropoietin as a stimulator. Small colonies, haemoglobinizing after about one week in culture (CFU-E) are derived from cells just proximal to early normoblasts. The size of this CFU-E cell population is regulated in vivo by erythropoietin[9]. After 2–3 weeks in culture, at higher erythropoietin levels, blood and marrow give rise to large haemoglobinized colonies (up to 50 000 cells) known as erythroid bursts (BFU-E). Bursts are so named because they frequently consist of several subcolonies, presumably indicating the mobile nature of the early progenitor cells. Although erythropoietin is required for the terminal differentiation and haemoglobinization of the progeny of BFU-E, it has been shown that the early divisions of BFU-E in vitro are independent of erythropoietin[10]. They appear to require a specific factor known as burst promoting activity (BPA). The cellular origins of BPA have stimulated much interest and controversy and are discussed in more detail in a later section of this chapter.

Megakaryocyte progenitor cells can similarly be induced to form megakaryocytes in vitro[11]. Although erythropoietin has been used as a stimulatory source, it is likely that there is a distinct megakaryocyte colony stimulating factor (Mega CSA) found in high levels in the serum of patients with aplastic anaemia[12].

Multipotential colonies of granulocytes, erythrocytes, macrophages and megakaryocytes (CFU-GEMM) and possibly T-cells[13], can also be grown in vitro. The multipotentiality of these colony forming cells suggests that they are very primitive cells, but most do not self replicate, and should be considered as progenitor cells and not true stem cells. Long term Dexter type cultures have been adapted to human marrow and such systems may provide more information about true stem cell regulation. The lack of clonality in such systems however makes it very difficult to even semiquantitatively enumerate stem cell numbers.

Bone marrow morphological analysis and cell culture studies have thus provided an outline of haemopoietic differentiation. In an effort to further define myeloid stem cells and progenitor cells, several new techniques have been investigated. One of these, the production of monoclonal antibodies to differentiation associated cell surface antigens promises to have considerable impact on our ability to identify and purify progenitor cells and to compare the surface structure of normal progenitor cells with their leukaemic cell counterparts.

MONOCLONAL ANTIBODIES TO MYELOID CELLS

Introduction

Although the first monoclonal antibodies to myeloid associated antigens were described only 5 years ago[14,15,16] there has since been a profusion of antibodies reported in the world literature. Many of the different antibodies described are certainly directed to the same antigenic structures, and the First International Workshop on Human Leukocyte Differentiation (November 1982) took the first steps to clarify this situation[17]. Anti-myeloid antibodies from different investigators were submitted to a central laboratory where they were coded and redistributed to other test laboratories. These antibodies were screened for reactivity against peripheral blood T-cells, granulocytes, monocytes, bone marrow cells, acute myeloid leukaemia (AML) cells, chronic myeloid leukaemia (CML) cells and with leukaemic cell lines. The pattern of reactivity with the normal and leukaemic cells was then used to identify clusters of antibodies with similar reactivities against each cell type. Data from all the cell types was then pooled and five overall clusters

Table 10.1 Simplified representation of first international workshop on human leukocyte differentiation cluster analyses of anti-myeloid antibodies

| Cluster No. | Example Antibodies | Reactivity with different cell types | | | | | | References |
		Monocytes	Granulocytes	Bone marrow cells	AML	AML-5	CGL	
CD 11	MO 1	++	++	+	+	+	+	18
	B2.2			(40–50%)				17
CDw12	M 67	+	+	–	–	–	±	17
	20.2	(60–65%)	(70–75%)					17
CDw13	MY 7	+	+	–		+	+	19
	MCS.2	(60–65%)	(70–75%)					20
CDw14	5F 1	++			+	+		21
	MO 2	+ (71%)	–	–	–	–	–	18
	MY 4	++			–	+		19
	FMC 17	++			–	+		20
CDw15	80H 3				–	–		22
	FMC 12				–	–		23
	FMC 10	–	++	+	–	–	+	23
	TG 1		(30–65%)		+	+		15
	VIM D5				+	+		24
	IG 10				+	+		21
Non clustered	FMC 11	–	+ (90%)	–	–	–	+	23
	MY 8	+ (68%)	+ (67%)	+ (37%)	+	+	–	19

Antibodies reacting with T-cells or B-cell lines were excluded from analysis.

++ = clustering with positive controls

 – = clustering with negative controls. This does not necessarily imply that no cells reacted with this antibody. TG-1, (CDw15) for instance reacted with 23% of monocytes and yet clustered with the negative controls.

 + = cluster intermediate between positive and negative controls. For some cell types several intermediate clusters were identified. The mean number of cells stained positively with the different antibodies giving intermediate reactivity are shown in parentheses.

Discordant reactivity within a given cluster is shown by the boxes.

identified. These are shown with example antibodies in Table 10.1. Six antibodies did not conform to any cluster and FMC 11 and MY 8 are shown as examples. Such cluster analyses are of course only preliminary observations. Some antibodies in the same cluster had different ranges of reactivity, especially when tested against acute leukaemic cells, e.g. CDw14 and CDw15. The First International Workshop did not attempt to characterize the antigenic structures defined by the different antibodies, but the report of Second International Workshop will provide information on the biochemical nature of these antigens. This will hopefully clarify the situation further, and allow appropriate comparisons of data from different laboratories, which have used different antibodies that are reactive with the same antigenic structures. Biochemical characterization of antigens may not always be simple. Most antibodies will precipitate one or two proteins of distinct molecular weight but this is not invariable. Some antibodies precipitate no specific protein and these antibodies presumably react with carbohydrate or glycolipid antigens.

Monoclonal antibodies reacting with granulocytes and monocytes

The specificity of a variety of well characterized monoclonal antibodies against granulocytic and monocytic cells is shown in Figure 10.2. Several of these antibodies are worthy of further note.

FMC 10 and FMC 11 are specific for granulocytes in the peripheral blood. FMC 11 stains granulocytes weakly and only stains metamyelocytes and granulocytes in the bone marrow. FMC 10 stains cells from the myelocyte stage onwards[23]. MY-1 refers to a granulocytic series specific differentiation antigen[25]. Civin and colleagues have produced 18 separate antibodies using the (HL60) cell line as immunogen, all of which react with this same antigen. This antigen is the carbohydrate structure lacto N fucopentuose III[32]. Despite the fact that all 18 antibodies recognize the same parent antigen, they do not all have precisely the same cellular specificity. Whereas they all react with granulocytic cells from the promyelocyte stage onwards, only 2 of

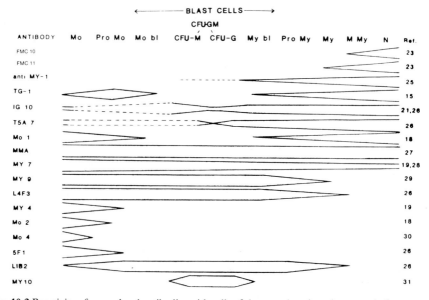

Fig. 10.2 Reactivity of monoclonal antibodies with cells of the granulocytic and monocytic lineage.

6 antibodies tested reacted with granulocytic progenitor cells. The antibody IG-10 described by Bernstein and colleagues[21] similarly reacts with the Gal 1-4 (Fuc 1-3) Glc N Ac determinant of lacto N fucopentuose III[33]. IG-10 reacts with granulocytic cells and their precursors and a small proportion of monocytes. It also reacts with day 7 CFU-GM and some day 14 CFU-GM (derived from more primitive progenitor cells)[26]. Progenitor cells express this antigen weakly and different results with the different anti-MY-1 antibodies may reflect differences in antibody affinity. The presence or absence of this antigen is not directly coded by a given gene; the relevant gene presumably codes for a particular glycosyl transferase enzyme. The expression of the lacto N fucopentuose III antigen is however not just dependent on the presence of the correct glycosyl transferase enzymes. Many non-granulocytic cells including common ALL cells become reactive with anti-MY-1 antibodies after treatment with neuraminidase, indicating that the antigen was present in these cells but was masked by salicylic acid. This group of antibodies thus illustrate clearly the complexity of antigen expression by haemopoietic cells. Finally it should be noted that all of the antibodies described to the MY-1 antigen are of the IgM class; the reason for this is not clear.

Several other antibodies have similar specificity to the anti-MY-1 antibodies including PMN-6 and PMN-29 described by Ball & Fanger[34] and FMC 12 and FMC 13 described by Zola and colleagues[23].

TG-1 is also an IgM antibody reacting with the granulocytic cells from the promyelocyte onwards. It also reacts with about 20% of monocytes and probably most promonocytes. It does not react with progenitor cells. This antibody differs from the anti-MY-1 antibodies in that it precipitates a protein molecule of approximately 150 000 daltons. TG-1 reacts with eosinophils as well as neutrophils[15]. This is similar to other anti-neutrophil antibodies such as FMC 10–13[23] but is in contrast to antibodies such as 28[35] IB5 and 4D1[36] which react with neutrophils and their precursors but not eosinophils. Most reports of anti-myeloid antibodies have not reported on the reactivity with eosinophils.   T5A7 described by Andrews et al[26] reacts strongly with granulocytes and metamyelocytes and more weakly with early granulocytic precursor cells. It reacts with a proportion of day 7 granulocytic/monocytic colony forming cells and virtually no day 14 colony forming cells. It also reacts with approximately 50% of peripheral blood monocytes. Although it does not react with T-cells and B-cells it must be noted that it does react with about 30% of PHA stimulated T-lymphocytes.

Mol[18] and OKM1[11] react with granulocytes and their precursors and also the large majority of monocytes. These antibodies also react with null cells and E$^+$T3$^-$ lymphocytes, many of which bear Fc receptors for IgG and have the properties of natural killer cells[37].

MMA also reacts with most monocytes and granulocytes and their precursors but in addition appears to react with nearly all bone marrow granulocytic/monocytic progenitor cells[27]. MMA is unreactive with B-cells and T-cells including those expressing γ Fc receptors, but the antigen is expressed by activated T-cells.

The antigen detected by MY 7 which has a MW (molecular weight) of approximately 160 kDa is expressed by monocytes and a proportion of granulocytes[19,28] but not other blood cells. In the bone marrow the percentage of cells expressing the MY 7 antigen is variable, with more cells expressing this antigen in regenerative states, e.g. post chemotherapy. A proportion of CFU-C are MY 7 positive, and these appear to be those in S phase. Peripheral blood CFU-C do not react with MY 7. Thus MY 7 is related to the proliferative state of a cell as well as its stage of differentiation.

MY 9 reacts with monocytes in the peripheral blood but not with granulocytes or lymphocytes[29]. In the marrow MY 9 antigen is expressed on about 30% of cells and these include myeloblasts, promyelocytes and myelocytes but not more mature granulocytic cells. Erythroid precursor cells and lymphoid cells are not reactive with MY 9. Over 90% of marrow CFU-GM react with MY 9, as do the majority of peripheral blood CFU-GM. Approximately 50% of the BFU-E express MY 9 whereas CFU-E are MY 9 negative. The distribution of the antigen detected by L4F3 appears very similar to that of MY 9[26], and biochemical characterization of the respective antigens is required. Anti-MY 9 precipitates a broad band of approximately 68–74 kDa. The antibody D5D6 described by Linker-Israeli and colleagues[38] also reacts with monocytes, 90% of CFU-GM and not granulocytes. The reactivity with erythroid precursor cells has not been reported. MY 11 has only been described in a preliminary form[39]. It does react with monocytes but not granulocytes, and 50% of CFU-GM. BFU-E are negative. Lymphoid cells in blood and marrow are also MY 11 positive so the antibody is clearly not detecting a restricted differentiation antigen.

MY 4 reacts strongly with monocytes and weakly with granulocytes. Only monocytes are positive in the bone marrow[19]. The antigen has a MW of 55 kDa. Mo2 is expressed by monocytes exclusively in blood and bone marrow and also has a MW of 55 kDa. Mo4 reacts with 40–80% of monocytes but also reacts with platelets and megakaryocytes. The molecular weight of the Mo4 antigen is 100 kDa[30]. The 5FI antibody raised by Andrews et al[26] also reacts with monocytes but not granulocytes, lymphocytes or CFU-GM. This antibody also reacts with platelets, nucleated red cells and CFU-E but not BFU-E.

L1B2 reacts with virtually no peripheral blood cells[26]. In the marrow it reacts with nearly all myeloid precursor cells and CFU-GM. Erythroid progenitor cells do not react with this antibody. MY 10 also reacts with no peripheral blood cells and its reactivity is far more restricted than L1B2 within the bone marrow. Only 2% of low density bone marrow cells are MY 10 positive and the majority of these cells are blasts. Over 90% of CFU-GM and BFU-E are MY 10 positive[31]. The antigen recognized by MY 10 is a glycoprotein with an apparent MW of 115 kDa. Its expression is probably not limited to myeloid progenitor cells as about 30% of cases of ALL react with this antibody. Nonetheless, its range of reactivity is unique and this antibody will be of immense value for the purification of myeloid progenitor cells and the study of early myeloid differentiation.

Neutrophil heterogeneity and functional studies
The majority of monoclonal antibodies that react with neutrophils react with virtually all such cells[15,16,23]. Several antibodies have been described, however, that react with only a subpopulation of neutrophils. PMN 6 is reported to react with only 58%–95% of neutrophils[34]. The FACS profiles reveal that the staining is fairly weak however and there are not two distinct populations. The antibodies 1B5 and 4D1, by contrast, react with just over half the neutrophils and FACS profiles show two

clearly separate populations, one strongly positive and one negative[36]. Such phenotypic heterogeneity has not yet been correlated with functional heterogeneity.

Cotter and colleagues have reported two interesting antibodies that inhibit various aspects of neutrophil function. NCD1 reacts with virtually all neutrophils and inhibits neutrophil degranulation to a wide range of stimuli including C5a, f Met–Leu–Phe, and soluble aggregated immunoglobulin, but does not inhibit enzyme release in response to the calcium ionophore A23138 or to phorbol myristate acetate. Chemotaxis to f Met–Leu–Phe and zymosan-activated plasma is also inhibited by this antibody. Superoxide formation in response to f Met–Leu–Phe, opsonized zymosan and phorbol myristate acetate is not affected. The inhibitory action of this antibody was present with F(ab) fragements but not F(ab) single fragments, indicating that the inhibition was probably not due to competition for ligand binding[40]. NCD3 also inhibits chemotaxis to f Met–Leu–Phe but has far less inhibitory activity to chemotaxis in response to C5a or zymosan activated plasma. NCD3 does not inhibit phagocytosis, granule enzyme release or superoxide formation. As with NCD1, NCD3 is only inhibitory in the divalent state suggesting that cross linking of antigenic structures is required to produce inhibition[41]. This data suggests that the mechanism of f Met–Leu–Phe chemotaxis is different from other forms of chemotaxis, and that degranulation can occur by several mechanisms. These antibodies should be highly useful to dissect the precise mechanisms of neutrophil activation. It is likely that more antibodies will be described that block specific functions, as in future, antibodies will often be primarily screened in functional rather then phenotypic assays.

Monocyte/macrophage heterogeneity and functional studies

Many monoclonal antibodies to monocyte antigens react with approximately 70–80% of circulating monocytes. These include OKM1[14], Mo1[18], Mo2[18], Mo4[19], UCHM1, Smθ[35], 63D3[16], Mo P-9, Mo S-1, Mo S-39 and Mo P-15[42] FM 17, FM 32 and FM 33[43]. UCHM1 and Smθ both react with the same 80% of monocytes but it is not clear whether the other antibodies recognize the same major monocyte subset. Adherent monocytes not expressing the UCHM1 or Smθ antigens appear identical to those that express those antigens, contain non specific esterase, and express fibrinectin receptors and HLA-Dr antigens[35]. No functional heterogeneity has yet been reported with these major subset antibodies.

The antigen detected by Mo1 is a cell surface molecule consisting of two non covalently linked glycoproteins, an α chain of 155 kDa and a β chain of 94, kDa. Mo1 reacts with the α chain, which is closely associated with the C3bi receptor[44].

The binding of Mo1 to granulocytes and monocytes blocks C3bi binding and inhibits the phagocytosis of opsonized particles. Several patients have now been described in whom this membrane protein complex is deficient[45,46,47]. The β chain of the Mo1 antigen complex appears to be common to the lymphocyte function antigen, LFA-1, (composed of an α chain of 180 kDa and a β chain of 94 kDa) and this LFA-1 antigen is also deficient in these patients (both α and β chains). Phagocytes from these patients have defective C3 and IgG dependent phagocytosis and their lymphocytes have deficient cytotoxic activity. There may be a heterogeneity of this condition with some patients having complete absence of the C3bi receptor and some an incomplete deficiency[45,47]. All patients suffer from recurrent bacterial infections and infants with the complete form of the disease may have delayed separation of the cord and death in early childhood[47].

Various other antibodies react with only a small subset of monocytes. TG-1 reacts with only 20% of circulating monocytes[35] although it appears to react with nearly all marrow NSE positive cells[48]. Mo P-7 and Mo 17 react with approximately 35% of circulating monocytes[42] but the antigens detected by these antigens are expressed at very low densities and there may not be two distinct populations. Of great interest is the Mac 120 antibody which reacts with about 40% of total circulating monocytes. Monocytes expressing the Mac 120 antigen and HLA-DR are able to present antigens to T-cells in a genetically restricted manner, whereas HLA-DR⁺ Mac 120⁻ monocytes are not[49].

Circulating monocytes are at an intermediate stage in the differentiation pathway between the progenitor cells and the tissue macrophage, and the reactivity of various antibodies with different types of macrophages is not identical to that with blood monocytes. Mo 3 for instance, reacts with <20% of virgin monocytes but with nearly 80% of monocytes after 16 hours in culture at 37°C. This antigen increase can be partially inhibited by puromycin and is probably due to increased antigen synthesis rather than to uncovering of covert antigen[30]. Peritoneal macrophages which are presumably at a later stage of differentiation do not express the Mo 3 antigen, suggesting that Mo 3 antigen expression is a transient phenomenon in macrophage development. Several groups have now reported on the reactivity of anti-monocyte antibodies with tissue macrophages and simplified patterns of reactivity are shown in Table 10.2. Antibodies such as PHM3 and TG-1 react with a proportion of circulating monocytes but barely react with any tissue macrophages. Other antibodies reacting with monocytes react particularly with macrophages in specific sites. For instance, FMC 34 reacts strongly with Kupffer cells but not with most other macrophages and FMC 17 reacts particularly strongly with alveolar macrophages and only few macrophages from other sites. Within the lymphoid tissue FMC 32 and FMC 33 reacted with interdigitating reticulum cells as well as macrophages whereas UCHM1 reacted only with the macrophages. It is not yet clear whether these phenotypic differences in different sites represent differences in cell populations or function, and this difficult area of research will be a focus of great activity in the future.

Table 10.2 Expression of myeloid cell surface antigens on tissue macrophages

Percentage circulating monocytes stained	Lymph Node	Spleen	Tonsil.	Thymus	Peritoneal	Alveolar	Liver	Breast milk	Ref.
PHM 3 – 65%	0	0	NR	0	+/−	0	+/−	NR	50
FMC 17 – 82%	0	+/−	NR	+	0	++	0	NR	43, 50
FMC 32 – 79%	++	++	NR	++	++	++	++	NR	43, 50
FMC 33 – 70%	++	++	NR	++	++	++	++	NR	43, 50
FMC 34 – 25%	0	0	NR	0	+/−	0	++	NR	50
OKM 1 – 80%	++	++	NR	++	++	++	0		50
63D3 – 80%	++	++	NR	++	++	++	++	NR	50
UCHMI – 80%	+	+	++	+	++	+/−	0	++	35
Smθ – 80%	0	0	+	0	+	+/−	0	+	35
TG-1 – 20%	0	0	0	0	0	0	0	0	35

Erythroid series

The specificity of several antibodies for cells at different stages of erythroid differentiation is shown in Figure 10.3. The antibodies R10 and R6A produced by Edwards and colleagues[51] react with erythrocyte specific antigens that are expressed on recognizable erythroid precursor cells but not erythroid progenitor cells[52]. R10 reacts with the trypsin sensitive portion of glycophorin A[51]. Other monoclonal antibodies to the trypsin resistant portion of glycophorin A have been produced and several react with the red cell Wr^b antigen[51,55,56]. These antibodies block invasion of red cells with Plasmodium falciparum indicating that this antigenic structure is involved in parasite entry[56]. R6A was initially described as reacting with Band III protein but more recent evidence suggests this may not be so.

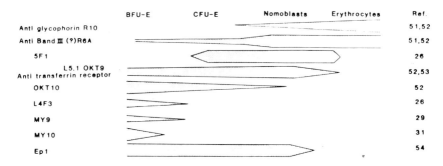

Fig. 10.3 Reactivity of monoclonal antibodies with cells of the erythroid lineage.

Antibody 5F1 reacts with nucleated red cells and CFU-E but is not erythroid specific; it also reacts with monocytes and platelets. Interestingly, this antibody will inhibit CFU-E proliferation in the absence of complement[57]. Antibodies to the transferrin receptor, as expected, react with nucleated red cells and reticulocytes but not mature red cells. In addition they react with erythroid progenitor cells. This progenitor reactivity is not erythroid specific as these antibodies also react with a proportion of myeloid progenitor cells, some thymocytes and many malignant cell line. The expression of transferrin receptors is thus strongly associated with cell proliferation in general. OKT10 similarly defines an antigen present on most primitive haemopoietic cells; BFU-E, GM-CFC and thymocytes[52,57]. L453 and MY9 react with a proportion of BFU-E and no CFU-E. They react with virtually all GM-CFC but not with cells of the lymphoid series[29,26]. There appears to be individual variation in the density of the MY 9 antigen on BFU-E. In some individuals nearly all BFU-E are negative, though in other individuals a majority are positive albeit weakly. MY 10 reacts with both BFU-E and GM-CFC. EP1 has only been reported in preliminary form but appears to react with all committed erythroid cells except mature red cells[54].

Expression of 'Ia-like' antigens of haemopoietic progenitor cells

The human HLA-D region on chromosome 6 is analogous to the I region of the murine histocompatibility complex. In both mouse and man these regions code for a series of polymorphic bimolecular glycoprotein complexes with MW's of approximately 29 000 and 34 000. The 'Ia-like' antigens are characteristically expressed on B-cells, monocytes and activated T-cells. Except for myeloblasts and promonocytes, myeloid and erythroid precursor cells do not express Ia-like antigens. The myeloid progenitor cells and myeloblasts do however react with heterologous anti-Ia sera[59,60].

Three distinct genetic loci coding for distinct Ia-like molecules have now been identified in man: DR (equivalent to mouse I E/C), DQ (previously known as DC and equivalent to mouse I-A) and DP (previously known as SB[61,62]).

Alloantisera have been used to define additional polymorphisms of Ia-like antigens, but their exact nature remains uncertain. Several of these antibodies react with clusters of DR specificities, and are thus often called 'supertypic'. MB1, MT1 and LB12 antisera, for instance all react with cells expressing DR1, 2 and W6 and they almost certainly react with the antigen which is in strong linkage disequilibrium with these DR antigens. The antigen MT2 associated with DR3, 5, W6 and W8 cells, by contrast, does appear to be coded in the DR region[61].

Monoclonal antibodies have been raised to these Ia-like antigens, and DR antigens can be demonstrated on GM-CFC, granulocytic and monocytic cluster forming cells, BFU-E and CFU-E[63,64]. Several groups have suggested that BFU-E express DR antigens whereas CFU-E do not[64], but this probably indicates weaker DR expression on CFU-E rather than complete absence. In the mouse DR is not expressed on the CFU-S and the human pluripotent stem cell may also be DR⁻. Human GEMM-CFC's do express DR antigen[65] but such multipotential progenitor cells are not true stem cells. The DP antigen as detected by the I-LR1 monoclonal antibody is also expressed on granulocytic/monocytic and erythroid progenitor cells, although the percentage of positive cells determined by immune separation techniques (40–70%) is less than with anti-DR monoclonal antibodies (>90%)[66]. This difference probably represents relatively weak DP antigen expression rather than distinct subpopulations of positive and negative progenitor cells. DQ antigen expression is of considerable interest. Seiff and colleagues found that the monoclonal antibody Genox 3.53 which recognizes the DQ1 antigens was not reactive with progenitor cells from DQ1 positive individuals[52]. These observations are difficult to interpret because DQ expression is generally weak relative to DR expression on B-cells and monocytes. There is considerable individual variation however, and Linch and colleges showed in selected individuals with high DQ expression on monocytes and B-cells, that all the haemopoietic progenitor cells were still DQ negative as determined by the Leu 10 antibody[66].

This suggests that DQ is not only antigenically distinct from other Ia-like antigens but probably also has a different function. The function of such antigens on haemopoietic progenitor cells is unknown but it is tempting to speculate that they mediate cell interactions regulating haemopoiesis, as in the generation of the immune response. Pelus has reported that only progenitor cells expressing DR antigens are susceptible to suppression by soluble inhibitors[67], and T-cell mediated suppression by both normal T-cells and those from a patient with T-cell lymphocytosis and red cell aplasia, has been shown to be genetically restricted[68,69]. The detailed mechanisms of such suppression have yet to be determined.

Platelet series

A limited number of monoclonal antibodies have been described that react with surface determinants on platelets. McMichael and colleagues described two antibodies, AN51 and J15 that were specific for platelets and megakaryocytes[70]. AN51 recognizes an antigen on glycoprotein Ib that is expressed during megakaryocyte maturation and J15 recognizes an antigen on the glycoprotein IIb/IIIa complex that is probably expressed at an earlier stage in the megakaryocyte differentiation pathway. The phenotype of Mega-CFC was not reported. The AN51 antibody does not react with platelets from patients with the Bernard Soulier syndrome and J15 antibody does not react with platelets from patients with Glanzmann's thrombocythaemia in which the glycoproteins Ib, IIb, IIa respectively are defective. Another antibody produced by Coller et al[71] also reacts with the platelet glycoprotein Ib, at or near the membrane receptor for von Willebrand factor. This antibody thus blocks the binding of von Willebrand factor to platelets and inhibits aggregation in response to von Willebrand factor and ristocetin. Minno and colleagues have described another interesting antibody, B59.2, which also precipitates the IIb/IIIa complex[72]. Incubation of platelets with this antibody inhibited secretion and aggregation but not thromboxane synthesis in response to collagen, arachidonic acid and ADP. This inhibition of aggregation appears to be mediated in part by the blocking of fibrinogen binding to activated platelets.

Other antibodies have been described that react with platelets and other haematological cells. These include Mo4[30] and Smθ[35] that react with monocytes and platelets, and CALL 1[73] and J2[74] that react with platelets, megakaryocytes and acute lymphoblastic cells. Studies with J2 have shown that the J2-antigen is not expressed on Mega-CFC (Lipton & Linch, unpublished observations).

CELL LINES AND MONOCLONAL ANTIBODIES

Cultured human myeloid cell lines have been widely used as immunogens for the production of monoclonal antibodies[25,27,31]. This is because they represent a relatively homogenous population of cells with the phenotype of immature haemopoietic cells. The cell lines can also be used for the initial screening and characterization of any antibodies produced. The distribution of myeloid antigens defined by a variety of monoclonal antibodies is shown in Table 10.3. Lymphoid cell lines are also widely used during the screening process for anti-myeloid antibodies, to detect antibodies which react with both myeloid and lymphoid cells. A certain amount of caution must be exercised however as the phenotype of cultured mature cells may not correspond precisely to normal cells. TG-1 for instance reacts only with normal myeloid cells from the promyelocyte stage onwards, and yet it reacts with the myeloid cell line K562 and some lymphoid cell lines[35].

Studies of cell lines can also be informative as some lines can be induced to undergo terminal differentiation. HL60 for instance, a promyelocytic cell line, can be induced by DMSO, or retinoic acid, to undergo granulocytic differentiation[75,76] or by phorbol ester and cytosine arabinoside to monocyte like cells[76,77]. Thus HL60 can be induced by DMSO or retinoic acid to express the antigens detected by OKM1 and S5.25 which are normally present on both granulocytes and monocytes and also

Table 10.3 Expression of myeloid cell surface antigens on human leukaemic cell lines

Antibody	HL 60 (Promyelocyte)	KG 1 (Myeloblast)	U 937 (Promonocyte)	K 562 (Pluripotent stem cell)	Ref.
FMC 11	+/-	NR	-	+	23
FMC 10	+	NR	-	+	23
MY 1	+	-	+	+	25
TG 1	+	+	+	+	15
8 OH.3	+	-	-	-	22
FMC 12	+	NR	-	+	23
1 G 10	+	NR	NR	-	21
VIM D5	+	NR	+	+	24
MO 1	+/-	+	+/-	-	18
FMC 17	-	NR	-	-	43
FMC 32	-	NR	-	-	43
FMC 33	-	NR	-	-	43
MMA	NR	NR	+	+	43
MY 7	+	+	+	+/-	19
MY 9	+	+	+	+	29
MY 4	-	-	-	-	19
Mo 2	-	-	-	-	18
5F 1	-	NR	NR	-	26
UCHM 1	-	NR	+	-	?§
Sm θ	-	NR	+	+/-	35
28	+	NR	+	+	35
MY 10	NR	+(KG-1a)	-	NR	31

L12.2 which is normally expressed only on granulocytic cells[76]. Phorbol ester induces expression of the monocyte specific antigens Mo2 and MY 4[78]. Similar studies of antigen induction have also been reported with the KG-1 cell line[76]. Ferrero et al[76] used a large panel of antibodies in their studies and concluded that such in vitro induced differentiation only partly mimics the changes observed during myeloid differentiation in vivo. Nonetheless, such models of differentiation may prove to be valuable tools in the determination of the molecular events involved in antigen expression and differentiation in general.

STUDY OF AML CELLS

A large range of monoclonal antibodies have been used to study myeloid leukaemic blast cells. Several individual antibodies are of value in differentiating between AML and ALL (Table 10.4). MY 7 reacted with 70% and D5D6 and MY 9 over 80% of cases of AML;[19,29,38] all reacted with <1% of ALL's. Other anti-myeloid antibodies

Table 10.4 Monoclonal antibodies differentiating between AML and ALL

	AML			ALL		
	No. tested	No. pos.	% pos.	No. tested	No. pos.	% pos.
MY7	70	59	70	109	0	0
MY9	97	80	82	109	1	<1
D5D6	50	44	88	15	0	0

may be equally effective in differentiating between AML and ALL but only small studies have so far been published. The combined use of anti-lymphocyte antibodies in conjunction with the anti-myeloid antibodies increases the discriminating power of the immunological typing further. Among the most useful panel of non-myeloid antibodies for this purpose are anti-HLA-DR (positive in >90% AML)[79] anti-CALLA (positive in <1% AML)[80], B4 (positive in <1% AML)[81] and WT1 (positive in 6% AML)[82]. It should of course be noted however that the vast majority of cases of AML can be identified by conventional morphology and cytochemistry.

Anti-myeloid monoclonal antibodies may also be useful to identify subgroups of AML. One approach has been to compare immunological phenotypes with the FAB classification. The FAB classification is based on the degree and type of differentiation shown by leukaemic cells as defined by standard morphology and cytochemistry. Van der Reijden et al reported on 55 patients with AML studied with a panel of monoclonal antibodies[83]. There was a tendency for antibodies which reacted only with granulocytes to react with more differentiated subgroups of AML, both granulocytic and monocytic.

Antibodies reactive with both granulocytes and monocytes such as B2.12 and OKM1 tended to react equally with all types of AML. In agreement with other observers[84] it was shown that monoclonal antibodies to HLA-DR reacted with most AML cells except acute promyelocytic leukaemia. The immunological phenotype thus in general reflected the level of differentiation of the AML cells as determined by conventional criteria, but the correlation with the FAB classification was very imperfect. Correct prediction of the FAB classification by immunological phenotyping was only possible after computer analysis in 69% of cases.

Several other groups have also found that antibodies which are granulocyte specific do not always give the expected profile with leukaemic cells. Thus PMN-6 and PMN-29 which react with granulocytes and their precursors but not monocytes, did not react with the granulocytic (M1 and M2) variants of AML and reacted strongly with M4 leukaemias[85]. The antibody TG-1 which reacts with all granulocytes and only about 20% of monocytes in the peripheral blood, reacts with virtually all cases of M4 and M5 leukaemic and less than half of M1 and M2 leukaemias[86]. These three antibodies all react with recognizable granulocyte precursors but not GM-CFC and the lack of reactivity with M1 and M2 leukaemias probably indicates that the blast cells are at a primitive level of differentiation prior to the expression of the antigens detected by these antibodies. Reactivity with the monocytic leukaemias probably indicates that normal monoblasts and promonocytes express these antigens although peripheral blood monocytes do not. Various other antibodies which react with both normal granulocytic and monocytic cells, such as Mo 1, MY 7 and MY 9 show little subtype preference in their reactivity[29,87]. Antibodies specific for monocytes and not granulocytes have also been used to detect the AML monocytic variants. Mo 2 reacted with 46% of cases of M4 and M5 leukaemia but also with 9/57 of M1 and M2 leukaemias. MY 4 reacted with over 60% of M4/M5 leukaemias but also with 9/36 of M1/M2 leukaemias. Mo 3 reacted with 0/27 cases of M1 and M2 leukaemia but only 3/21 cases of M4/M5 leukaemia. A greater degree of discrimination has been reported with the antibodies UCHM1 and UCHALF[86]. These two antibodies react only with monocytes in normal blood and marrow. UCHM1 reacted with 38/40 cases of M4/M5 leukaemia and 1/17 cases of

M1/M2 leukaemia. The antibody UCHALF detects surface bound lactoferrin and thus indirectly detects the lactoferrin receptor. It similarly reacted with38/40 cases of M4/M5 leukaemia and 1/17 cases of M1/M2 leukaemia. Another antibody of interest in this study was E11. This antibody detects the C3/C4b receptor[80]. This antibody also reacted with most cases of monocytic leukaemia but not with M1/M2 leukaemias although it reacts with about 50% of normal granulocytes. This confirms previous studies using rosetting techniques that M1/M2 leukaemias do not in general express C3b receptors whereas these are detected on blasts showing monocytic differentiation[89]. These studies with UCHM1, UCHALF and E11 have included relatively few cases of M1/M2 leukaemias but the results are encouraging as the recognition of monocytic variants may have prognostic implications. Furthermore, it appears that some cases without monoblast morphology or non-specific esterase staining may be of monocytic origin although it must be noted that there is no final arbitrator of monocytic cell lineage.

Several of the anti-erythroid antibodies may be valuable probes in the diagnosis of erythroleukaemia (M6) variants. Greaves and colleagues have shown that an anti-glycophorin antibody R10, reacted with blasts from 21/27 cases of overt erythroleukaemia[90]. Interestingly it also reacted with 2/329 cases of apparent ALL, 8/205 cases of AML and 8/109 blast crises of Ph' positive chronic myeloid leukaemia. These cases may well represent occult erythroleukaemia although abberrant gene expression can not be excluded. Some of the anti-platelet antibodies may similarly be of value in detecting the rare megakaryoblastic leukaemias[70,91].

From the viewpoint of leukaemia classification, to show that the immunological phenotype corresponds to conventional subtyping is not particularly informative. The crucial issue is whether the immunological phenotyping provides any further information. Civin and colleagues studied 33 cases of AML for the expression of the anti-myeloid antibody MY 1 and MY 10 antigens[92]. 13 out of 13 (100%) cases in which the myeloblasts expressed the MY 1 antigen achieved a complete remission (CR) whereas only 12/19 (63%) cases not expressing MY 1 achieved a CR. The MY 10 antigen which is present on normal progenitors but not on recognizable myeloid precursor cells, was expressed on 3/18 cases; only 1 of these 3 obtained a CR (33%). In contrast, 13/15 MY 10 patients entered CR (87%). Although the numbers of cases in this preliminary study were small, the differences for both MY-1 and MY 10 were reported as statistically significant. In another small study Blazar et al have examined the prognostic implications of the expression of the antigens detected by BA-1 and BA-2[93]. These antibodies are not myeloid specific and also react with normal lymphoid cells and some cases of ALL. Six of 35 cases were positive with BA-1 and five of these (83%) achieved CR compared to 66% in the BA-1 negative cases. A more striking difference in CR rates was observed between the BA-2 positive and negative populations, the CR rates being 75% (21/36 cases positive) and 25% (15/36 cases negative) respectively. These differences in CR rates were also matched by differences in the median survival. There was little difference in the CR rate in this study between the DR+ and DR- cases, although the median survival was longer in those cases with cells expressing DR antigens.

Griffin and colleagues have analysed 70 cases of AML with a panel of monoclonal antibodies including anti HLA-DR, MY 4, MY 7, MY 8, MY 9 and Mo 1[87]. Four patterns of reactivity were observed which corresponded to stages of normal differentiation determined by fluorescent activated cell sorting and culture studies of normal marrow (Fig. 10.4): 62 of the 70 cases corresponded to one of these four categories; 13 cases had the most immature cell phenotype corresponding to the GM-CFC; 10 of these were classified as M1/M2 by conventional criteria; 16 cases were in group II corresponding to 'late myeloblasts'; 12 were classified as M1/M2 and 4 as M4. Group III corresponding to the normal promyelocyte contained 5 cases; this included the three cases of acute promyelocytic leukaemia and also one case of HLA DR⁻ AML and one case of DR⁻ M4 leukaemia. Twenty-eight patients were in group IV corresponding to the normal promonocyte; 23 were classified as M4/M5 leukaemia and 5 as M1/M2. The immunological phenotypes were thus related to the morphological appearances, although the correspondence was not

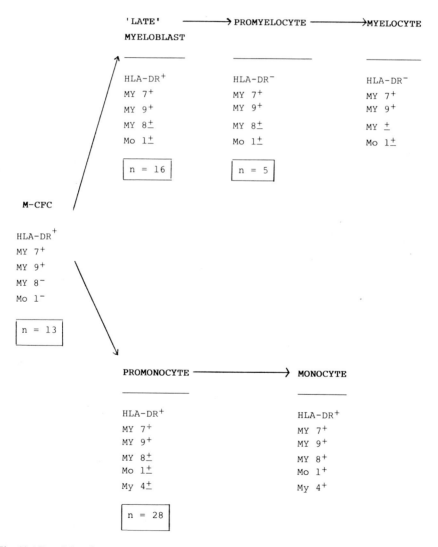

Fig. 10.4 Reactivity of monoclonal antibodies in 70 cases of AML.

perfect. The CR ratio in the different groups were not significantly different although there was a tendency for patients in Group II to have a higher remission rate.

Such studies of acute leukaemic cells provide valuable information about normal cells. Thus the investigations reported by Griffin et al serve to confirm their scheme of normal antigen expression during early myeloid differentiation. Leukaemic cells are particularly useful in the study of early monocytic development as the normal monoblast and promonocyte cannot readily be identified. It is largely by inference from such studies that one can conclude that the antigens recognized by UCHM1, UCHALF, EII, TG-1, Mo1, MY 4, MY 7, MY 9 and HLA-DR are expressed on 'promonocytes'. In a combined study of the immunological phenotype and the non-specific esterase (NSE) isoenzymes in monocytic leukaemias, Scott and colleagues have further suggested that the monocyte antigens detected by UCHM1, UCHALF and EII are expressed at an earlier stage of differentiation than the monocyte specific NSE isoenzymes[94]. It was also suggested in this study that the monocytic cells in the M4 leukaemias were in general more primitive than those in the M5 leukaemias. Although M4–M5 leukaemic blasts had the same immunological phenotype with the antibodies used, this is not true with other antibodies. PMN6 and PMN29 described by Ball & Fanger thus react with blast cells from most cases of M4 leukaemia, but not M1/M2 leukaemias or M5 leukaemias[85].

The extrapolation of data obtained from leukaemic cells is based on the concept that most leukaemic cells have the same phenotype as their normal counterpart. Although, this in general appears to be true, individual cases may display abberrant gene expression. Indeed, Smith et al have suggested that abberrant phenotypes are very common in acute leukaemia[95].

We and others have not observed such a high incidence of unexpected immunological phenotypes although we have observed apparent discordance between normal and malignant myeloperoxidase and TG-1 antigen expression. In normal marrow, TG-1 positive myeloblasts are nearly all myeloperoxidase negative. In M1/M2 leukaemias 60% of cases do not express TG-1 antigen and many of these cases are peroxidase positive (Table 10.5). This may indicate that many cases of AML have the phenotype of a rare (small differentiation window) cell. In one case in which only a proportion of blast cells were TG-1 positive however the peroxidase activity was no higher in these isolated TG-1 positive cells than in the negative cells. This may suggest that either TG-1 is abberrantly missing in many cases of AML or that myeloperoxidase is abberrantly expressed at an earlier stage of differentiation. Abnormal granule formation (Auer rods) is well recognized in AML and if granule myeloperoxidase expression is relatively advanced in AML, this might account for the great reliability of peroxidase cytochemistry in delineating AML.

SEROTHERAPY IN AML

Leukaemia specific monoclonal antibodies have not been described. Such antibodies would have obvious potential in the serotherapy of AML, but are, we believe, unlikely to materialize. Ball and colleagues have used anti-myeloid antibodies to treat three patients with AML[96]. The antibody or antibodies used were shown to react

Table 10.5 TG1 antigen expression and myeloperoxidase in M1/M2 leukaemias % Cells positive

Patient No.	TG–1	Peroxidase
1	+++	0
2	++	+++
3	+	+
4	+	+
5	+	+
6	+	+++
7	+	+
8	0	+++
9	0	+++
10	0	0
11	0	++
12	0	0
13	0	0
14	0	+
15	0	+++
16	0	+++
17	0	+++
18	0	++

0   = <10%
+   = 10–30%
++ = 30–60%
+++ = >60%

with the majority of leukaemic cells, although such findings may not be fully relevant when serotherapy is considered. Leukaemic colonies can be grown in vitro and there is some evidence that the leukaemic colony forming cells (L-CFC) are the precursors of those cells that are the major blast cell population in the blood and marrow. These L-CFC do not necessarily have the same phenotype as the majority of blast cells and it is these highly proliferative leukaemic stem cells at which therapy must be directed. In M4 leukaemias for instance, the monocytic blast cells express Mo 2 and MY 4 antigens but cell sorting experiments have shown that L-CFC are invariably MY 4 negative[97].

In a further study Griffin and colleagues examined the expression of HLA-DR and MY 9 antigen on L-CFC in seven patients with AML. The majority of blast cells expressed these antigens in each case, but in two instances, either HLA-DR or MY 9 antigen was not present on the large majority of L-CFC[29]. More pronounced discrepancies between the phenotypes of L-CFC and the major blast cell population have been reported by Lange et al[98]. With the panel of antibodies used in this study, there was in general a greater reactivity with L-CFC than the majority of blast cells, but this again emphasises the importance of determining the L-CFC phenotype prior to serotherapy or cleansing of bone marrow autografts with monoclonal antibodies in AML. The latter study showed that whereas some L-CFC had the same phenotype as 'late progenitor cells' which react with antibodies such as RIB19, other cases had the phenotype of early RIB19 negative progenitors. The authors thus suggest that the former category of patients may be suitable for serotherapy or autologous bone marrow transplantation with marrow cleansing. It has also been suggested that cleansing of bone marrow with anti-HLA-DR may be appropriate in AML. This is because, while most leukaemic blasts, L-CFC, and normal progenitor cells are DR$^+$, the normal primitive stem cells responsible for regeneration may be DR$^-$. In a marmoset model, marrow treated with anti-HLA-DR and complement, although severely depleted of GM-CFC will still lead to normal haemopoietic regeneration[99]. Even if this is true in man, however the use of anti-HLA-DR antibodies to treat AML marrows must still be viewed with caution. Just as the major blast cell population may not represent the leukaemic stem cell, this may also be true for the L-CFC. Fialkow and colleagues[100] have in fact shown in G6PD heterozygotes with AML that this disease may affect the multipotential stem cell with involvement of all myeloid cell lines. The ultimate leukaemic stem may have the same phenotype therefore as the normal stem cell (presumed DR$^-$) responsible for successful regeneration. There is a suggestion that the leukaemic 'hit' may be at a later stage of differentiation in some forms of childhood AML but these cases can not be identified in the large majority of cases[100].

PURIFICATION OF HAEMOPOIETIC PROGENITOR CELLS

The purification of haemopoietic progenitor cells was one of the first reported uses of anti-myeloid monoclonal antibodies. Beverley, Linch & Delia used the two antibodies TG-1 and anti-HLe-1 (anti common leukocyte antigen) for this purpose[15]. If low density bone marrow cells are stained with anti-HLe-1, three populations of cells are apparent on FACS analysis; (1) small brightly staining cells; (2) dimly stained cells; (3) negatively stained cells (Fig. 10.5). The brightly stained cells are lymphocytes, the dimly stained cells are cells of the granulocytic series and the negative stained cells are erythroblasts. All of the progenitor cells both myeloid and erythroid are in the dimly stained fraction. When the marrow was first treated with TG-1 and complement which lyses all the recognizable granulocytic cells, subsequent staining with anti-HLe-1 revealed very few dimly stained cells. Sorting of this fraction showed them to be undifferentiated blasts and up to 25% of this fraction were capable of clonal growth into myeloid or erythroid colonies. In addition this fraction contained 3–15% Tdt positive cells which were presumably the lymphoid progenitor cells.

Griffin et al used monoclonal antibodies and immune rosetting to purify leukaemic colony forming cells from the blood of patients with chronic granulocytic leukaemia[101]. Lymphocytes, monocytes and most immature myeloid cells were simultaneously depleted from the bone marrow using the antibodies T11, B1, Mo 1 and MY 8. Cells expressing HLA-DR antigens were then further selected by a second immune rosetting procedure with the I-2 antibody. Up to 92% of cells in this final DR+ fraction were undifferentiated blast cells with up to 42% capable of forming colonies or clusters in agar cultures. These purified CGL colony forming cells showed an absolute requirement for exogenous colony stimulating factors (CSF). In the absence of CSF there was no proliferation event in short term cultures. This has enabled Griffin and colleagues to develop a rapid and sensitive assay for CSA, using purified CGL progenitor cells and tritiated thymidine uptake at 24–48 hours[102].

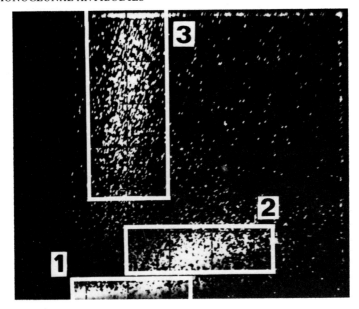

Fig. 10.5 Normal bone marrow stained with anti-HLe-1.
Cell size is shown on the x axis and fluorescence intensity on the y axis.
1. Small negatively stained cells.
2. Large dimly stained cells.
3. Small brightly stained cells.

A similar technique of negative selection with monoclonal antibodies and immune rosetting was used by Linch & Nathan to purify BFU-E from normal blood[103]. The antibodies used are shown in Table 10.6. Approximately 10% of the low density antibody depleted cells were BFU-E and a further enrichment was obtained by selecting for HLA-DR positive cells from this fraction. The growth in culture of these highly purified BFU-E was dependent on an added source of burst promoting activity (BPA) or accessory cells. Although some growth was obtained without the addition of BPA (other than that contaminating the serum and crude erythropoietin used), there were few BFU-E derived colonies and these were small and poorly

Table 10.6 Monoclonal antibodies used in the purification of BFU-E from peripheral blood

Antibody	Specificity
UCHT1	Pan T (CD 3)
Leu 5	Pan T (CD 2)
Leu 2a	'Suppressor' T-cells (CD 8)
Leu 3a	'Helper' T-cells (CD 4)
BA1	B-cells and granulocytes
B1	B-cells
Leu M1	Monocytes, granulocytes and NK-cells
Leu M2	Some monocytes
Leu M3	Some monocytes
TG1	Granulocytes, some monocytes
Leu 7	NK-cells, some T-cells

haemoglobinized. It was further possible to show that BFU-E colony growth was supported by conditioned media from two T-cell lines and a monocytoid cell line (Fig. 10.6). As the BFU-E were highly purified and the cells were cultured at only 5×10^2/ml, this indicated that BPA derived from both monocytoid and T-cell lines acted directly on the progenitor cell. Further proof of this was obtained by showing that these conditioned media could support BFU-E colony growth when plated at cell concentrations approaching one cell per well. Previous studies had suggested that T-cells mainly produced factors that augment BPA production by monocytes. They may produce such factors but they clearly also produce direct-acting BPA.

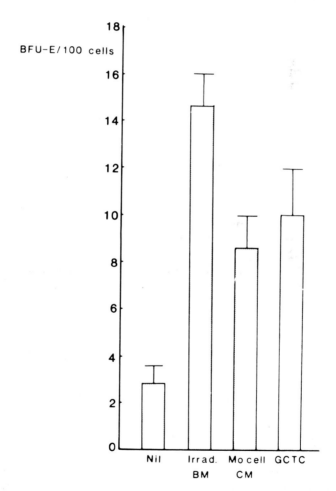

Fig. 10.6 Effects of irradiated bone marrow cells and conditioned media on the growth of highly purified BFU-E.
Nil = No conditioned medium.
Irrad BM = Irradiated bone marrow cells.
Mo Cell CM = A human T-cell line conditioned medium. Similar results were also obtained with the gibbon ape T-cell line MLA-144.
GCTC = A human monocytoid cell line conditioned medium.

Interestingly it was also shown that a bone marrow conditioned medium which had potent burst promoting activity against crude BFU-E populations, had virtually no activity against the highly purified BFU-E. This conditioned media contained indirect-acting factors. The cells producing such factors was not determined. These studies clearly demonstrate the importance of purified progenitor populations in studies to dissect the cellular interactions that regulate haemopoiesis and monoclonal antibodies will continue to be a major tool for this purpose.

REFERENCES

1. Barrett S G, Hansen K S, Bainton D F 1981 Differentiation of cell surface receptors on normal human bone marrow myeloid precursors. British Journal of Haematology 48: 491-500
2. Till J E, McCulloch E A 1961 A direct measurement of the radiation sensitivity of normal mouse bone marrow cells. Radiation Research 14: 213-222
3. Wu A M, Till J E, Siminovitch L, McCulloch E A 1968 Cytological evidence for a relationship between normal haemopoietic colony forming cells and cells of the lymphoid system. Journal of Experimental Medicine 127: 455-463
4. Fialkow P J, Jacobsen R Y, Papayanopoulou T 1977 Chronic myelocytic leukaemia; clonal origin in a stem cell common to the granulocyte erythrocyte platelet and monocyte/macrophage. American Journal of Medicine 63: 125-130
5. Pike P L, Robinson W A 1970 Human bone marrow colony growth in agar gel. Journal of cell Physiology 76: 77-84
6. Johnson G R, Dresch C, Metcalf D 1977 Heterogeneity in human neutrophil macrophage and eosinophil progenitor cells demonstrated by velocity sedimentation. Blood 50: 823-831
7. Dao C, Metcalf D, Bilski Pasquier G 1977 Eosinophil and neutrophil colony forming cells in culture. Blood 50: 833-839
8. Broxmeyer H E, Lu Li, Bognacki J 1983 Transferrin derived from an OKT8 positive sub-population of T-lymphocytes suppresses the production of granulocyte-macrophage colony stimulation factors from mitogen activated T-lymphocytes. Blood 62: 37-50
9. Iscove N N 1977 The role of erythropoietin in regulation of population size and cell cycling of early and late erythroid precursors in mouse bone marrow. Cell and Tissue Kinetics 10: 323-334
10. Iscove N N 1978 Erythropoietin independent stimulation of early erythropoiesis in adult marrow cultures by conditioned medium from lectin stimulated mouse spleen cells. ICN-UCLA Symposium on Haemopoietic Cell Differentiation. In: Golde D W, Cline M J, Metcalf D, Fox C F (eds) Moleculare and Cell Biology, Academic Press, New York, p 37-82
11. Vainchenker W, Bouget J, Guichard J, Breton Gorius J 1979 Megakaryocyte colony formation from human bone marrow precursors. Blood 54: 940-945
12. Hoffman R, Mazur E, Bruno E, Floyd V 1981 Assay of an activity in the serum of patients with disorders of thrombopoiesis that stimulates formation of megakaryocyte colonies. New England Journal of Medicine 305: 533-538
13. Fauser A A, Messner H A 1978 Granuloerythropoietic colonies in human bone marrow peripheral blood and cord blood. Blood 52: 1243-1246
14. Breard J, Reinherz E L, Kung P C, Goldstein G, Schlossman S F 1980 A monoclonal antibody reactive with human peripheral blood monocytes. Journal of Immunology 124: 1943-1948
15. Beverley P C L, Linch D C, Delia D 1980 Isolation of human haematopoietic progenitor cells using monoclonal antibodies. Nature 287: 332-333
16. Ugolini V, Nunez G, Smith R G, Stastny P, Capra J D 1980 Initial characterization of monoclonal antibodies against human monocytes. Proceedings of the National Academy of Sciences, USA 77: 6764-6768
17. Joint Report of the First International Workshop on Human Leucocyte Differentiation Antigens by the Investigations of the Participating Laboratories: M2 Protocol 1984 In: Bernard A, Boumsell L, Dausset J, Milstein C, Schlossman S F (eds) Leucocyte typing, Springer Verlag, Berlin, p 82-108
18. Todd R F, Nadler L M, Schlossman S F 1981 Antigens on human monocytes identified by monoclonal antibodies. Journal of Immunology 126: 1435-1441
19. Griffin J D, Ritz J, Nadler L M, Schlossman S F 1981 Expression of myeloid differentiation antigens on normal and malignant myeloid cells. Journal of Clinical Investigations 68: 932-941

20. Tatsumi E, Sagawa K, Mirro J, Civin C I, Preisler H D, Henderson E S, Minowda J 1981 Immunological membrane phenotypes in human myeloid leukaemia by monoclonal antibodies. Proceedings of the American Association of Cancer Research 22: 717

21. Bernstein I D, Andrews R G, Cohen S F, McMaster B E 1982 Normal and malignant human myelocytic and monocytic cells identified by monoclonal antibodies. Journal of Immunology 128: 876–881

22. Mannoni P, Janowska-Wieczorek A, Turner A R, McGann L 1982 Monoclonal antibodies against human granulocytes and myeloid differentiation antigens. Human Immunology 5: 309–323

23. Zola H, McNamara P, Thomas M, Smart I J, Bradley J 1981 The preparation and properties of monoclonal antibodies against human granulocyte membrane antigens. British Journal of Haematology 48: 481–490

24. Majdic O, Liszka K, Lutz D, Knapp W 1981 Myeloid differentiation antigen defined by a monoclonal antibody. Blood 58: 1127–1133

25. Civin C I, Mirro J, Banquerigo M L 1981 MY-1 a new myeloid specific antigen identified by a mouse monoclonal antibody. Blood 57: 842–844

26. Andrews R G, Torok Storb B, Bernstein I D 1983 Myeloid associated differentiation antigens on stem cells and their progeny identified by monoclonal antibodies. Blood 62: 124–132

27. Hanjan S N S, Kearney J F, Cooper M D 1982 A monoclonal antibody (MMA) that identifies a differentiation antigen on human myelomonocytic cells. Clinical Immunology and Immunopathology 23: 172–188

28. Griffin J D, Ritz J, Beveridge R P, Lipton J M, Daley J F, Schlossman S F 1983 Expression of MY 7 antigen on myeloid precursor cells. International Journal of Cell Cloning 1: 33–48

29. Griffin J D, Linch D C, Sabbath K, Larcom P, Schlossman S F 1984 A monoclonal antibody reactive with normal and leukaemic human myeloid progenitor cells. Leukaemia Research Vol 8 No 4: 521–534

30. Todd R F, Schlossman S F 1982 Analysis of antigenic determinants on human monocytes and macrophages. Blood 59: 775–786

31. Strauss L C, Civin C I 1983 MY 10, a human progenitor cell surface antigen identified by a monoclonal antibody. Experimental Haematology 11: (suppl 14) 370a

32. Huang L C, Civin C I, Magnani J L, Shaper J H, Ginsburg V 1983 MY 1, the human myeloid specific antigen detected by mouse monoclonal antibodies is a sugar sequence found in lacto N fucopentuose III. Blood 61: 1020–1023

33. Urdal D L, Brentnall TA, Bernstein I D, Hakomori S I 1983 A granulocyte reactive monoclonal antibody, Ig10, identifies the Gal B1-4 (Fuc 1-3), Glc NAc (× determinant) expressed in HL 60 cells on both glycolipid and glycoprotein molecules. Blood 62: 1022–1026

34. Ball E D, Graziano R F, Shen Li, Fanger M W 1982 Monoclonal antibodies to novel myeloid antigens reveal human neutrophil heterogeneity. Proceedings of the National Academy of Sciences, USA 79: 5374–5378

35. Hogg N, McDonald S, Slusarenko M, Beverley P C L 1984 Monoclonal antibodies specific for human monocytes, granulocytes and endothelium. Immunology 53: 753–768

36. Clement L T, Lehmeyer J E, Gartland G L 1981 Identification of neutrophil subpopulations with monoclonal antibodies. Blood 61: 326–332

37. Beverley P C L, Callard R E 1981 Distinctive functional characteristics of human T-lymphocytes defined by E rosetting or a monoclonal anti T-cell antibody. European Journal of Immunology 11 (4): 329–334

38. Linker-Israeli M, Billing R J, Foon K A, Terasaki P I 1981 Monoclonal antibodies reactive with acute myelogeneous leukaemia cells. Journal of Immunology 127: 2473–2476

39. Strauss L C, Fackler M, Brovall C, Civin C I 1983 MY 11, a normal lymphohematopoietic surface antigen expressed by myelomonocytic but not erythroid progenitor cells (Abstr) Blood 62 (Suppl 1): 469

40. Cotter T G, Spears P, Henson P M 1981 A monoclonal antibody inhibiting human neutrophil chemotaxis and degranulation. Journal of Immunology 127: 1355–1360

41. Cotter T G, Keeling P J, Henson P M 1981 A monoclonal antibody inhibiting FMLP induced chemotaxis of human neutrophils. Journal of Immunology 127: 2241–2245

42. Dimitriu Bona A, Burmester G R, Waters S J, Winchester R J 1983 Human mononuclear phagocyte differentiation antigens. Journal of Immunology 130: 145–152

43. Brooks D A, Zola H, McNamara P J, Bradley J, Bradstock K F, Hancock W W, Atkins R C 1983 Membrane antigens of human cells of the monocyte/macrophage lineage studied with monoclonal antibodies. Pathology 15: 45–56

44. Arnaout M A, Todd R F, Dana N, Melamed J, Schlossman S F, Colten H R 1983 Inhibition of phagocytosis of complement C3 on IgG coated particles and of C3bi binding by monoclonal

antibodies to a monocyte granulocyte membrane glycoprotein (Mol). Journal of Clinical Investigation 72: 171–179

45.   Dana N, Todd R F, Pitt J, Springer T A, Arnaout M A 1983 Deficiency of a surface membrane glycoprotein (Mol) in man. Journal of Clinical Investigation 73: 153–159

46.   Beatly P G, Ochs H D, Harlan J M, Price T H, Rosen H, Taylor R F, Hansen J A, Klebanoff S J 1984 Absence of monoclonal antibody defined protein complex in a boy with abnormal leukocyte function. Lancet i: 535–537

47.   Seger R, Fischer A, Durandy A, Bohler M C, Virelizier J L, Kazatchkina M, Deschamps B, Triang P H, Grospierre B, Griscelli C Adhesive protein deficiency resulting in abnormal phagocytic functions and impaired cytotoxicities. Progress in immunodeficiency research and therapy I. Griscelli C, Vossen J Excerpta Medica 83–90

48.   Linch D C, Boyle D, Beverley P C L 1982 T-cell and monocyte requirements for erythropoiesis. Acta Haematologica 67: 324–328

49.   Raff H V, Picker L J, Stobo S D 1980 Macrophage heterogeneity in man. A subpopulation of HLA-DR bearing macrophages required for antigen induced T-cell activation also require stimulators for autologous reactive T-cells. Journal of Experimental Medicine 152: 581–589

50.   Hancock W W, Zola H, Atkins R C 1983 Antigenic heterogeneity of human mononuclear phagocytes: immunohistological analysis using monoclonal antibodies. Blood 62: 1271–1279

51.   Anstree D J, Edwards P A W 1982 Monoclonal antibodies to human erythrocytes. European Journal of Immunology 12: 228–232

52.   Sieff C, Bicknell D, Caine G, Robinson J, Lam G, Greaves M F 1982 Changes in cell surface antigen expression during haemopoietic differentiation. Blood 60: 703–713

52.   Lebman D, Trucco M, Bottero L, Lange B, Pessano S, Rovera G 1982 A monoclonal antibody that detects expression of transferrin receptor in human erythroid precursor cells. Blood 59: 671–676

54.   Das Gupta A, Yokochi T, Brice M C, Papayannopoulou Th, Stamatoyannopoulos G 1983 New erythroid lineage specific and myeloid lineage specific determinants identified by two different monoclonal antibodies (Abstr). Blood 62 (Suppl 1) 287

55.   Adamo J, Broviak M, Brooks W, Johnson N T, Issih P D 1971 An antibody in the serum of a Wr (a⁺) individual reacting with an antigen of very high frequency. Transfusion 11: 290–291

56.   Pavsol G, Jungery M, Weatherall D J, Parsons S F, Anstee D J, Tanner M J A 1982 Glycophorin as a possible receptor for Plasmodium falciparum. Lancet ii: 947–950

57.   Andrews R G, Brentnall T A, Torok Storb B, Bernstein I D 1984 Stages of myeloid differentiation identified by monoclonal antibodies. In: Bernard A, Boumsell L, Dausset J, Milstein C, Schlossman S F (eds) Leucocyte typing, Springer Verlag, Berlin, p 398–403

58.   Crawford D H, Francis G E, Wing M A, Edwards A J, Janossy G, Hoffbrand A V, Prentice H G, Secher D, McConnell I, King D C, Goldstein G 1981 Reactivity of monoclonal antibodies with human myeloid precursor cells. British Journal of Haematology 49: 209–215

59.   Winchester R J, Meyers P A, Broxmeyer H E, Wang C Y, Moore M A S, Kunkel H G 1978 Inhibition of erythropoietic colony formation in culture by treatment with Ia antisera. Journal of Experimental Medicine 148: 613–622

60.   Janossy G, Francis G E, Capellano D, Goldstone A H, Greaves M F 1978 Cell sorter analysis of leukaemia associated antigens on human myeloid precursors. Nature 276: 176–178

61.   Bodmer J, Bodmer W 1984 Histocompatibility. Immunology Today 5: 251–254

62.   Auffray C, Kuo J, De Mars R, Strominger J L 1983 A minimum of four human class II-chain genes are encoded in the HLA region of chromosome 6. Nature 304: 214

63.   Belzer M B, Fitchen J H, Ferrone S, Foon K A, Billing R J, Golde D W 1981 Expression of Ia like antigens on human erythroid progenitor cells as determined by monoclonal antibodies and heteroanti-serum to Ia-like antigens. Clinical Immunology Immunopathology 20: 111–122

64.   Robinson J C, Sieff C, Delia D, Edwards P A W, Greaves M 1981 Expression of cell surface HLA-DR, HLA ABC and glycophorin during erythroid differentiation. Nature 289: 68–72

65.   Fitchen J H, Cline M J 1979 Human myeloid progenitor cells express HLA antigens. Blood 53: 794–798

66.   Linch D C, Nadler L M, Luther E A, Lipton J M 1984 Discordant expression of human Ia-like antigens on haematopoietic progenitor cells. Journal of Immunology 132: 2324–2329

67.   Pelus L M 1982 Association between colony forming units-granulocyte macrophage expression of Ia-like (HLA-DR) antigen and control of granulocyte and macrophage production. A new role for prostaglandin E. Journal of Clinical Investigation 70: 568–578

68.   Tork Storb B J, Hansen J A 1982 Modulation of in vitro BFU-E growth by normal Ia-positive T-cells in restricted by HLA-DR. Nature 298: 473–476

69.   Lipton J M, Nadler L M, Canellos G P, Kudisch M, Reiss C S, Nathan D G 1983 Evidence for genetic restriction in the suppression of erythropoiesis by a unique subset of T-cells in man. Journal of Clinical Investigation 72: 694–706

70. Vainchenker W, Deschamps J F, Bastin J M, Guichard J, Titeux M, Breton Gorius J, McMichael A J 1982 Two monoclonal anti-platelet antibodies as markers of human megakaryocyte maturation: immunogluorescent staining and platelet peroxidase detection in megakaryocyte colonies and in in vivo cells from normal and leukaemic patients. Blood 59: 514–521

71. Coller B S, Peerschke E I, Scudder L E, Sullivan C A 1983 Studies with a murine monoclonal antibody that abolishes ristocetin induced binding of von Willebrand factor to platelets: additional evidence in support of Gplb as a platelet receptor for von Willebrand factor. Blood 61: 99–110

72. Di Minno G, Thiagarajan P, Perussia B, Martinez J, Shapiro S, Trinchieri G, Murphy S 1983 Exposure of platelet fibrinogen-binding sites by collagen, arachidonic acid and ADP: inhibition by a monoclonal antibody to the glycophorin IIb-IIa complex. Blood 61: 140–148

73. Deng C T, Terasaki P I, Iwaki Y, Hofman F M, Koeffler P, Cahan L, El Awar N, Billing R 1983 Monoclonal antibody cross reactive with human platelets, megakaryocytes and common acute lymphocytic leukaemia cells. Blood 61: 759–764

74. Herchend T, Nadler L M, Pesando J M, Reinherz E L, Schlossman S F, Ritz J 1981 Expression of a 26 000 dalton glycoprotein on activated human T-cells. Cell Immunology 64: 192

75. Collins S J, Ruscetti F W, Gallagher R E, Gallo R C 1979 Normal functional characteristics of cultured human promyelocytic leukaemia cells (HL60) after induction of differentiation by dimethyl suphoxide. Journal of Experimental Medicine 149: 969–973

76. Ferrero D, Pessano S, Pagliardi G L, Rovera G 1983 Induction of differentiation of human myeloid leukaemias: surface changes probed with monoclonal antibodies. Blood 61: 171–179

77. Griffin J D, Major P P, Monroe D, Kufe D 1982 Inducation of differentiation of human myeloid leukaemia cells by inhibitors of DNA synthesis. Experimental Haematology 10: 774–781

78. Todd R F, Griffin J D, Ritz J, Nadler L M, Abrams J, Schlossman S F 1981 Expression of normal monocyte – macrophage differentiation antigens on HL60 promyelocytes underoing differentiation induced by leukocyte conditioned medium or phorbol diester. Leukaemia Research 5: 491–495

79. Newman R A, Greaves M F 1982 Characterization of HLA-DR antigens on leukaemic cells. Clinical Experimental Immunology 50: 41–50

80. Ritz J, Pesando J M, Notis-McConarty, Lazarus H, Schlossman SF 1980 A monoclonal antibody to human acute lymphoblastic leukaemia antigen. Nature 283: 583–585

81. Nadler L M, Anderson K C, Marti G, Bates M, Park E, Daley J F, Schlossman S F 1983 B4, a human B lymphocyte associated antigen expressed on normal, mitogen activated and malignant B lymphocytes. Journal of Immunology 131: 244–250

82. Vodinelich L, Tax W, Bai Y, Pegram S, Capel P, Greaves M F 1983 A monoclonal antibody (WTI) for detecting leukaemias of T-cell precursors (T-ALL) Blood 62: 1108–1113

83. Van der Reijden H J, van Rhenen D J, Lansdorp P M, van't Veer M B, Langenhuijsen M M A C, Englefriet C P, Von dem Borne A E G K 1983 A comparison of surface marker analysis and FAB classification in acute myeloid leukaemia. Blood 61: 443–448

84. McVerry B A, Goldstone A H, Janossy G 1979 Acute promyelocytic leukaemia: further evidence of the differentiation linked expression of Ia-like (p28,33) antigens on leukaemic cells. Scandinavian Journal of Haematology 22: 53–56

85. Ball E D, Fanger M W 1983 The expression of myeloid specific antigens on myeloid leukaemia cells: correlations with leukaemic subclasses and implications for normal myeloid differentiation. Blood 61: 456–463

86. Linch D C, Allen C, Beverley P C L, Bynoe A G, Scott C S, Hogg N 1984 Monoclonal antibodies differentiating between monocytic and non-monocytic variants of AML. Blood 63: 556–573

87. Griffin J D, Mayer R J, Weinstein H J, Rosenthal D S, Coral F S, Beveridge R P, Schlossman S F 1983 Surface marker analysis of acute myeloblastic leukaemia: identification of differentiation associated phenotypes. Blood 62: 557–563

88. Hogg N, Ross G D, Jones D B, Slusarenko M, Walport M J, Lachman P J 1984 Identification of an anti-monocyte monoclonal antibody that is specific for membrane complement receptor type I (CR1) European Journal of Immunology (In press)

89. Scott C S, Bynoe A G, Linch D C, Allen C, Hough D, Roberts B E 1983 Membrane Fc-IgG and C3b receptors on myeloid leukaemia cells: a comparison with cytoplasmic acid naphthyl acetate esterase cytochemistry. Journal of Clinical Pathology 36: 555–558

90. Greaves M F, Sieff C, Edwards P A W 1983 Monoclonal antiglycophorin as a probe for erythroleukaemias. Blood 61: 645–646

91. Griffin J D, Todd R J, Ritz J, Nadler L M, Canellos G P, Rosenthal D, Gallivan M, Beveridge R P, Weinstein H, Karp D, Schlossman S F 1983 Differentiation patterns in the blastic phase of chronic myeloid leukaemia. Blood 61: 85-91

92. Civin C I, Vaughan W P, Strauss L C, Schwartz J F, Karp J E, Burke P J 1983 Diagnostic and prognostic utility of cell surface markers in acute non-lymphocytic leukaemia (ANLL) Experimental Haematology 11 (Suppl 14) 152a

93. Blazar B R, Bloomfield C D, Robison L L, Nesbit M E, Kersey J H 1983 Prognostic significance of monoclonal antibody phenotypes in acute non-lymphocytic leukaemia (Abstr) Blood 62: Suppl 1 568

94. Scott C S, Linch D C, Bynoe A G, Allen C, Hogg N, Ainley M J, Hough D, Roberts B E 1984 Alpha napthyl acetate esterases in acute myeloid leukaemia: assessment by isoelectric focussing and cytochemistry and relationship to the expression of monocyte specific antigens and the receptor for IgG. Blood 63: 517-526

95. Smith L J, Curtis J E, Messner H A, Senn J S, Furthmayr H, McCulloch E A 1983 Lineage infidelity in acute leukaemia. Blood 61: 1138-1145

96. Ball E D, Bernier G M, Cornwall G G, McIntyre O R, O'Donnell J F, Fanger M W 1983 Monoclonal antibodies to myeloid differentiation antigens: in vivo studies of three patients with acute myelogeneous leukaemia. Blood 62: 1203-1210

97. Griffin J D, Larcom P, Schlossman S F 1983 Use of surface markers to identify a subset of acute myelomonocytic leukaemia cells with progenitor cell properties. Blood 62: 1300-1303

98. Lange B, Ferrero D, Pessano S, Hubbell H, Palumbo A, Lai S K, Giovanni R 1984 Discrimination between normal hemopoietic stem cells and myeloid leukaemia cells using monoclonal antibodies. In: Lowenberg B, Hagenbeek A (eds) Minimal residual disease in acute leukaemia Martinus Nijhoff Publishers, p 55-65

99. Heatherington C M, Crawford D H, Blacklock P A, Leach G, Janossy G, Francis G E, Crawford T, Prentice H G 1981 Successful bone marrow transplantation with whole marrow and CFU-C depleted marrow in the Marmoset (Callithrix Jacchus). Bone Marrow Transplantation in Europe Vol III Touraine J L, Gluckman E, Griscelli C (eds) Excepta Medica Amsterdam, Oxford, Princeton, p 274-279

100. Fialkow P J, Singer J W, Adamson J W, Vaidya K, Dow L W, Odis J, Moohr J W 1981 Acute non-lymphocytic leukaemia: heterogeneity of stem cell origin. Blood 57: 1068-1073

101. Griffin J D, Beveridge R P, Schlossman S F 1982 Isolation of myeloid progenitor cells from peripheral blood of chronic myelogenous leukaemia patients. Blood 60: 30-37

102. Griffin J D, Sullivan R, Beveridge R P, Schlossman S F 1984 Induction of proliferation of purified human myeloid progenitor cells: a rapid assay for granulocyte and monocyte colony stimulating factors. Blood 63: 904-911

103. Linch D C, Nathan D G 1984 T cell and monocyte-derived burst promoting activity directly act on erythroid progenitor cells. Nature 312: 775-777

11

Clinical and biological studies with monoclonal antibodies

P. C. L. Beverley

INTRODUCTION

In the 9 years since Kohler & Milstein[1] published their procedure for derivation of specific monoclonal antibodies (Mabs) by the hybridization of antibody secreting cells to a myeloma cell line, it has provided reagents for investigations in almost every field of biology. Probably because it was developed by immunologists, cells of the haemopoietic system were among the first immunogens and a very large number of antibodies reacting with them have been produced[2]. In addition haemopoietic cells are readily available and amenable to study with serological methods such as immunofluorescence or complement mediated lysis, unlike cells of most other tissues which cannot easily be obtained in single cell suspension. Progress in applying Mabs to haematological problems has therefore been rapid. Methods developed for using Mabs to study the haemopoietic system are now being applied to other tissues and can be expected to yield a great deal of information on the processes of differentiation, of cellular function and malignant transformation in non-haemopoietic cells, as they have in the haemopoietic system.

In this chapter I shall not consider in any detail the technical advances which have contributed so greatly to understanding of the haemopoietic system since these are covered extensively in other chapters. Instead I shall discuss areas in which Mabs have been applied to gain new insight into cellular and molecular function within the haemopoietic system. In the long term it is this understanding of cellular and molecular function which will lead to the development of major new forms of therapy but in the short terms Mabs are also being used as diagnostic and therapeutic agents. Some examples of these more practical uses will be discussed but it is a principal theme of this chapter that while the first use of new Mabs has often been in the identification and separation of different cell types, in the longer term their main importance is in providing reagents which identify individual molecules. Mabs can be used to isolate them, to study their distribution but above all to investigate their function.

In this chapter I shall adopt the terminology of the first[2] and second international workshops on human leukocyte differentiation antigens in which large panels of Mabs were used to study a wide variety of cell types. The reactivities of the sera were studied by cluster analysis and Mabs reacting similarly grouped together to identify clusters of differentiation (CD). Immunochemical analysis has provided additional evidence for the reality of these clusters by showing that antibodies which cluster together on serological analysis also immunoprecipitate identical molecules. Table

11.1 shows the old and new terminologies for T-cell antigens. The CD terminology has the advantage that it does not imply that antigens are cell type or lineage specific but merely gives the cell type in which expression is most obvious. This has become more relevant as with increasing study fewer and fewer antigens appear to be completely restricted in expression to a single cell type.

THE FUNCTION OF T-CELL SURFACE MOLECULES

T-cell receptors and activation

Because the surface antigens of human thymus derived (T) lymphocytes have been particularly well studied I shall discuss these most extensively to illustrate the uses of monoclonal antibodies.

Monoclonal antibodies have made an important contribution to the resolution of one of the major problems of immunology, the nature of the T-cell receptor for antigen and mechanisms of activation of T-lymphocytes. It has become clear that the initial signal is delivered by antigen via a complex of surface glycoproteins consisting of idiotype bearing molecules associated with the non-polymorphic component CD3. Historically CD3 was identified first and the sequence of studies of this molecule illustrate the ways in which monoclonal antibodies have been utilised.

The first anti-CD3 antibody, OKT3[3], was derived during attempts to produce antibodies which distinguish T-cell subsets. The procedure was the commonly employed 'shotgun' method. Thus mice were immunized with human T-cells and supernatants of hybrids were screened on T- and non-T-cells. More extensive testing on lymphoid cells and cell lines was used to confirm the initial results. Antibodies derived in this fashion were then used to separate antigen positive and negative cells for functional studies. CD3 positive cells were shown to function in a fashion very similar to E rosette forming cells. They could respond to mitogens, provide help for pokeweed mitogen driven immunoglobulin synthesis and included cytotoxic and mixed lymphocyte culture responding T-cells[4,5]. Studies with other anti-CD3 antibodies have amply confirmed these initial results while revealing additional details. We have shown for example that CD3 is not detectable on all cells

Table 11.1 Terminology for human T-cell antigens

New terminology	Old name	Reactivity	Typical antibodies
CD1 (Thy, gp45, 12)*	T6	Cortical Thymocytes	NA1/34, OKT6
CD2 (T, gp50)	T11	E receptor	9.6, OKT11, Leu5
CD3 (T, gp19–29)	T3	Pan T	OKT3, UCHT1
CD4 (T, gp55)	T4	Helper/Inducer	OKT4, Leu3a
CD5 (T, gp67)	T1	Pan T + B CLL	OKT1, UCHT2, Leu1
CD6 (T, gp120)	T12	Pan T	Tu33, MBG6
CD7 (T, gp41)	—	Pan T	3A1, Leu9
CD8 (T, gp32)	T8	Suppressor/cytotoxic	OKT8, Leu2a, UCHT4
CD25 (T, gp55)	Tac	IL2 receptor	anti-Tac
CD26 (T, gp120)	—	T activation	T1119-4-7, 4ELIC7

*CD stands for Cluster of Differentiation. The following letters and numbers in brackets indicate first the main cell type displaying the antigen (e.g. T for thymus derived lymphocytes), second the nature of the antigen (gp indicates glycoprotein) and third the approximate molecular weight in kilo daltons.

which can form E rosettes[6]. While E+ CD3+ cells function as T-cells in several assays including the provision of help for a specific antibody response, the E+ CD3- cells (5–10% of E+ cells) are inactive in assays of T-cell function. These cells have the characteristic large granular lymphocyte morphology of natural killer (NK) cells and indeed have high NK activity in vitro[6]. Expression of CD3 antigen thus seems to be highly correlated with functional T-cell activity. Similarly the acquisition of maturity in the T-cell lineage is associated with expression of CD3, thymocytes and immature T-cell tumours (Thy-ALL) showing low CD3 expression while peripheral T-cells and mature T-cell tumours (T-CLL, Sezary cells) shows high expression[7]. Additional support for the close correlation between CD3 expression and T-cell function was provided by immunohistological studies. In lymphoid tissues CD3 positive cells are localized predominantly in the paracortical zones while only a few positive cells are seen within follicles. The thymus contains mainly antigen positive cells with the strongest staining seen in the medulla[8].

Thus the early data on CD3 firmly associated expression of the antigen with T-cell function but this association was not unique since antibodies to the CD5 antigen and to CD2 (the E rosette receptor) gave very similar results. Progress in understanding the role of CD3 came from the use of the monoclonal antibodies in two further types of study. These are interference with cell function and biochemical characterisation of the molecule. While both aspects have progressed further in the case of CD3 than for many other monoclonal antibody defined molecules, the studies of CD3 illustrate general principles in the application of monoclonal antibodies and will therefore be considered in some detail.

Anti-CD3 antibodies were early on shown to have two, at first sight, paradoxical effects on the function of T-lymphocytes. These were that on the one hand they were powerful mitogens[9,10] and on the other that they could block T-cell responses including the mixed lymphocyte reaction, proliferative responses to soluble antigens and T-cell mediated cytotoxicity[10-13]. The interpretation of the inhibition of a proliferative response to soluble antigens or alloantigens is unclear when the inhibiting agent is itself a mitogen since the peak proliferative response to soluble or alloantigens are measured at 6–7 days. Thus it is likely that anti-CD3 'pre-empts' the proliferative response so that cell division has returned to the baseline level by day 6–7. Obviously similar arguments do not apply to the blocking of cytotoxicity since this is a short term (4–6 hour) assay. On this somewhat ambiguous evidence it was proposed that anti-CD3 might recognize a component of the T-cell receptor[11]. Whether or not this might be the case remains to be proved but clearly a reagent defining a molecule associated with the proliferative and other functions of T-cells was likely to be a useful probe for understanding immunoregulation. Subsequent studies have borne this out, particularly the elegant work of the Boston group on T-cell clones.

A problem of the earlier studies using anti-CD3 (and other monoclonal antibodies) was the heterogeneity of the cell population employed. Since anti-CD3 binds to all T-cells the functional outcome might be the net effect of activating or inhibiting several different T-cell types. The use of T-cell clones responding to alloantigens overcomes these problems though it should be borne in mind that interleukin-2 (IL2) dependent T-cells must be maintained consistently in a partially activated state (always expressing IL2 receptors for example). Thus experiments performed on these cells may not be informative with respect to the processes of activation or regulation of resting small lymphocytes.

In their studies of cytotoxic T-cell clones, Reinherz, Schlossman and their colleagues investigated the effects of antibodies to several T-cell antigens CD2, CD3, CD4, CD5, CD8 etc. as well as raising antibodies to clone specific antigens (anti-clonotypes). The principal findings of these studies can be summarized as follows. Both anti-clonotype and anti-CD3 inhibit T-cell cytotoxicity when added directly to the assay[14]. Furthermore these molecules were shown to be associated at the cell surface by co-modulation experiments[15], thus cells exposed overnight to anti-clonotype or anti-CD3 and then examined by indirect immunofluorescence for the presence of either molecule have lost both. Cells pre-treated with either antibody in this way are also unable to kill allogeneic target cells nor can they respond to alloantigen by proliferation but they remain perfectly well able to proliferate in response to IL2.

Analogous results were obtained with influenza virus haemagglutinin specific clones in that pre-exposure to anti-CD3 led to loss of responsiveness to antigen presented by accessory cells. In addition these experiments provided direct evidence that CD3 was associated with the antigen binding T-cell receptor (Ti) since pre-exposure of the T-cells to a high dose of their specific antigen, a 24 amino acid haemagglutinin peptide, led both to loss of surface CD3 antigen and induction of unresponsiveness to specific antigen. As for alloantigen responding T-cells the influenza specific cells retained responsiveness to IL2[16].

These experiments thus imply that the T-cells receptor and CD3 are associated at the cell surface although the exact nature of the association is yet not clear nor is the role of CD3. That anti-CD3 antibodies are mitogenic implies however that CD3 may be important in transmission of signals across the cell membrane. In order to clarify the role of CD3 in T-cell activation we have studied one of the earliest events in cell activation using the calcium sensitive dye Quin 2. We have shown that the mitogenic lectins phytohaemagglutinin (PHA) and concanavalin A (Con A) can induce a rapid rise of intracellular free calcium concentration (Ca^{2+}) in human T-lymphocytes. The anti-CD3 antibodies UCHT1, Leu 4 and WT-32 produced a similar change[17,18]. Interestingly the antibody WT-31 which is thought to identify a determinant on the constant portion of the T-cell receptor[19], was unable to stimulate the mobilization of Ca^{2+} in resting peripheral blood T-cells. WT-31 is nevertheless mitogenic for T-cells.

Intriguingly the effect of WT-31 was not the same on all T-cells since although it could not trigger directly IL2 dependent T-cell clones or lines, when these were pretreated with WT-31 the response to subsequent stimulation with UCHT1 was more rapid. Similarly WT-31 could trigger directly a response in some T-cell tumour lines[18]. The interpretation of results with WT-31 antibody is complicated by the finding that antibodies to clonotypic determinants can trigger strongly a rise in $(Ca^{2+})i$ in the T-ALL line HPB-ALL while WT-31 has only a very weak effect on the same tumour cells[20]. Since the epitopes identified by WT-31 and anti-clonotypic antibodies are mostly likely both on the polypeptide chains of Ti these data suggest that while antibodies to particular epitopes may initiate mobilisation of Ca^{2+} others do so less effectively. If interaction between Ti and CD3 is required for transmission of signals delivered to Ti (see below) it may be that some anti-Ti Mabs interfere with signal transmission by steric hindrance. In any case these data suggest that the relationship of the receptor and CD3 may vary in T-cells at different stages of differentiation or activation and that activated T-cells may be more readily triggered to mobilise Ca^{2+}. On the other hand it is clear that a rise in $(Ca^{2+})i$ is not sufficient to induce cell division since while peripheral blood T-cells of all individuals tested showed a change in $(Ca^{2+})i$ on stimulation with UCHT1, approximately a quarter failed to respond in proliferation assays[18]. This non-responsiveness to IgG_1 mouse Mabs to CD3 has been shown to be due to a polymorphism of accessory cell Fc receptors. Non-responder monocytes failed to bind mouse IgG_1[21]. It has therefore been suggested that immobilisation of surface CD3 or Ti by crosslinking may be a pre-requisite for T-cell triggering[21]. This suggestion is supported by the finding that IgG_1 anti-CD3 antibodies on sepharose beads will trigger a mitogenic response in non-responder T-cells or in T-cell clones which are rendered unresponsive by soluble anti-CD3[21,22].

In sum the data suggest that binding of ligands to CD3 or Ti can trigger a rise in $(Ca^{2+})i$. While we have as yet investigated the effects of few ligands which bind directly to the T-cell receptor the data are consistent with the view that signals delivered via this receptor are transmitted via CD3. Biochemical data (see below) suggest that CD3 and the T-cell receptor are associated but the exact nature of this complex is not yet clear, nor is the relationship of other cell surface antigens to the CD3– receptor complex. Nevertheless monoclonal antibodies to several other cell antigens also affect T-cell function and the possible roles of these will be considered in the next section.

Surface antigens and T-cell function

The sheep red blood cell receptor. While the data discussed in the previous section firmly link the CD3-T receptor complex to recognition and triggering of T-lymphocytes by antigen, CD3 is by no means the only surface component implicated in these processes. In this section therefore I shall discuss the role of other surface components. In all cases the evidence for the role of particular antigens derives from studies similar to those detailed above for CD3. Thus antibodies derived usually from 'shotgun' immunizations and generally with a cell and tissue distribution limited to haemopoietic organs, have been tested for their effect in a variety of lymphocyte function assays. Several types of monoclonal antibody consistently block various T-cell functions but so far only anti-CD3/Ti and anti-CD2 Mabs have been shown to be stimulatory.

A number of studies of the effect of antibodies to the sheep red blood cell (E) receptor (anti-CD2) have shown that these can block proliferative responses to mitogens, alloantigens and soluble antigens as well as T-cell mediated cytotoxicity[23,25]. This led to suggestions that CD2 antigen delivered only an 'off' signal to cells. Recent data however shows as with Ti the situation may be more complex. Most of the earlier anti-CD2 Mabs defined an antigen of 55 kd and could block the binding of sheep red cells to T-cells[26] however it became clear that several epitopes on the molecule could be distinguished[25,27]. Recently Meuer and his colleagues[28] have shown that two anti-CD2 Mabs, which do not block E rosette formation and define new epitopes ($T11_2$ and $T11_3$), when used in combination are strongly mitogenic. Interestingly the $T11_3$ epitope is not detectable on resting T-cells but rapidly appears following stimulation with PHA, suggesting that ligand binding to CD2 may alter the orientation of the molecule in the membrane. That PHA binds to CD2 and may indeed activate cells via CD2 is strongly suggested by experiments showing that treatment of T-cells with anti-CD2 can prevent subsequent mobilization of Ca^{2+} by PHA but the response to anti-CD3 is unaffected[29]. Conventional anti-CD2 antibodies do not themselves trigger a rise in $(Ca^{2+})i$ but the combination of anti-T11$_2$ and T11$_3$ does so (Reinherz personal communication) suggesting that calcium mobilization is an early event in the activation either via CD2 or CD3.

Other functionally important molecules

Five groups of antibodies (Table 11.2) are able consistently to block responses both of resting and activated T-cells. While anti-CD4, CD8, CD2 and LFA-1 antibodies all block proliferative responses stimulated by alloantigens, and anti-CD2 and LFA-1 also to soluble antigens[23-24,30-31], interpretation of these data is made difficult because of the length of incubation required and the complex series of cellular interactions involved in these responses. Furthermore recent data suggests that some antibodies to cell surface components may form soluble immune complexes which profoundly modulate accessory cell and hence T-cell function[21]. Thus interpretation of the data from short term assays is easier and much information has been obtained using T-cell cytolysis especially with cloned IL2 dependent populations of effector cells and homogeneous target cells.

The results of these studies show that anti-T monoclonal antibodies inhibit cytotoxicity at different stages of the process. In single cell assays where it is possible to isolate target binding and lytic steps anti-CD3[32] does not prevent target binding whereas anti-CD4 or CD8 do. Anti-LFA-1 also appears to inhibit target binding[33] while it is not known at what stage anti-CD2 is effective. Thus in this system anti-CD3 appears to block signal transmission although whether this is because the T-cell has been triggered by binding of anti-CD3 prior to encountering a target cell and is therefore refractory to further stimulation, remains unclear. Since the other antibodies block at the stage of target cell recognition it is possible that these molecules are receptors for antigens on other cell types.

The CD4 and CD8 antigens are mutually exclusive on peripheral T-cells and CD4+ and CD8+ cells have been designated 'helper/inducer' or 'suppressor/

Table 11.2 Blocking of function by anti-T cell Mabs

| Target antigen | Proliferation induced by | | Soluble antigen | Cell-mediated cytotoxicity |
	Mitogens	Alloantigens		
CD2	+[1]	+[1]	+[1]	+
CD3	mitogenic	+	+	+
CD4	–	+[2]	–	+[2]
CD8	–	+[2]	–	+[2]
LFA-1	+	+	+	+

+indicates blocking of function and – no blocking. [1]Conventional anti-CD2 Mabs block but certain combinations of anti-CD2 Mabs are mitogenic (see text). [2]Anti-CD4 and CD8 block responses to MHC class II and class I molecules respectively.

cytotoxic' on the basis of in vitro data[34]. In the mouse it was shown that Lyt2+ (homologous to CD8) cells recognised MHC Class I[35]. A number of authors have obtained data in man which supports the view that most CD4+ CTL are directed at MHC Class II leading to the suggestion that the CD8 molecule might recognise Class I antigens and CD4 Class II[36]. Direct evidence for this is lacking and several human and mouse clones have now been described which do not fit this hypothesis. Nevertheless it remains the case that CD8+ (Lyt2+) cells are biased toward recognition of MHC Class I and CD4+ (Lyt2-) cells to MHC Class II. The overall frequency of the exceptional clones in the repertoire of T-cells remains uncertain.

While anti-CD4 and CD8 identify molecules which seem associated in some way with recognition of MHC antigens and the function of the responding T-cells the role of the glycoproteins identified by anti-CD2 and LFA-1 antibodies is less clear. Antibodies to these molecules inhibit cytotoxicity of both CD4 and CD8+ cells and LFA-1 at least appears to be involved in the adherence of the cytolytic cells to their targets.

The data on T-cell recognition discussed above provides evidence for multiple interactions between T-cells and their targets. Overwhelming evidence favours the view that T-cells always 'see' antigen in association with self MHC molecules[37] (genetic restriction) and increasing evidence suggests that the exogenous antigen may be a small fragment perhaps processed by accessory cells[38,39]. The undoubted favourite as the recognition unit for such antigen-MHC complexes is the clonotypic structures associated with CD3 and indeed evidence from gene cloning studies strongly suggests that this molecule is a highly variable dimeric structure with obvious homology to immunoglobulin although not belonging to any of the known immunoglobulin gene families[40,41]. If the clonotypic structure recognizes antigen-MHC the role of CD4 and CD8 is less clear but these molecules could form low affinity interactions with MHC I and II antigens which help to stabilize the cell–cell interaction. LFA-1 may be a member of a family of molecules which also mediate cell–cell contacts. If the affinity of the T-cell receptor for antigen is high the other interactions of CD4 or CD8 and LFA-1 may be less important whereas with low affinity antigen receptors other interactions may be essential for triggering of T-cell functions. Experimental evidence supports such a concept since T-cell clones are markedly heterogeneous in their susceptibility to inhibition by anti-CD4 or 8[42]. Less easy to interpret however, is the heterogeneity in susceptibility to inhibition by anti-CD3 since this molecule does not appear to be directly involved in contact between the T-cell and its target.

Once adhesion and antigen specific recognition has occurred, the signal for activation of the T-cell to cell division or other functional activities appears to be transmitted via CD3. It should be borne in mind that for some of these processes further signals may be required. These are not necessarily mediated by cell–cell contact and often involve soluble mediators such as IL1 and IL2.

The foregoing discussion has made the simplistic assumption that the effects of monoclonal antibodies on short term assays are generally due to the direct effect of bound antibody in preventing binding of ligands to a surface antigen. This may not of course always be the case. Antibodies may have many other effects including triggering inhibition processes, preventing formation of multimolecular complexes in the cell membrane, modulation of antigens from the surface and triggering of cellular processes leading to a subsequent refractory state. Elucidation of the mechanism by which an antibody mediates its effect can only come about by a combination of the cell biological approaches discussed above and biochemical studies discussed in the following section.

BIOCHEMISTRY OF T-CELL ANTIGENS

Monoclonal antibodies have provided powerful tools for characterisation of molecules shown to play a role in functional assays. Initial fears that monoclonal antibodies might often have too low affinity or be poor in forming lattices so that they would fail to immunoprecipitate have not been borne out. Thus all of the antibodies discussed in the previous section have been used to precipitate from isotope labelled cells their target antigens which can then be separated by SDS PAGE. Table 11.3 summarizes published information.

The analysis of the structures precipitated by antibodies to the CD3-receptor complex is of particular interest in view of the extensive functional studies carried out with antibodies to this complex. There remain at present some difficulties in integrating all the data from different laboratories but there is agreement in at least some important areas. While the earliest studies with OKT3 antibody showed a single band only 19 kDa molecular weight, subsequent studies have revealed much greater complexity. The antigen precipitated from[125]I surface labelled cells has a prominent band of 19–20 kDa and further bands variously described as 23 and 26 kDa[43] or 25–28 kDa[44]. Studies using the inhibitor of N-glycosylation tunicamycin and digestion with the enzymes. Endo-H and Endo-F which remove respectively high mannose (immature) and complex (mature) N-linked sugars reveal further complexity. In the presence of tunicamycin anti-CD3 precipitates contain mainly a 19–20 kDa form with a weaker band at 16 kDa Endo-H and Endo-F digestions of anti-CD3 precipitates suggest that at least a part of the 19–20 kDa band has no N-linked sugar while the 21 kDa band has both mature and immature N-linked sugars and the 26 kDa band only mature sugars[43]. Endo-F digestion yields the 19–21 kDa bands and two polypeptides of 14 and 16 kDa.

Additional experiments using proteinase-K digestion of microsomal CD3 provide evidence that all of the major CD3 polypeptides have a transmembrane orientation with a cytoplasmic tail[43] and that the 19–20 kDa peptide which lacks N-linked sugars is predominantly an intramembrane protein since it can be labelled with hydrophobic reagents[44] (Kanellopoulos & Crumpton personal communication). The final observation which needs to be taken into account when building models to represent the CD3 structure is that immunoprecipitates with anti-CD3 monoclonal

Table 11.3 Biochemistry of T-cell surface antigens

Antigen	Molecular weight	Special features
CD2	50 kDa	Multiple epitopes, some only detected after activation
CD3	20, 25–28 kDa	Two 20 kDa chains, one glycosylated and one intra membrane
CD4	55 kDa	Several variants lacking Mab defined epitopes
CD8	32 kDa	Forms homopolymers in the cell surface
LFA-1	95, 160 kDa	Invariant 95 kDa chain associates with several 160 kDa chains

antibodies commonly contain additional higher molecular weight bands[19,43,44]. The intensity of these varies depending on the antibody used, the method of labelling, the cell type used and the technical details of the gel system but their consistent presence and absence from control precipitates strongly implies an association with CD3. These higher molecular weight polypeptides of molecular weights 37–41 and 44–53 kDa almost certainly represent the α and β chains of the T-cell receptor as identical polypeptides can be precipitated by anti-clonotypic antibodies[14]. The antibody WT-31, which shares many properties with anti-CD3 antibodies, precipitates predominantly 37 and/or 44 kDa bands but both this antibody and anti-clonotypes sometimes reveal weak 20 kDa (CD3) bands[29]. The data therefore suggest a rather variable association of the various CD3 and receptor polypeptides, a conclusion supported by the polydisperse nature of CD3 analysed by gel filtration in detergent (Kanellopoulos & Crumpton personal communication). Figure 11.1 illustrates possible models for assembly of CD3-receptor complexes.

By comparison with CD3 the other antigens in Table 11.3 present far fewer problems of interpretation in immunoprecipitation analysis. Antibodies to CD4 and CD2 identify glycoproteins of molecular weight 55 and 50 kDa respectively. Since reduction has no effect it appears that these molecules consist of a single polypeptide chain[25,26,45]. In contrast both CD8 and LFA-1 are multimeric proteins. The basic unit of the CD8 antigen appears to be a polypeptide of 32 kDa[19,46] which is seen under reducing conditions. When non-reduced gels are run a series of multimers are detectable of which the most obvious are bands of 67 and 76 kDa although higher molecular weight species are also seen. It has been suggested that some of the heterogeneity of apparent molecular weight may be due to differences in internal disulphide bonding[46]. An interesting feature of the CD8 antigen is the strong structural similarity between this antigen and the Lyt2,3 antigens of mice[45]. Recently also a mouse homologue of the CD4 antigen has been identified[47]. So far structural analysis of these antigens has not advanced sufficiently far to provide clues to their function but monoclonal antibodies have provided reliable tools for identification of the molecules. Leucocyte function antigens have been described in both mouse and man[24,33]. The antigens consist of heterodimers of 95 and 160 kDa.

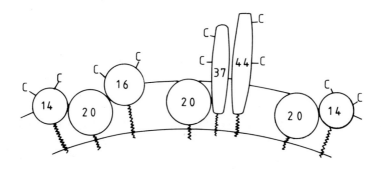

Fig. 11.1 Model for the structure of CD3-Tull receptor complexes.

FUNCTION OF MOLECULAR DOMAINS

The foregoing sections have attempted to convey how monoclonal antibodies have been used to define subsets of cells, to interfere with the function of cells and to identify the molecular structures involved in these functions. While these studies have defined molecular structures important in T-cell recognition and activation and allowed an initial biochemical analysis, there is as yet little data defining the way in which the molecules function. Although much information will no doubt come from sequence analysis of the molecules, as has been the case for the T-cell receptor[40,41], monoclonal antibodies have an important role to play in strategies for further analysis of molecular function.

The simplest method for attempting to dissect the function of different domains is to raise families of antibodies against a single molecule. This strategy has been applied to the sheep red cell receptor (CD2). Interestingly in deriving six new anti-CD2 antibodies no attempt was made to purify the molecule but the authors relied on immunisation with whole cells and screening to select anti-CD2 antibodies. Of 1369 growing clones, 452 secreted antibody reactive with the immunizing cells and 72 did not react with a B lymphobastoid line homologous to the immunizing T-cell. Six of the 72 T specific antibodies proved to react with the 50 kDa E rosette receptor defining at least three different epitopes on the molecule[28]. Antibodies to these three epitopes have distinct functional effects (see above) but since the sequence and three dimensional structure of CD2 are as yet unknown, these effects cannot yet be related to structural features of the molecule.

In the case of other T-cell surface molecules the shotgun approach to immunization, screening and identification of antisera has yielded less interesting data. Although evidence presented at the first international workshop on leucocyte differentiation antigens[2] indicated that the anti-CD8 and anti-CD5 antibodies submitted, detected multiple epitopes on their target molecules, the functional effects of most anti-CD8 or CD5 antibodies are similar. In the case of anti-CD3 all current anti-CD3 antibodies appear to have similar effects other than in accessory cell dependent proliferative assays. This is in spite of the fact that there is some evidence that more than one CD3 epitope is recognized[48] although existing sera may all react with the 20 kDa glycosylated chain (Terhorst personal communication). The conclusion that only this chain is functionally important is weakened by the lack of antibodies to other parts of the complex, a lack which highlights the weakness of the shotgun approach. In the case of some or perhaps many molecules, particular epitopes or domains may be immunodominant so that raising antibodies to other regions of the molecule may be difficult. Several strategies are being attempted to circumvent this problem. These include the use of plasma membrane fractions rather than whole cells, detergent solubilized membrane glycoproteins and in a more directed approach immunization with synthetic peptides.

The last obviously requires a knowledge of the protein sequence derived either from direct protein sequencing or gene cloning. While this approach has as yet been little used in the analysis of surface antigen function, synthetic peptides can be used to raise antibodies and identify functionally important domains of molecules as for example has been shown by studies of the influenza virus haemagglutinin molecule[49].

An important part of further analysis of molecular structure is the derivation of the amino acid sequence and monoclonal antibodies may play an important role in gene cloning procedures. An approach which relies on antibodies is the transfection of human genes into mouse L-cells and their detection in the transfected cells. High molecular weight fragments of human DNA are mixed with herpes virus derived DNA coding for the enzyme thymidine kinase (TK) and the mixture is introduced into TK- mouse fibroblasts (L-cells) by calcium phosphate precipitation[50]. The L-cells are then grown in selective medium so that only those cells which have taken up DNA (including TK genes) will survive. Since expression of any given gene in L-cells is a rare event, selection of the desired transfectant is necessary. This has been achieved by fluorescence activated cell sorting of cells stained with an antibody to the desired antigen. After two or more cell sorts antigen positive cells are usually sufficiently enriched to be able to clone the antigen positive cell population[50]. The antigen expressing cells can be used in a variety of ways. The first is the analysis of the transfected molecule in the absence of other human genes. Mouse L-cells expressing human Class I genes have been used in this way to show that lysis by human allocytotoxic T-cells requires not only expression of the target MHC Class I antigens but that other gene products are required on the target cells[51]. These may perhaps be molecules which can bind to those molecules such as CD8, CD2 and LFA-1 which have been shown to be important in the interaction of cytotoxic T-cells and their targets.

A second use of the transfected cells is in the cloning of the transfected human genes. Genes for the human molecule inserted by transfection can be recovered by hybridization of DNA from the mouse cells to a probe for human repeat sequences and then cloned in a conventional vector for subsequent sequencing. Alternatively, and especially if the transfected gene is amplified, it may be possible to clone it by subtraction. In this case cDNA from the transfected L-cells is hybridized to RNA of normal cells to remove all mouse genes. The resulting human enriched cDNA probe is then used to pull out clones from a library prepared from the transfected L-cells. These can then be sequenced[52].

Further manipulations of transfected and cloned molecules are possible either by inserting specific amino acid changes by site directed mutation[53] or by making hybrid molecules consisting of domains from two different molecules as has already been achieved for MHC antigens[54]. It is to be expected that these genetic engineering techniques will be very powerful in the analysis of the structure–function relationships of many of the T-cell antigens discussed above.

B LYMPHOCYTE ANTIGENS

Until recently B lymphocytes have been defined almost solely by their expression of surface immunoglobulin. Recently however, many Mabs defining B-cell associated antigens have been produced. The analysis of the structure and function of these molecules has not yet progressed so far as with T-cell antigens but a serological study performed as part of the second international workshop on human leucocyte differentiation antigens has produced an initial classification of B-cell antigens (Table 11.4). While the clusters of differentiation defined might only represent molecules which were particularly immunogenic in the mouse, experience with T-cell antigens suggest that this is not the case and that CD antigens are identified in screening after 'shotgun' immunization because they are lineage restricted and thus likely to be involved in lineage or cell type specific functions. Our own studies with the B-cell panel of sera from the workshop show that antibodies from three of the B-cell clusters (CD 19, 20 and 22) block the induction of immunoglobulin in both the CESS B lymphoblastoid line[55] and CLL or PLL cells[56]. In agreement with others[57] we also found that antibodies to CD 20 could activate B-cells. Thus it appears that antibodies to at least some non-Ig B-cell surface antigens can have profound effects on B-cell growth and differentiation in man as in the mouse (see Ch. 8).

Antibodies to well characterized B-cell associated antigens will also be important in understanding B-cell ontogeny and heterogeneity. While data from the mouse suggests that B-cell subsets with different functions may exist, this remains unproven. Phenotypic analysis of developing lymphoid organs[58] and of the in vitro function of B-cell subsets separated according to surface phenotype[59] will provide data to examine the nature of B-cell heterogeneity.

The development of well characterized anti-B-cell reagents is also potentially important both for diagnosis and therapy. The rational classification of lymphomas remains difficult and may be improved by the use of a panel of Mabs against well characterized B-cell antigens and the use of Mabs in the therapy of B-cell tumours is currently being explored (see below).

CURRENT CLINICAL USES OF MABS

In the first part of this chapter I have reviewed some aspects of the use of Mabs for analysis of the function of lymphocytes. It has been emphasized that Mabs are most useful not because they identify cells but because they identify and can be used to purify molecules. In the long term it is understanding of molecular function that will lead to new forms of therapy. For the present however, Mabs are being applied to diagnostic and therapeutic problems mainly because they identify cells. In the second part of this chapter I shall not attempt to review comprehensively the clinical uses of Mabs many of which are discussed elsewhere in this book (see Chs. 5, 7, 10) but rather will attempt to highlight some advantages and limitations of their use.

Table 11.4 Human B-cell antigens

Designation	Molecular weight	Distribution	Typical antibodies
CD9	24 kDa	Pre-B-cells PMN, platelets	BA 2
CD10	100 kDa	CALLA, Pre-B-cells, PMN (weak)	J 5, VILAI
CD19	95 kDa	Pan B	B 4
CD20	35 kDa	Pan B	B 1
CD21	140 kDa	B subset EVB/complement receptor	B 2
CD22	135 kDa	B subset	HD6
CD23	45 kDa	Activated B-cells	Blast 2
CD24	45, 55, 65 kDa	Pan B + PMN	BA 1

IMMUNODIAGNOSIS

Introduction

Monoclonal antibodies have found two main roles in haematology. The first is the use of Mabs to enumerate subsets of normal lymphocytes in a variety of diseases, the second to refine the diagnosis and classification of leukaemias and lymphomas. Methods for these types of diagnostic procedures are given in detail elsewhere (chs. 5, 7). Here I wish only to discuss some general features of these types of study.

Analysis of cell suspensions

When monoclonal antibodies to lymphocyte subsets became available it rapidly became fashionable to 'phenotype' peripheral blood mononuclear cells. In the earlier studies much attention was focussed on T-cells and T-cell subsets. The data was commonly presented as a helper/suppressor ratio. This ratio was disturbed in a variety of disease states[60,61]. While correlations between disease activity and helper/suppressor ratio continue to be reported the interpretation of data presented in this way is unclear and based on an oversimple view of immunoregulation. Several factors need to be considered in extracting information from counts of peripheral blood subsets.

The first and most obvious is that the peripheral blood may not be representative of the state of the remainder of the lymphoid organs. While few studies have yet correlated phenotypic data from blood and lymphoid organs, functional analysis of cells from blood and spleen has shown that certain subsets may be poorly represented in the circulation[62]. Sweeping generalizations as to helper or suppressor functions based on analysis of peripheral blood lymphocytes only, are therefore best avoided. A related point is that when changes are seen in peripheral blood these may well be secondary effects. Since the frequency of cells responding to any single antigen, or complex of antigens such as a micro-organism, is low (<1%) this would be expected to have an undetectable effect even if only one subset of cells in peripheral blood was affected. Thus it is unlikely when gross changes in numbers of CD4 or CD8+ cells are seen that these cen be directly related to a specific immune response in most cases.

A second relatively trivial, but often overlooked, point is that helper/suppressor ratios often obscure the actual nature of subset disturbances. An example will make this point clear. In both infectious mononucleosis (IM)[63] and acquired immunodeficiency syndrome (AIDS)[64] there is commonly a helper/suppressor ratio of <1 but the cause differs in the two diseases. In IM there is an increase in the absolute number of suppressor (CD8+) cells while helper (CD4+) cells remain approximately normal. In contrast in AIDS the striking feature is a depletion in absolute numbers of CD4+ cells. Clearly in these two diseases the underlying disturbance leading to a reduced or inverted CD4/CD8 ratio is very different. This provides two lessons; the first is that more diagnostic information can be gained by measuring absolute numbers of cells. This has become increasingly simple using whole blood procedures and directly fluorochrome labelled Mabs so that losses or inadvertent selection for or against particular subsets during separation and staining procedures are less likely.

The second lesson is that understanding of the immunopathology of different diseases will only come from a careful identification of which cell type is disturbed and an understanding of its physiology. In IM and AIDS the disturbances seen in the peripheral blood become more interpretable in the light of data showing that an important component of the response to the Epstein-Barr Virus (EBV) is the generation of CD8+ cytotoxic T-cells[65] while in AIDS it has been shown that the causative virus, LAV or HTLV3, has a restricted tropism for CD4+ cells[66]. Thus in IM the rise in CD8+ cells may represent a host protective response to virus infection while in AIDS the depletion of CD4+ cells occurs because HTLV3 is a lytic virus which can only readily enter CD4+ cells. It is interesting that the tropism of HTLV3 appears to be closely correlated with expression of CD4 and our own studies using Mabs to block infection in vitro, strongly suggest that CD4 is the receptor for the virus[67].

In the examples given above it is possible to hypothesize as to the cause of the phenotypic change seen in peripheral blood and conversely identification of these particular changes may provide prognostic or diagnostic information (for example a depressed absolute number of CD4+ cells in a patient with lymphadenopathy would be suggestive of pre-AIDS). In most cases however, changes in phenotype are less easy to understand. In part this is because equating CD4 and CD8 expression with helper and suppressor function is a gross oversimplification. In vitro data while far from perfect shows that both the major populations can be further subdivided into functionally distinct subsets. In the case of CD4, Mabs have been described which can distinguish cells which provide help for antibody responses from those which induce suppression in CD8+ cells[68,69]. Among CD8+ cells, cytotoxic T-cells and suppressor cells may be distinguishable using the 9.3 antibody[70]. Further heterogeneity is also revealed by analysis at a single cell level using IL2 dependent T-cell clones[71].

Finally it is clear that quantitation of antigen expression may be important. We have noted that in some neutropenic patients there is an excess of CD8+ T-cells in peripheral blood and a striking feature of these cells is their low expression of CD5 (T1) antigen[72]. In this case it is likely that the cells represent an expansion of a subset of cells with this phenotype present in normal peripheral blood, but we have also noted in samples from patients with a variety of diseases that expression of many cell surface antigens is quantitatively abnormal (Terry & Beverley, unpublished observations). As yet the exact significance of these abnormalities remains undetermined but as the function of cell surface antigens is unravelled such abnormalities will become interpretable.

Analysis of frozen sections

Elegant immuno-enzymatic and immunofluorescence methods for analysis of frozen sectins or cell smears are described in chapter 7. Here I wish only to make some general comments on the use of these methods and the nature of the information they provide. Their principal use has been in the identification and classification of haematological malignancies but the success of the method in this context will depend ultimately in the reliability of Mabs for this task. If Mabs with specificity for tumour antigens existed, identification of malignant cells would be greatly simplified but so far no such antibodies have been produced. Existing Mabs identify differentiation antigens and the distinction between normal and malignant cells may often be difficult to make (for example in remission bone marrow samples).

Nevertheless Mabs have proved useful in several circumstances. One such is in identifying the origin of undifferentiated tumours. In this case antibodies to the leucocyte common antigen and to cytokeratins or to epithelial membrane antigens can usually identify the tumour cells as of haemopoietic or epithelial origin[73]. Further identification of the cell type of the haemopoietic tumours may be difficult. In a recent series, 17% of high grade lymphomas were devoid of cytoplasmic or surface immunoglobulin, however using a panel of antibodies against non-immunoglobulin T- and B-cell antigens all of these were shown to express antigens of one or other of the lineages[74].

This study illustrates the point that identification of tumour cells often requires the use of a panel of Mabs because tumours may have unusual phenotypes. This may be because abnormal combinations of genes are expressed following malignant transformation or because the tumours represent cells which are rarely found under normal circumstances. Both C-ALL and CLL have phenotypes which are examples of the latter.

Until now most Mabs have been used in haematology as convenient tools for identifying cells but as the functions of the molecules identified by the Mabs becomes better understood, it will be possible to catalogue the functionally active gene products of tumour cells. Some Mabs already identify molecules of known function of which the transferrin receptor is known to be related to cell cycle and thus is a marker for cell proliferation. In a study of lymphomas the percentage of transferrin receptor bearing cells was shown to correlate with prognosis[75]. Other markers associated with cell division may be expected to provide similar prognostic information. In the long term cataloguing active genes may provide information for logical therapeutic strategies designed to interfere preferentially with tumour cells.

IMMUNOTHERAPY

Introduction
It is not the intention of this section to represent a comprehensive review of immunotherapy with Mabs but rather to present the problems and possibilities. While at present results of both in vitro and in vivo forms of therapy are preliminary but encouraging, as with all new therapeutic agents much work remains to be done in defining the diseases most amenable to this form of treatment, the correct way in which to administer the agent, how Mabs can be combined with other forms of therapy and how to overcome the problems associated with their use.

In vitro therapy
Mabs are being used in two ways in vitro. The first is for the prevention of graft–versus–host (GVH) reactions in the treatment of a variety of haematological disorders by allogeneic bone marrow transplantation and the second is in the treatment of leukaemia by autologous bone marrow transplantation. The problems posed by these two forms of treatment differ and will be discussed separately.

Prevention of GVH disease
Extensive animal experimental data has shown that when bone marrow is transplanted into an irradiated major histocompatibility complex (MHC)

mismatched recipient, GVH disease results. In early attempts at human bone marrow transplantation the same result was obtained. In mice it was shown that GVH disease can be prevented by removal of T-lymphocytes from the transplanted marrow[76,77], so that it was an obvious approach to attempt to remove T-cells from human bone marrow prior to transplantation. The practical problems then, are to find a method for T-cell removal which ensures preservation of stem cells and can be simply used on the relatively large volume of bone marrow required to reconstitute adult graft recipients. Several methods using conventional heteroantisera or lectins[78] have been used in humans but monoclonal antibodies have the advantage of well defined specificity and reproducibility. Two main methods have been used for the T-cell removal step, complement mediated lysis and Mab-toxin conjugates. In both cases an essential step in development of the procedure is to show that treated bone marrow still has stem cells and this has been demonstrated by in vitro assays detecting myeloid, erythroid and mixed colony forming cells. While none of these assays may detect cells as early in the haemopoietic lineage as the murine spleen colony forming cell, in practice colony forming activity detected in vitro does seem to correlate with the ability of a marrow sample to repopulate a recipient. With the wide range of anti-T-cell Mabs now available it has not been difficult to select panels of antibodies which do not damage stem cells. Most groups have chosen to use mixtures of antibodies in order to maximize the anti-T-cell effects and experimental data supports the view that mixtures may indeed be more effective[79].

Complement mediated lysis. The use of Mabs with complement has the advantage of simplicity since no chemical manipulation of the antibodies is necessary but on the other hand its effectiveness is intimately related to the potency of the complement. The more conventional strategy for the use of complement has been to use mouse Mabs of complement fixing immunoglobulin subclasses and to combine these with an optimal source of complement. In practice rabbit complement has been found to be most active with the majority of mouse Mabs. It is usually necessary to screen to find active and non-toxic (to stem cells) batches. If this is done the method appears to be simple, safe and effective in depleting T-cells. The results of preliminary trials in leukaemic patients suggest that this is also an effective procedure for GVH prophylaxis[80].

An elegant alternative strategy has been to develop rat Mabs with an appropriate specificity for T-cell removal which fix human complement[81]. An antibody of this type Campath 1 is now under trial in several centres and the initial results are promising. This method obviates the problem of selection of rabbit complement batches since either donor or recipient serum can be used.

Monoclonal antibody-toxin conjugates. A variety of agents have been conjugated to Mabs for use as 'magic bullets'[82] but as yet few of these have been assessed in clinical therapy. The monoclonal anti-T-cell Mab anti-Thy-1 was however shown to be effective in preventing GVH disease in mice when coupled to Ricin and used for T-cell depletion[77]. This result has been followed up first by in vitro studies in man, when either single anti-T-cell Mab-toxin conjugates or a cocktail of these reagents were used to test the effectiveness of T-cell removal and toxic effects on stem cells[79]. Subsequent clinical studies have shown that the cocktail is safe and appears to be effective in GVH disease prophylaxis[83].

So far the majority of studies using T-cell removal have been carried out on HLA matched transplants and although the results are preliminary it is becoming clear that GVH disease can be almost eliminated. The potential for bone marrow transplantation would be greatly extended if mismatched transplants could be carried out. While the techniques discussed above may well be capable of preventing GVH disease in mismatched transplants, these present additional problems. Failure of engraftment following T-cell removal has been reported although the cause of this is unclear[84]. Whether full reconstitution of immune functions can be expected in adult mismatched grafts also remains doubtful.

Treatment of leukaemia by autologous bone marrow grafting

Autologous bone marrow grafts avoid the problem of GVH disease but present a different problem; how to distinguish between normal and leukaemic cells. Few if any Mabs detect tumour specific antigens so that in practical terms it is necessary to find Mabs which detect differentiation antigens present on the leukaemic population but not on stems cells necessary for engraftment. The issue is complicated by the fact that in many tumours the clonogenic cell may not be identical to the most readily detected tumour population. Chronic myeloid leukaemia provides the most obvious example of this phenomenon since it has been shown that the characteristic Philadelphia chromosome may be present in other cell lineages as well as very early myeloid precursors. In the blast phase differentiation becomes blocked and the early cells then become the predominant population[85]. In most forms of leukaemia the phenotype of the clonogenic cell has not been clearly identified so that present strategy generally aims at removal of the phenotypically leukaemic population with sparing of the (hopefully) normal stem cells. Obviously the more closely related to the stem cell is the clonogenic leukaemic cell, the more difficult the task.

In spite of these problems, treatment of common acute lymphoblastic leukaemia (cALL) has been attempted using an anti-CALLA Mab and complement with some success[86]. When relapse does occur in such patients it is impossible to establish whether this was due to failure to eliminate leukaemic cells from the re-infused bone marrow or from the patient. Comparison with allografted patients suggests but does not prove the latter[86]. Extension of this methodology to a wider spectrum of haematological malignancies, particularly lymphomas, will be dependent not only on finding appropriate Mabs, which may be relatively simple for 'mature' phenotype tumours, but also on finding treatments capable of eradicating disease from extramedullary sites.

In vivo therapy

The use of antibodies in vivo presents additional problems to those encountered in vitro (Table 11.5). In vivo the precise specificity is more important since both the presence of the target antigen on non-tumour cells or crossreactivity with other molecules could have unfortunate consequences. Both phenomena have been documented in the haemopoietic system. Many antibodies to B lymphocyte antigens react with renal tissue[2] and some anti-CD3 Mabs crossreact with cerebellar Purkinje neurones[48]. Such extra reactivities do not necessarily cause problems as anti-CALLA, which reacts with the kidney and UCHT1 (anti-CD3) have both been used in vivo without ill effects[87,88]. This may be because the renal or brain antigens were

Table 11.5 Problems and possibilities for Mabs in vivo

Problems	Possibilities
1. Specificity	
Are there tumour specific antigens?	Idiotypes of B and T-cells are tumour specific but absolute specificity may not be necessary
2. Fate of antibody in vivo	
Antibody class affects clearance	Use Fab or F (ab) fragments
Antibody class affects anti-tumour effectiveness	Use toxin drug or radioisotope conjugates
Selective toxicity due to R E clearance	Block R E system before antibody administration
Immune response to foreign Mabs	Induce tolerance to Ig
	Use human Mabs
3. Target antigens	
Modulation	Choose non-modulating antigens or use monovalent antibody
Antigen negative cells	Use cocktails of Mabs
Free antigen in circulation	Use cytoreductive therapy or plasmapheresis before Mab

inaccessible to antibody but it does suggest that the reactivity of any antibodies to be used in vivo should be carefully assessed.

Given that antibodies with sufficient specificity for a particular tumour type can be obtained are they likely to be effective as therapy? In experimental model systems antibodies can undoubtedly cause regression of tumours, although in the majority of experimental models very few tumour cells are used and antibody is given at or around the time of tumour grafting, a situation very different from that in tumour patients. Nevertheless antibody therapy has been attempted in man in both leukaemia and lymphoma. Several factors affect the outcome. First the target antigen must be available for antibody binding. This may not always be the case because the target cells may be inaccessible, although at least in one case lymph node lymphoma cells were shown by biopsy to be coated by administered antibody[89]. Alternately, the antigen may become unavailable because it is internalized or shed from cells in the presence of antibody (modulation). This has been shown to occur when anti-CALLA antibody was administered and can also be demonstrated in vitro[87]. Thus selection of target antigens on the basis of their behaviour in the presence of antibody may be necessary. A second factor which may be important in determining the outcome is the nature of the target antigen itself. One patient with a lymphoma was treated with a Mab to the idiotye of the tumour surface immunoglobulin and has had a prolonged complete remission[90]. The reason for the success of the treatment is not entirely clear but it is possible that the use of anti-idiotype can call into play powerful immunoregulatory, and in this case anti-tumour, effects[91]. Finally the immunoglobulin class may be important. Certainly in mice bearing human tumours, IgG_{2a} anti-tumour antibody was effective while other classes were not[92]. In man, at least in vitro, different Ig classes can have profoundly different effects. For example IgG_{2a} anti-CD3 antibodies are mitogenic for all individuals, IgG_1 for 60–80% of individuals and IgG_{2b} for very few[18,21]. It is likely therefore that the biological effects of these antibodies in vivo would be very different.

Because of the uncertainties attendant on using antibodies alone it is an attractive idea to use their specificity to deliver drugs, radioisotoes or toxin to tumours (reviewed in reference[82]). Clearly the use of such agents may confer therapeutic advantage but may also lead to selective toxic effects. Mab-toxin conjugates administered to mice for example are selectively sequestered and damage the reticulo-endothelial system[93]. While the development of stable conjugates with low non-specific toxicity is technically possible, much more needs to be known about how these enter cells since it is clear, as in the case of unconjugated antibodies, that not all antigens are equally good targets. In spite of these difficulties the striking therapeutic effects sometimes obtained in model systems[94] suggest that clinically useful reagents will be produced.

CONCLUSION

In this chapter I have reviewed briefly some current uses of Mabs in clinical haematology, and much more extensively their use in the investigation of the function of cells and molecules. This imbalance has been deliberate in that it is my conviction that understanding of molecular functions will lead to new and effective forms of therapy for many haematological diseases.

REFERENCES
1. Kohler G, Milstein C 1975 Continuous cultures of fused cells secreting antibody of predetermined specificity. Nature 256: 495–497
2. Bernard A, Boumsell L, Dausset J, Milstein C, Schlossman S F (eds) Leucocyte typing, Springer Verlag, Berlin
3. Kung P C, Goldstein G, Reinherz E, Schlossman S F 1979 Monoclonal antibodies during distinctive human T-cell surface antigens. Science 206: 347–349
4. Reinherz E L, Kung P C, Goldstein G, Schlossman S F 1979 A monoclonal antibody with selective reactivity with functionally mature thymocytes and all peripheral human T-cells. Journal of Immunology 123: 1312–1317
5. Reinherz E L, Schlossman S F 1980 The differentiation and function of human T-lymphocytes. Cell 19: 821–827
6. Beverley P C L, Callard R E 1981 Distinctive functional characteristics of human 'T' lymphocytes defined by E rosetting or a monoclonal anti-T-cell antibody. European Journal of Immunology 11: 329–334
7. Catovsky D C, Linch D C, Beverley P C L 1982 T-cell disorders in haematological disease. Clinics in Haematology 11: 661–695
8. Beverley P C L 1982 The application of monoclonal antibodies to the typing and isolation of lymphocreticular cells. Proceedings of the Royal Society of Edinburgh 816: 221–232
9. Van Wauve J, D Mey J, Gossens J 1980 OKT3: a monoclonal anti-human T-lymphocyte antibody with potent mitogenic properties. Journal of Immunology 124: 2708–2713
10. Burns G F, Boyd A W, Beverley P C L 1982 Two monoclonal anti-human T-lymphocyte antibodies have similar biologic effects and recognize the same cell surface antigen. Journal of Immunology 129: 1451–1458
11. Chang T W, Kung P C, Gingras P, Goldstein G 1981 Does OKT3 monoclonal antibody react with an antigen recognition structure on human T-cells. Proceedings of the National Academy of Sciences 78: 1805–1808
12. Reinherz E L, Hussey R E, Schlossman S F 1980 A monoclonal antibody blocking T-cell function European Journal of Immunology 10: 758–765
13. Spits H, Keizer G, Borst J, Terhorst C, Hekman A, de Vries J E 1983 Characterization of monoclonal antibodies against cell surface molecules associated with cytotoxic activity of natural and activated killer cells and cloned CTL lines Hybridoma 2: 423–437
14. Meuer S C, Acuto O, Hussey R E, Hodgson J C, Fitzgerald K A, Schlossman S F, Reinherz E L 1983 Evidence for the T3-associated heterodimer as the T-cell antigen receptor Nature 303: 808–810
15. Reinherz E L, Meuer S C, Fitzgerald K A, Hussey R E, Lavine H, Schlossman S F 1982 Antigen recognition by human T-lymphocytes is linked to surface expression of the T3 molecule complex. Cell 30: 735–745

16. Zanders E D, Lamb J R, Feldmann M, Green N, Beverley P C L 1983 Tolerance of T-cell clones is associated with membrane antigen changes. Nature 303: 625–627

17. O'Flynn K, Linch D C, Tathan P E R 1984 The effect of mitogenic lectins and monoclonal antibodies on intracellular tree calcium concentrations in human T-lymphocytes. Biochemical Journal 219: 661–666

18. O'Flynn K, Zanders E D, Lamb J R, Beverley P C L, Wallace D L, Tatham P E R, Tax W J M, Linch D C 1985 Investigation of early T-cell activation: analysis of the effect of specific antigen IL-2 and monoclonal antibodies on intracellular free calcium concentration. European Journal of Immunology 15: 7–11

19. Terhorst C 1984 Cell surface structures which are involved in human T-lymphocyte specific functions. Receptors and Recognition 16: (In press)

20. Beverley P C L, O'Flynn K, Wallace D L, Lamb J R, Boylston A W, Linch D C 1984 Regulation of activation and proliferation in T-cells. Proceedings of the Second International Workshop on Human Leucocyte Differentiation Antigens (In press)

21. Tax W J M, Hermes F F M, Willems R W, Capel P J A, Koene R A P 1984 Fc receptors for mouse IgG on human monocytes: polymorphism and role in antibody-induced T-cell proliferation Journal of Immunology 133: 1185–1190

22. Meuer S C, Hodgson J C, Hussey R E, Protentis J P, Schlossman S F, Reinherz E L 1983 Antigen like effects of monoclonal antibodies directed at receptors on human T-cell clones. Journal of Experimental Medicine 158: 988–993

23. Palacios R, Martinex-Maza D 1982 Is the E receptor on human T-lymphocytes a 'negative signal receptor'? Journal of Immunology 129: 2479–2485

24. Krensky A M, Sanchez-Madrid F, Robbins E, Nagy J A, Springer T A, Buraoff S J 1983 The functional significance, distribution and structure of LFA-1, LFA-2 and LFA-3: cell surface antigens associated with CTL target interactions. Journal of Immunology 131: 611–616

25. Martin P J, Longton G, Ledbetter J A, Newman W, Brann M P, Beatty P A, Hansen J A 1983 Identification and functional characterization of two distinct epitopes on the human T-cell surface proteiiin Tp50. Journal of Immunology 131: 180–185

26. Verbi W, Greaves M F, Schneider C, Koubek K, Janossy G, Stein H, Kung P, Goldstein G 1982 Monoclonal antibodies OKT11 and OKT11A have pan-T reactivity and block sheep erythrocyte receptors. European Journal of Immunology 12: 81–86

27. Bernard A, Gelin C, Raynal B, Pham D, Gosse C, Boumsell L 1982 Phenomenon of human T-cells rosetting with sheep erythrocytes analyzed with monoclonal antibodies. Journal of Experimental Medicine 155: 1317–1333

28. Meuer S C, Hussey R E, Fabbi M, Fox D, Acuto O, Fitzgerald K A, Hodgdon J C, Protentis J P, Schlossman S F, Reinherz E L 1984 An alternative pathway of T-cell activation: functional role for the 50kd T11 sheep erythrocyte receptor protein. Cell 36: 897–906

29. O'Flynn K, Krensky A M, Beverley P C L, Burakoff S J. Linch D C 1985 Phytohaemagglutinin activation of T cells through the sheep red blood cell receptor. Nature 313: 686–687

30. Hildreth J E K, Gotch F M, Hildreth P D K, McMichael A J 1982 A human lymphocyte function-associated antigen involved in cell mediated lympholysis. European Journal of Immunology 13: 202–208

31. Engelman E G, Benike C J. Glukman E, Evans R L 1981 Antibodies to membrane structures that distinguish suppressor/cytotoxic and helper T-lymphocyte subpopulations block the mixed leukocyte reaction in man. Journal of Experimental Medicine 153: 193–201

32. Landegren U, Ramstedt U, Axberg I, Ullberg M, Jondal M, Wigzell H 1982 Selective inhibition of human T-cell cytotoxicity at levels of target recognition or initiation of lysis by monoclonal OKT3 and Leu 2a antibodies. Journal of Experimental Medicine 155: 1579–1584

33. Pierres M, Gorides G, Goldstein P 1982 Inhibition of murine T-cell-mediated cytolysis and T-cell proliferation by rat monoclonal antibody immunoprecipitating two lymphoid cell surface polypeptides of 94 000 and 180 000 molecular weight. European Journal of Immunology 12: 60–69

34. Beverley P C L 1984 Hybridomas, monoclonal cells and the analysis of the immune system. British Medical Bulletin 40: 213–217

35. Swain S L 1981 Significance of Lyt phenotypes: Lyt-2 antibodies block activities of T-cells that recognize class I major histocompatibility complex antigens regardless of their function. Proceedings of the National Academy of Sciences 78: 7101–7108

36. Biddison W E, Rao P E, Talle M A, Goldstein G, Shaw S 1982 Possible involvement of the OKT4 molecule in T-cell recognition of Class II HLA antigens. Journal of Experimental Medicine 156: 1065–1076

37. Zinkernagel R M, Doherty P C 1975 H-2 compatability requirement for T-cell-mediated lysis of

target cells infected with lymphocytic choriomen-n ingitis virus. Different cytotoxic T-cell specificities are associated with structures coded for in H-2K of H-2D. Journal of Experimental Medicine 141: 1426–1438

38.   Lamb J R, Eckels D D, Lake P, Woody J N, Green N 1982 Human T-cell clones recognize chemically snthesized peptides of influenza haemagglutinin. Nature 300: 66–68

39.   Matis L A, Longo D L, Hedrick S M, Hannum C, Margoliash E, Schwartz R H 1873 Clonal analysis of the major histocompatability complex restriction and the fine specificity of antigen recognition in the T-cell proliferative response to cytochrome C. Journal of Immunology 130: 1527–1535

40.   Yanagi Y, Yoshika Y, Leggett K, Clark S P, Aleksander I, Mak T W 1984 A human T-cell specific cDNA clone encodes a protein having extensive homology to immunoglobulin chains. Nature 308: 145–148

41.   Hedrick S M, Cohen D I, Nielsen E A, Davis M M 1984 Isolation of cDNA clones encoding T-cell-specific membrane-associated proteins. Nature 308: 149–152

42.   Moretta A, Pantaleo G, Mingari M C, Moretta L, Cerottini J C 1984 Clonal heterogeneity in the requirement for T3, T4 and T8 molecules in human cytolytic T-lymphocyte function. Journal of Experimental Medicine 159: 921–934

43.   Kanellopoulos J M, Wigglesworth N M, Owen M J, Crumpton M J 1983 Biosynthesis and molecular nature of the T3 antigen of human T-lymphocytes. EMBO Journal 2: 1807–1814

44.   Borst J, Alexander S, Elder J, Terhorst C 1983 The T3 complex on human T-lymphocytes involves four structurally distinct glycoproteins. The Journal of Biological Chemistry 258: 5135–5141

45.   Ledbetter J A, Evans R L, Lipinski M, Cunningham-Rundles C, Good R A, Herzenberg L A 1981 Evolutionary conservation of surface molecules that distinguish T-lymphocyte helper/inducer and cytotoxic/suppressor populations in mouse and man. Journal of Experimental Medicine 153: 310–323

46.   Snow P M, Terhorst C 1983 The T8 antigen is a multimeric complex of two distinct subunits on human thymocytes but consists of homomultimeric forms on peripheral blood T-lymphocytes. Journal of Biological Chemistry 258: 14675–14681

47.   Dialynas D P, Wilde D B, Marrack P, Pierres A, Wall K A, Havran W, Otten G, Loken M R, Pierres M, Kappler J, Fitch F W 1983 Characterization of the murine antigenic determinant, designated L3T4a, recognized by monoclonal antibody GK-1.5: expression of L3T4a by functional T-cell clones appears to correlate primarily with Class II MHC antigen reactivity. Immunological Reviews 74: 29–56

48.   Garson J A, Beverley P C L, Coakham H B, Harper E I 1982 Monoclonal antibodies against human T-lymphocytes label Purkinje neurones of many species. Nature 298: 375–377

49.   Green N, Alexnader H, Olson A, Alexander S, Shinnick T M, Sutcliffe J G, Lerner R A 1983 Immunogenic structure of influenza virus haemagglutinin. Cell 28: 477–491

50.   Kavathas P, Herzenberg L A 1983 Stable transformation of mouse L cells for human T-cell differentiation antigens, HLA and β2-microglobulin: selection by fluorescence-activated cell sorting. Proceedings of the National Academy of Sciences 80: 524–528

51.   Bernabeu C, Van de Rijn M, Finlay D, Maziarz R, Biro A, Spits H, De Vries J, Terhorst C 1983 Expression of the major histocompatability antigens HLA-A2 and HLA-B7 by DNA-mediated gene transfer. Journal of Immunology 131: 2032–2037

52.   Kavathas P, Sukharme V P, Herzenberg L A, Parnes J R 1984 Isolation of the gene coding for the human T-lymphocyte differentiation antigen Leu-2 (T8) by gene transfer and cDNA subtraction. Proceedings of the National Academy of Sciences (In press)

53.   Zoller M J, Smith M 1983 Oligonucleotide directed mutagenesis of DNA fragments cloned into M13 derived vectors. Methods in Enzymology 100: 468–500

54.   Arnold B, Burgert H-G, Hamann U, Hammerling G, Kees U, Kvist S 1984 Cytolytic T-cell recognize the two amino-terminal domains of H-2 antigens in tandem in influenza A infected cells. Cell 38: 79–87

55.   Muragushi A, Kishimoto T, Miki Y, Kuritani T, Kaedi T, Yoshisaki K, Yamamura Y 1981 T-cell replacing factor (TRF) induced IgG secretor in a human lymphoblastoid cell line and demonstration of acceptors for TRF. Journal of Immunology 127: 412–418

56.   Golay J, Rawle F, Beverley P C L 1984 B lymphocyte surface antigens involved in the regulation of immunoglobulin secretion. Proceedings of The Second International Workshop on Human Differentiation Antigens (In press)

57.   Clark E A, Shu G, Ledbetter J A 1984 Expression and function of the pan B-cell surface polypeptide Bp32. Proceedings of The Second International Workshop on Human Leucocyte Differentiation Antigens (In press)

58.   Bodger M P, Janossy G, Bollum F J, Burford G D, Hoffbrand A V 1983 The ontogeny of terminal deoxynucleotide transferase positive cells in the human foetus. Blood 61: 1006–1010

59. Kuritani T, Cooper M D 1982 Human B-cell differentiation. II Pokeweed mitogen-responsive B-cells belong to a surface immunoglobulin D-negative subpopulation. Journal of Experimental Medicine 155: 1561–1566

60. McMichael A J, Fabre J W (eds) 1982 Monoclonal antibodies in clinical medicine. Academic press, London

61. Janossy G, Prentice H G 1982 T-cell subpopulations, monoclonal antibodies and their therapeutic applications. Clinics in Haematology 11: 631–660

62. Souhami R L, Babbage J, Sigfusson A 1983 Defective in vitro antibody production to varicella zoster and other virus antigens in patients with Hodgkin's disease. Clinical and Experimental Immunology 53: 297–307

63. Reinherz E L, O'Brien C, Rosenthal P, Schlossman S F 1980 The cellular basis for viral-induced immunodeficiency: analysis by monoclonal antibodies. Journal of Immunology 125: 1269–1274

64. Schroff R W, Gottlieb M J, Prince H E, Chai L L, Fahey J L 1983 Immunological studies of homosexual men with immunodeficiency and Kaposi's sarcoma. Clinical Immunology and Immunopathology 27: 300–314

65. Crawford D H, Iliescu V, Edwards A J, Beverley P C L 1983 Characterization of Epstein Barr Virus-specific memory T-cells from the peripheral blood of seropositive individuals. British Journal of Cancer 47: 681–686

66. Klatzmann D, Barre-Sinoussi F, Nugeyre M T, Daugnet C, Vilmer E, Griscelli C, Brun-Vezinet F, Rouzioux C, Gluckman J C, Chermann J C, Montagnier L 1984 Selective tropism of lymphadenopathy associated virus (LAV) for helper–inducer T-lymphocytes. Science 225: 59–63

67. Dalgleish A G, Beverley P C L, Clapham P R, Crawford D H, Greaves M F, Weiss R A 1985 The CD4 (T4) antigen is an essential component of the receptor for the AIDS retrovirus (HTLV-3). Nature 312: 763–765

68. Gatenby P A, Kansas G S, Xian C Y, Evans R L, Engleman E G 1982 Dissection of immunoregulatory subpopulations of T-lymphocytes within the helper and suppressor sublineages in man. Journal of Immunology 129: 1997–2000

69. Reinherz E L, Morimoto C, Fitzgerald K A, Hussey R E, Daley J F, Schlossman S F 1982 Heterogeneity of human T4+ inducer T-cells defined by a monoclonal antibody that delineates two functional subpopulations. Journal of Immunology 128: 463–468

70. Lum L G, Orcutt-Thordarson N, Seigneuret M C, Hansen J A 1982 In vitro regulation of immunoglobulin synthesis by T-cell subpopulations defined by a new human T-cell antigen (9.3). Cellular Immunology 72: 122–129

71. Feldmann M, Schrier M (eds) 1982 Lymphokines 5. Academic Press, New York

72. Callard R E, Smith C M, Worman C, Linch D C, Cawley J C, Beverley P C L 1981 Unusual phenotype and function of an expanded population of T-cells in patients with haemopoietic disorders. Clinical and Experimental Immunology 43: 59–55

73. Gatter K C, Abdulaziz Z, Beverley P C L, Ford C, Lane E B, Mota M, Pulford K, Stein H, Taylor-Papadimitriou J, Woodhouse C, Mason D Y 1982 The use of monoclonal antibodies for the histopathological diagnosis of human malignancy. Journal of Clinical Paahology 35: 1253–1267

74. Pallesen G, Beverley P C L, Lane E B, Madsen M, Mason D Y, Stein H 1984 Nature of non-B, non-T lymphomas: an immunohistological study on frozen tissues using monoclonal antibodies. Journal of Clinical Pathology 37: 911–918

75. Habershaw J A, Lister T A, Stansfeld A G, Greaves M F 1983 Correlation of transferrin receptor expression with histological class and outcome in non-Hodgkin lymphoma. Lancet 1: 498–501

76. Vallera D A, Soderling C C B, Carlson G J, Kersey J H 1981 Bone marrow transplantation across major histocompatibility barriers in mice: the effect of elimination of T-cells from donor grafts by treatment with monoclonal Thy 1.2 plus complement or antibody alone. Transplantation 31: 218–222

77. Vallera D A, Youle R J, Neville D M, Kersey J H 1982 Bone marrow transplantation across major histocompatibility barriers. V. Protection of mice from lethal GVHD by pretreatment of donor cells with monoclonal anti-thy-1.2 coupled to the toxic lectin ricin. Journal of Experimental Medicine 155: 949–954

78. Reisner Y, Kapoor N, Pollack M J, Dupont B, Chagant R S K, Good R A, O'Reilly R J 1981 Transplantation for acute leukaemia with HLA-A and —B non-identical parental marrow cells fractionated with soybean agglutinin and sheep red blood cells. Lancet 2: 327–331

79. Vallera D A, Ash R C, Zanjani E D, Kersen J H, Le Bien T W, Beverley P C L, Neville D M, Youle R J 1983 Immunotoxins for human allogeneic bone marrow transplantation. Science 222: 512–515

80. Prentice H G, Blacklock H A, Janossy G, Gilmore M J M L, Price-Jones L, Tidman N,

Trejdosiewics L K, Skeggs D B L, Panjwani D, Ball S, Graphakos S, Patterson J, Ivory K, Hoffbrand A V 1984 Depletion of T-lymphocytes in donor marrow prevents significant graft–versus–host disease in matched allogeneic leukaemic marrow transplant recipients. Lancet 1: 472–476

81. Hale G, Bright S, Chumbley G, Hoang T, Metcalf D, Munro A, Waldmann H 1983 Removal of T-cells from bone marrow for transplantation: a monoclonal anti-lymphocyte antibody which fixes human complement. Blood 62: 873–882

82. Moller G (ed) 1982 Antibody carriers of drugs and toxins in tumour therapy. Immunological Reviews 62

83. Filipovitch A H, Vallera D A, Youle R J, Quinones R R, Neville D M, Kersey J H 1984 Ex-vivo treatment of donor bone marrow with anti-T-cell immunotoxins for prevention of graft–versus–host disease. Lancet 1: 469–472

84. Powles R L, Morgenstein G R, Kay H E M, McEewain T J, Clink H M, Dady P J, Barrett A, Jameson B, Depledge M H, Watson J G, Sloane J, Leigh M, Lumley H, Hedley D, Lawler S D, Filshie J, Robinson B 1983 Mismatched family donors for bone-marrow transplantation as treatment for acute leukaemia. Lancet 1: 612–615

85. Greaves M F, Janossy G 1978 Patterns of gene expression and the cellular origins of human leukaemias. Biochimica and Biophysica Acta 56: 193–230

86. Ritz J, Sallan S E, Blast R C, Lipton J M, Nathan D G, Schlossman S F 1983 In vitro treatment with monoclonal antibody prior to autologous bone marrow transplantation in acute lymphoblastic leukaemia. Haematologie und Bluttransfusion 28: 117–123

87. Ritz J, Pesando J M, Sallan S E, Clavell L A, Notis-McConarty J, Rosenthal P, Schlossman S F 1981 Serotheray of acute lymphoblastic leukaemia with monoclonal antibody. Blood 58: 141–152

88. Linch D C, Beverley P C L, Newland A, Turnbull A 1983 Treatment of a low grade T-cell proliferation with monoclonal antibody. Clinical and Experimental Immunology 51: 133–140

89. Miller R A, Levy R 1981 Response to cutaneous T-cell lymphoma to therapy with hybridoma monoclonal antibody. Lancet 2: 226–229

90. Miller R A, Maloney D G, Warnke R, Levy R 1982 Treatment of B-cell lymphoma with monoclonal anti-idiotype antibody. New England Journal of Medicine 306: 517–522

91. Jerne N K 1974 Towards a network theory of the immune system. Annals of Immunology of the Pasteur Institute 1256: 373–389

92. Herlyn D, Koprowski H 1982 IgG 2a Monoclonal antibodies inhibit human tumour growth through interaction with effector cells. Proceedings of the National Academy of Sciences 79: 4761–4765

93. Jansen F K, Blythman H E, Carriere D, Casellas P, Gros O, Gros P, Laurent C, Paolucci F, Pau B, Poncelet P, Richer G, Vidal H, Voisin G A 1982 Immunotoxins: hybrid molecules combining high specificity and potent cytotoxicity. Immunological Reviews 62: 185–216

94. Thorpe P E, Detre S I, Mason D W, Cumber A J, Ross W C 1983 Monoclonal antibody therapy: 'model' experiments with toxin-conjugated antibodies in mice and rats. Haematologie und Bluttransfusion. 28: 107–111

Index